In Clinical Practice

Taking a practical approach to clinical medicine, this series of smaller reference books is designed for the trainee physician, primary care physician, nurse practitioner and other general medical professionals to understand each topic covered. The coverage is comprehensive but concise and is designed to act as a primary reference tool for subjects across the field of medicine.

More information about this series at http://www.springer.com/series/13483

Said Abdallah Al-Mamari

Urolithiasis in Clinical Practice

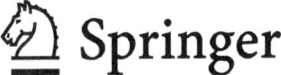 Springer

Said Abdallah Al-Mamari
The Royal Hospital
Muscat, Oman

ISSN 2199-6652   ISSN 2199-6660   (electronic)
In Clinical Practice
ISBN 978-3-319-62436-5   ISBN 978-3-319-62437-2   (eBook)
DOI 10.1007/978-3-319-62437-2

Library of Congress Control Number: 2017953039

Printed on acid-free paper

This Springer imprint is published by Springer Nature
The registered company is Springer International Publishing AG
The registered company address is: Gewerbestrasse 11, 6330 Cham, Switzerland

In Memoriam

My father Abdallah

While I still needed his wisdom, guidance, and inspiration, he unexpectedly left our world to meet his Creator since that sorrowful sunset of February 6th 2014.

To him I dedicate this book as a fruit of the continuous effort, sacrifice, patience, and altruism he taught me.

May he eternally rest in peace within the paradise of our Lord, the Almighty.

Said

"If there's a book that you want to read, but it hasn't been written yet, then you must write it"

Toni Morrison (1931–)
(Nobel Prize in Literature in 1993)

Foreword

It is a privilege to write the Foreword to this wonderful book on Urolithiasis by Dr. Said Abdallah Al-Mamari from the Royal Hospital of Muscat, in the Sultanate of Oman. This handbook will be a very useful resource for urologists in practice as well as other physicians interested in the common condition of urolithiasis.

This manual is both comprehensive in its scope and current in all aspects of medical and surgical diagnosis and treatment of urinary stone disease. Each chapter begins with a memorable historic quote that immediately engages the interest of the reader. The figures, illustrations, and tables are tremendous in their quality and variety. All of the chapters are well supported with suitable references that are current and, in the case of historic material, interesting and valuable. The chapters related to surgical management are particularly notable in capturing the shifting landscape in the relative role of shock-wave lithotripsy versus various forms of endoscopic surgery for renal and ureteral stones.

While many textbooks of urology can be rather dry and factual, I found this book to be easy to read, concise in the delivery of relevant information, and engaging all in one package. For a resident with a query surrounding patient care or preparing for certification examinations, it will be a very useful reference with easy to find answers to common questions. Indeed, as an academic urologist with a strong subspecialty interest in urolithiasis I fully expect to be referring to this book myself, both for patient care questions and for purposes related to teaching students and residents.

Dr. Al-Mamari is to be congratulated for the production of this excellent work for which he is the sole author. One has the sense that production of this text has been a labor of love for Dr. Al-Mamari and he can be very proud of the final product.

Urolithiasis in Clinical Practice is an excellent contribution to our existing resources on urolithiasis.

John Denstedt, MD, FRCSC, FACS, FCAHS
Department of Surgery
Schulich School of Medicine and Dentistry
Western University, London, ON, Canada

Preface

Books are inherently confined within the human limits of their authors and no single manual contains all that is needed by the readers. Nevertheless no effort has been spared in the present publication to provide the essential information in all aspects of the urinary stone disease. These include the history, the etymology, the epidemiology, the pathophysiology, the etiology, the symptomatology, the differential diagnoses, as well as the latest diagnostic means and treatment options of urinary lithiasis.

The most recent and relevant publications in the medical literature have been meticulously decorticated and harmonized to produce a manual with the most up-to-date information. International guidelines have also been referred to when applicable and controversial issues raised whenever present. Although the concern of producing a digestible reading material was constantly kept in my mind, I did not hesitate to dig deeper whenever details were deemed necessary in order to avoid truncated information.

Accounts on the various surgical techniques performed for the urinary stone disease have been provided in this book with the intention to accompany the Urological Surgeon inside the operating room. However these are by no means intended to replace more comprehensive manuals on operative techniques that the reader is encouraged to consult for detailed information.

I believe this book will fit the needs of the resident in a urology training program as well as the Registrar and the Senior Consultant, serving as a pocket guide in their daily practice. I hope also it will be an excellent memory refreshing reference for the medical student and the urology trainee preparing for examinations.

Said Abdallah Al-Mamari
Urology Department
The Royal Hospital
Muscat, Oman

Acknowledgements

I'm deeply grateful to:
- **Dr. John Denstedt**, Professor of Urology, Department of Surgery, Schulich School of Medicine and Dentistry, Western University, London, Canada: for reviewing this book and for his expert Foreword.
- **Dr. Salim Said Al-Busaidy**, Senior Consultant and Head, Urology, The Royal Hospital, Muscat, Oman: for reviewing the content of this book, enhancing the accuracy of the information, and amending the manuscript in the English language.
- **Dr. Qais Mohamed Al-Hooti**, Consultant, Urology, The Royal Hospital, Muscat, Oman: for his comprehensive review of this book and his pertinent suggestions to improve its content.
- **Dr. Issa Salim Al-Salmi,** Senior Consultant and Head, Nephrology, The Royal Hospital, Muscat, Oman: for reviewing the chapters and paragraphs on metabolic causes, investigations, and medical treatment of urinary stones.
- **Dr. Santhosh Narayana Kurrukal**, Senior Specialist, Urology, The Royal Hospital, Muscat, Oman: for his contribution to the bibliographic documentation.
- **Dr. Sanmukh Das Bhagia**, Specialist, Urology, The Royal Hospital, Muscat, Oman: for his contribution to the illustration of this book.

Contents

Abbreviations

ADPKD	Autosomal dominant polycystic kidney disease
AGA	Alanine-glyoxylate aminotransferase
AHA	Acetohydroxamic acid
AUA	American Association of Urologists
BMI	Body mass index
CaOx	Calcium oxalate
CaP	Calcium phosphate
CECT	Contrast-enhanced computed tomography scan
CLU	Club della litiasi Urinaria
CT scan	Computed tomography scan
DECT	Dual-energy computed tomography
DJ stent	Double-J stent
DM	Diabetes mellitus
DMSA	Dimercaptosuccinic acid
DTPA	Diethylenetriaminepentaacetic acid
DTS	X-ray digital tomosynthesis
EAU	European Association of Urologists
EHL	Electrohydraulic lithotripsy
EKL	Electrokinetic lithotripsy
EPA	Eicosapentaenoic acid
EPN	Emphysematous pyelonephritis
ESRD	End-stage renal disease
ESWL	Extracorporeal shock wave lithotripsy
FTIR	Fourier transform infrared spectroscopy
GA	General anesthesia
HM3	(Dornier) human model 3
HN	Hydronephrosis

Ho:YAG laser	Holmium-yttrium aluminum garnet laser
HSK	Horseshoe kidney
HTN	Hypertension
HU	Hounsfield unit
IUCD	Intrauterine contraceptive device
IV	Intravenous
IVU (or IVP)	Intravenous urography (or pyelography)
KUB (CT, X-ray, or ultrasound)	Kidney-ureter-bladder (CT, X-ray, or ultrasound)
LP	Laparoscopic pyelolithotomy
LU	Laparoscopic ureterolithotomy
LUTS	Lower urinary tract syndrome
MAG3	Mercaptoacetyltriglycine
MAP	Magnesium ammonium phosphate
MET	Medical expulsive therapy
MOC cyst	Milk-of-calcium cyst
MRI	Magnetic resonance imaging
MS	Metabolic syndrome
NCCT	Non-contrast-enhanced CT scan (synonymous of UHCT: Unenhanced helical CT scan)
NSAIDs	Nonsteroidal anti-inflammatory drugs
OAN	Open anatrophic nephrolithotomy
OIH	Ortho-iodohippurate
OT	Operating theater
PHO	Primary hyperoxaluria
PCN	Percutaneous nephrostomy
PCNL	Percutaneous nephrolithotomy
PCS	Pelvicalyceal system
PTFE	Polytetrafluoroethylene
PUJ	Pelvi-ureteric junction
RGP	Retrograde pyelogram
RIRS	Retrograde intrarenal surgery
ROKS	The Recurrence of Kidney Stone nomogram
RTA	Renal tubular acidosis
SEM	Scanning electron microscopy

SSD	Skin-to-stone distance
UA	Uric acid
UAS	Ureteral access sheath
UHCT	Unenhanced helical CT scan (synonymous of NCCT: Non-contrast-enhanced CT scan)
URS	Ureteroscopy
US	Ultrasonography
UTI	Urinary tract infection
VUR	Vesico-ureteral reflux

Chapter 1
Introduction

"One must be reasonable in one's demands on life. For myself, all that I ask is: (1) accurate information; (2) coherent knowledge; (3) deep understanding; (4) infinite loving wisdom; (5) no more kidney stones, please."

Edward Abbey (1927–1989)

Humans are afflicted by the urinary stone disease since the dawn of time. Today this ailment is considered as the third most frequent urological pathological condition after infections and prostatic diseases, and statistics show a worldwide increase in its incidence and prevalence.

In 1994 data from the US National Health and Nutrition Examination Survey (NHANES) estimated the prevalence of stone disease at 5.2% of the American population, marking a significant increase compared to the year 1980 when a prevalence of only 3.2% has been observed [1]. A more recent study performed in 2010 suggested a further increase reaching 8.8% prevalence, roughly equivalent to 1 in 11 people [2]. The same trends have been observed all over the world and the highest prevalence of urinary stones was reported in Saudi Arabia with an estimated value of 20% [3].

Inexorably, urolithiasis treatment costs have dramatically increased and constitute a heavy economic burden today. In the United States alone, urinary stones have caused two million outpatient visits in the year 2000, corresponding to a 40% increase compared to 1994 [4]. The management cost in emergency departments alone varies from over 400 US$ per patient merely for diagnostic procedures (formal ultrasound

© Springer International Publishing AG 2017
S.A. Al-Mamari, *Urolithiasis in Clinical Practice*,
In Clinical Practice, DOI 10.1007/978-3-319-62437-2_1

in the X-ray Department, point-of-care ultrasound, or CT-scan) to around 1000 US$ for the total visit cost [5]. The estimated annual cost of acute management of urolithiasis in the USA varies from US$ 1.83 to 2.1 billion [4, 6], reaching a total of US$5.3 billion when including the direct costs of stone-related management and the indirect costs of productivity time lost [7]. These values are very close to those calculated by a comprehensive study conducted by the Canadian Agency for Drugs and Technologies in Health which estimated the overall economic burden of urinary stone treatment at approximately five billion US$ in 2005, including direct and indirect costs [8].

Furthermore, due to the agonizing pain and the tendency of repeated renal colic on the one hand, and the multiple possible complications of urolithiasis on the other hand, kidney stone formers have been found to have a worse health-related quality of life than the standard American population, with the greatest impact seen in cystine stone patients [9].

In the last three decades, significant progress has been made in the surgical management of stone disease, while a relatively small amount of new information has been learnt in the preventive and conservative measures. The successive introduction of percutaneous nephrolithotomy (PCNL), extracorporeal shockwave lithotripsy (ESWL), and flexible ureteroscopy in the Urologist's armamentarium as well as the subsequent development of retrograde intrarenal surgery (RIRS) and Holmium Laser fragmentation has led to a new era in the treatment of renal stones. This has resulted in minimally invasive approaches being performed in the majority of cases as opposed to open surgery.

Undoubtedly a better understanding of the pathology, a rational approach to investigative methods, a judicious use of conservative and preventive measures, and skillful surgery are essential to reduce the cost and optimize efficacy in the management of this disease.

References

1. Stamatelou KK, Francis ME, Jones CA, Nyberg LM, Curhan GC. Time trends in reported prevalence of kidney stones in the United States: 1976–1994. Kidney Int. 2003;63:1817–23.
2. Scales CD Jr, Smith AC, Hanley JM, Saigal CS, Urologic Diseases in America Project. Prevalence of kidney stones in the United States. Eur Urol. 2012;62(1):160–5.
3. Ramello A, Vitale C, Marangella M. Epidemiology of nephrolithiasis. J Nephrol. 2000;13:S45–50.
4. Pearle MS, Calhoun EA, Curhan GC, Urologic Diseases of America Project. Urologic diseases in America project: urolithiasis. J Urol. 2005;173(3):848–57.
5. Melnikow J, Xing G, Cox G, et al. Cost analysis of the STONE randomized trial: can health care costs be reduced one test at a time? Med Care. 2016;54(4):337–42.
6. Trinchieri A. Epidemiological trends in urolithiasis: impact on our health care systems. Urol Res. 2006;34:151–6.
7. Saigal CS, Joyce G, Timilsina AR. Direct and indirect costs of nephrolithiasis in an employed population: opportunity for disease management [quest]. Kidney Int. 2005;68:1808–14.
8. Treatment strategies for patients with renal colic: a review of the comparative clinical and cost-effectiveness [Internet]. Ottawa: Canadian Agency for Drugs and Technologies in Health; 2014 Nov. CADTH Rapid Response Reports. http://www.ncbi.nlm.nih.gov/books/NBK263317/
9. Modersitzki F, Pizzi L, Grasso M, Goldfarb DS. Health-related quality of life (HRQoL) in cystine compared with non-cystine stone formers. Urolithiasis. 2014;42(1):53–60.

Chapter 2
History of Stone Disease

"If you don't know history, then you don't know anything. You are a leaf that doesn't know it is part of a tree."

Michael Crichton (1942–2008) (Edgar Award in 1969)

"Calculus" is a Latin word meaning "small pebble". It is the diminutive form of calx (genitive: calcis) which means limestone or chalk. Pebbles were used in the Antiquity and Middle-age for counting of goods, animals, and slaves (Fig. 2.1). By synecdoche, the use of the word calculus progressed to refer to the whole counting operation as well as to more complex mathematical analyses.

In 1901, the English Archaeologist Elliott Smith discovered a stone in the pelvis of a mummy preserved inside a prehistoric Egyptian tomb. C^{14}-isotope studies helped dating the mummy at 4800 BC [1]. Since then paleopathology has revealed many other prehistoric and ancient cases of stone disease in various continents of the globe [2] (Table 2.1).

Stone disease has been described in all civilizations throughout the antiquity, including India, China, Persia, Greece, and Rome, as well as in the medieval European and Islamic period [2–4].

Perineal lithotomy was reported as earlier as around 600 BC by **Sushruta**, an ancient India surgeon, and this procedure continued to be performed later on in the Greco-Roman period [4]. Nevertheless it was rightly considered a very dangerous and delicate operation, being reserved exclusively to specialized surgeons as stated by **Hippocrates** (460–370 BC) in his oath: *"…I will not use the knife, even upon those*

© Springer International Publishing AG 2017

S.A. Al-Mamari, *Urolithiasis in Clinical Practice*,
In Clinical Practice, DOI 10.1007/978-3-319-62437-2_2

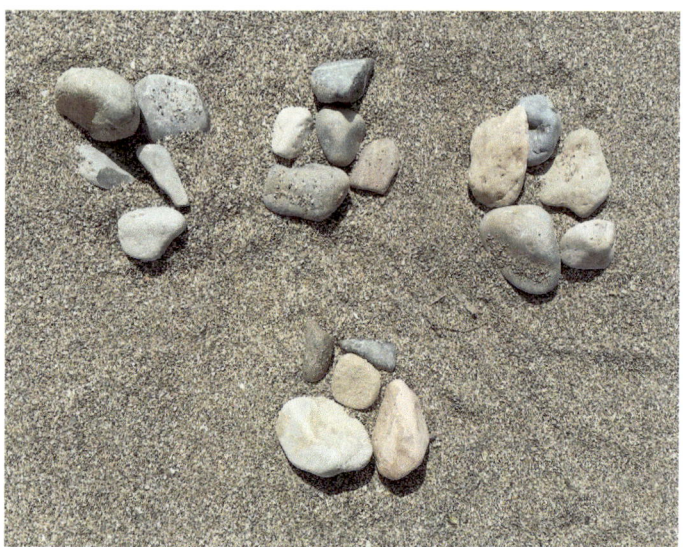

FIGURE 2.1 Counting with small pebbles

suffering from stones, but I will leave this to those who are trained in this craft." The term "lithotomy" was coined in 276 BC by the Greek surgeon Ammonius of Alexandria and was later on described by the Roman surgeon **Aulus Cornelius Celsius** (25 BC-50 AD) [5]. This so-called "celsian method of cystolithotomy" remained unchanged for centuries and was a particularly terrifying and often fatal procedure [5].

By the year AD 1000, the Arab surgeon **Abul-Qasim Khalaf Ibn Abbas Alzahrawi** (mostly known in western countries as **"Albucasis"**) from Cordova (Al-Andalus) revolutionized the technique of perineal lithotomy (Fig. 2.2). In a 30-volume encyclopaedia of medical information called "*Kitab Al-Tasreef*"[1], he described the operative steps aiming at improving the technique and reducing

---

[1] The complete title in Arabic "كتاب التصريف لمن عجز عن التأليف " is difficult to be exactly translated in the English language. However it can be meaningfully paraphrased as follows: "A book providing enough information to whoever cannot make further research", or simply "A sufficient book for researchers".

TABLE 2.1 Urinary stones and some relevant paleopathology findings

	Geographic area	Date	Finding
Europe	Italy, Sicily	6.500 B.C.	Bladder stone
	Southern France	2.100 B.C.	Bladder stone
	United Kingdom, Yorkshire	2.000–700 B.C.	Bladder stone
	Hungary	Bronze age	Bladder stone
	Germany	500–250 B.C.	Bladder stones (probably)
	United Kingdom, Somerset	450–1.000 A.D.	Bladder stones
	Hungary	Sixth to seventh century A.D.	Bladder stone
	Denmark	1.300–1.500 A.D.	Renal stone
	Italy	Early nineteenth century	Bladder stone
Africa	Predynastic skeleton	3.900–3.100 B.C.	Three bladder stones
	Abido, Egypt	3.500 B.C.	Bladder stone
	Helouan, Egypt	3.100 B.C.	Renal stones (several individuals)
	Naga-el-Deir, Egypt	2.800 B.C.	Four renal stones
	Mummy, Old Kingdom, Egypt	2.650–2.150 B.C.	Renal stone
	Mummy, XXI dynasty, Egypt	1.069–945 B.C.	Triangular stone located into the naris
	Jebel Moya, Sudan	1.000–100 B.C.	Bladder stones (several individuals)

(continued)

TABLE 2.1 (continued)

	Geographic area	Date	Finding
America	Kentucky	3.500–3.000 B.C.	Renal and bladder stones (three individuals)
	Illinois	1.500 B.C.	Renal stone
	Arizona	100 B.C.–500 A.D.	Bladder stone (mummy)
	Utah	950–1.100 A.D.	Bladder stone
	Chile	1.000 A.D.	Urethra stone (mummy)
	Arizona	1.100–1.250 A.D.	Bladder stone
	Indiana	1.500 A.D.	Bilateral renal stones
	West Virginia	1.600–1.700 A.D.	Renal stone

From Manfredini R et al. [2]. With permission from Verduci Editore S.r.l.

the complications. He notoriously invented new instruments such as *"nechil"* lithotomy scalpel, *"Al-Kalaleeb"* forceps to crush large bladder stones and *"Al-Mishaab"* to drill and fragment an impacted urethral stone, and greatly influenced surgery in Europe from the Middle-Age up to the renaissance period [6].

Further steps were achieved in the renaissance period when a bladder stone removal was performed on a criminal by **Germain Collot** in 1475 and various urological surgical instruments were introduced [3]. **Pierre Franco** (1505–1578) published the first case of cystolithotomy in a child in 1556, but only to surprisingly preach against its reproducibility because of the extreme hazards of his technique [7]. "The Physicians and Surgeons can defend themselves when unfortunate, but if we lithotomists have a mishap, we must run for our lives", he wrote.

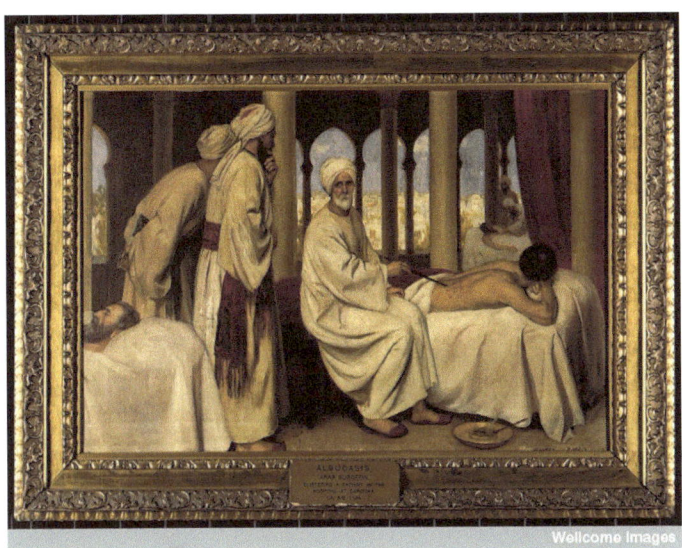

FIGURE 2.2 Albucasis (Al-Zahrawi) blistering a patient in the hospital at Cordova. By Ernest Board. Credit: Wellcome Library, London

Before the nineteenth century, bladder stones were only managed by open approaches, either through perineal route (Fig. 2.3) or suprapubically, or even trans-rectally, each technique carrying a very high mortality rate. The French Surgeon **Jean Civiale** (1792–1867) was the first to introduce a lithotrite transurethrally in 1832 to crush a bladder stone [4, 8] (Fig. 2.4). Later on this approach was popularized in the UK by one of his students, **Sir Henry Thompson** (1820–1904) who successfully treated the Belgian King Leopold I in 1862. In his book "*Parallèle des divers moyens de traiter les calculeux*"[2], Civiale published encouraging results of the new "Lithotripsy" technique in comparison with the "Lithotomy" approach, showing mortality rates of 2.2 and 18.8% respectively. He was then granted the Montyon Prize

---

[2]Free translation: "Comparison of the various methods to treat stone patients."

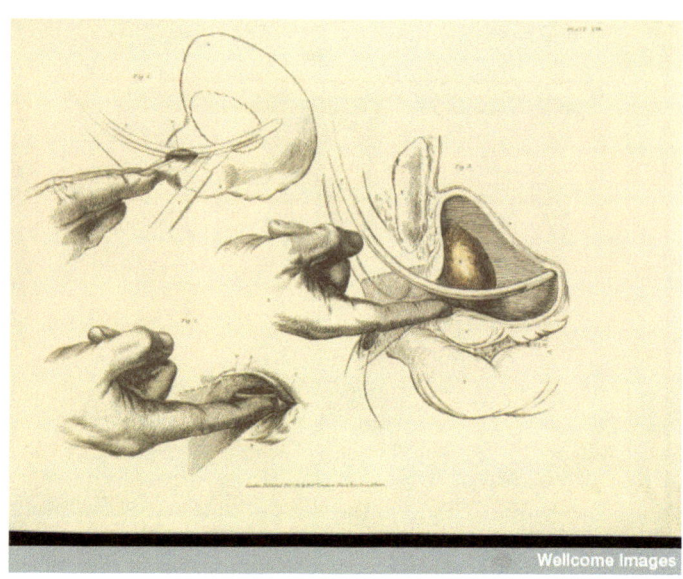

FIGURE 2.3 Surgical removal of a stone from the bladder. By Charles Bell (1821) **Credit:** Wellcome Library, London

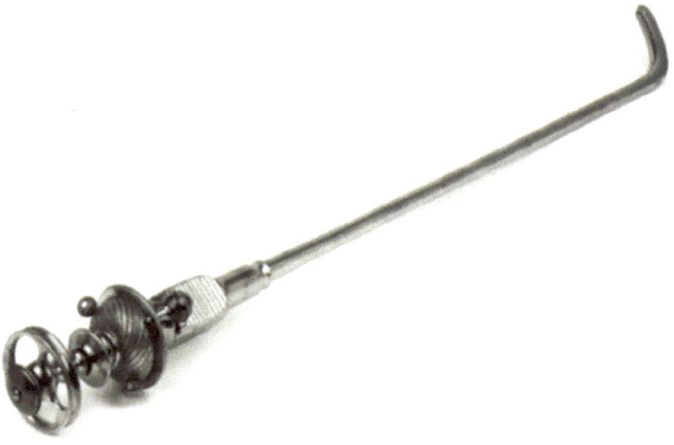

FIGURE 2.4 The lithotrite invented by Jean Civiale. From Karamanou M et al. [8]. With permission from Elsevier

(a nineteenth century precursor of the Nobel Prize) by the French Academy of Sciences in Paris in 1836 and is also recognized as a pioneer of evidence-based medicine [8, 9]. After the successful introduction of transurethral lithotripsy, one can better understand over 2400 years later why Hippocrates was so reluctant to use the knife upon stone patients.

In 1874, the American Surgeon **Henry Jacob Bigelow** (1818–1890) developed a stronger and harder lithotrite that was introduced into the bladder under anaesthesia to successfully perform in a single session a rapid lithotrity with evacuation of the stone. This procedure, called since then "litholapaxy" (from Greek lithos: stone, and lapassein: to clear, to empty, to washout), resulted in a dramatic improvement of the mortality rate from 25 to 2.4% compared to lithotomy [4, 10].

Further advances were realized in Western Europe in the second half of the nineteenth century, especially in France where many researchers, chiefly **Félix Guyon** (1831–1920) **and Joaquín Albarrán** (1860–1912) initiated and organized specialized management of urinary tract disease. The devotion of these Surgeons and of their companions and subsequent disciples made France to be rightly regarded today as the cradle of modern Urology [8, 11]. **Urology became a separate specialty from General Surgery in 1890 with Felix Guyon as the first Professor of Urology in Paris**. Herein a credit should also be given to the French Master Cutler and metallic tools designer **Joseph-Frédéric-Benoît Charrière** for his great contribution to the development of urological instruments (Fig. 2.5) [12].

Both Civiale lithotripsy and Bigelow litholapaxy were performed blindly being merely guided by the stone click on the metallic sound until **Hugh Hampton Young**[3] (1870–1945) **and**

---

[3]Among other accomplishments HH Young also performed the first perineal radical prostatectomy at the age of 33 years in 1903. He is also considered a pioneer in pediatric urology being the first to recognize and surgically treat posterior urethral valves, the first to perform a surgical correction of incontinence in patients with the epispadias-exstrophy complex, and the first to propose bilateral subtotal adrenalectomy to overcome the virilization syndrome in congenital adrenal hyperplasia [17]. For his outstanding contribution to modern Urology, HH Young is considered as the father of American Urology by many authors [18–20].

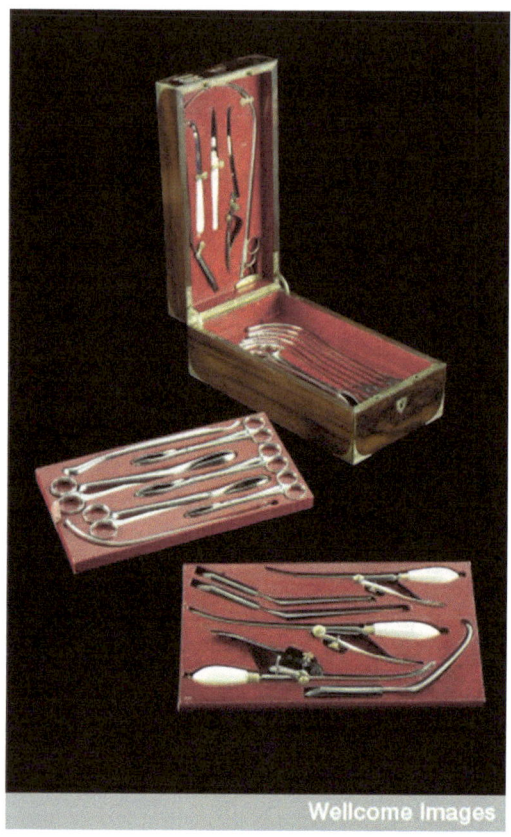

FIGURE 2.5 A set of Charrière instruments. Credit Science Museum, London, Wellcome Images (1820–1860). The name "Charrière" is linked to the measurement unit of endoscopes and catheters caliber: 1 Charrière = 1 mm outer circumference (approximately 1/3 mm outer diameter). So 3 Charrière = 1 mm outer diameter, and 12 Charrière = 4 mm outer diameter. In English speaking countries, the unit "French" is used in lieu of "Charrière" [12]

RW MacKay developed their cystoscopic lithotrite in 1904, based on the first modern diagnostic cystoscope introduced by the German Urologist **Maximilian Nitze** in 1877 [4, 13].

Young and MacKay opened a further perspective by performing the first ureteroscopy using a 9.5 Fr Cystoscope in a child with megaureter and posterior urethral valve in 1912 [4, 14].

However active stone treatment through ureteroscopic approach became a reality only in the 1970th after the experiences performed by **Goodman TM and Lyon ES** et al. [15, 16].

The many advances which arose in the twentieth century in open and minimally invasive surgeries (laparoscopic ureterolithotomy, percutaneous nephrolithotomy, rigid and flexible ureteroscopies with Laser stone ablation) as well as the advent of the Extracorporeal Shockwave Lithotripsy are still the mainstay of the active management of urinary stone disease in the twenty-first century and will be discussed later in the Treatment section.

Throughout history many famous personalities reportedly suffered from urinary stones. These include the French Emperors Napoleon Bonaparte and Napoleon III, Kings Leopold I of Belgium, Peter the Great of Russia, Louis XIV of France, and George IV of the United Kingdom, the English military and political leader Oliver Cromwell, the American Politician and Scientist Benjamin Franklin, the English scientist Isaac Newton, the physicians Harvey and Boerhaave, the anatomist Scarpa, the philosopher Bacon, and the artist Michelangelo [2, 4, 21] (Table 2.2).

TABLE 2.2 Some of the historical personalities documented to be kidney stone formers

Emperors, kings, popes, presidents	Politicians, religious persons, statesmen	Artists, philosophers, physicians, scientists, writers	Performers (music, cinema)
Caesar Augustus (63 b.C.–14a.D.)	Martin Luther (1483–1546)	Epicurus (341–270 b.C.)	Cole Porter (1891–1964)
James I Stuart (1566–1625)	John Calvin (1509–1564)	Michelangelo Buonarroti (1475–1564)	Alfred Hitchcock (1899–1980)

(continued)

TABLE 2.2 (continued)

Emperors, kings, popes, presidents	Politicians, religious persons, statesmen	Artists, philosophers, physicians, scientists, writers	Performers (music, cinema)
Innocent XI (1611–1689)	Oliver Cromwell (1599–1658)	Michele de Montaigne (1533–1592)	Bing Crosby (1903–1977)
Luois XIV (1638–1715)	Cardinal Jules Mazarin (1602–1661)	Francis Bacon (1561–1626)	Ava Gardner (1922–1990)
Peter the Great (1672–1725)	Samuel Pepys (1633–1703)	William Harvey (1578–1657)	Roger Moore (1927–)
Anna of Russia (1693–1740)	Benjamin Franklin (1706–1790)	Thomas Sydenham (1624–1689)	Burt Reynolds (1936–)
George IV (1762–1830)	Mother Teresa (1910–1997)	Robert Boyle (1627–1691)	Billy Joel (1949–)
Napoleon I (1769–1821)	Indira Ghandi (1917–1984)	Isaac Newton (1642–1727)	Tim Burton (1958–)
Leopold I of Belgium (1790–1865)		Gottfried von Leibnitz (1646–1716)	
Napoleon III (1808–1873)		Antonio Scarpa (1752–1832)	
Lyndon B. Johnson (1908–1973)		Jack London (1876–1916)	

From Manfredini R et al. [2]. With permission from Verduci Editore S.r.l.

Did Urinary Stone Disease Change the Course of the Modern Human History?

This question could appear supererogatory at first sight. However it soon becomes pertinent when considering the two French Emperors alone and the deleterious effect of intense pain and uraemia on humans' judgments and decisions. One can then imagine how much the agonizing pain suffered by Napoleon Bonaparte from a bladder stone, combined with piles and dysuria caused by his prostatic adenoma, might have influenced the outcome of his Russian campaign in 1812. Historians may also be wondering what would have happened in the battlefield of Sedan (France) in 1870 had an effective stone treatment be given to Napoleon III [22]. Perhaps the French sovereign would have resisted Otto von Bismarck's troops and the epilogue of the Franco-Prussian war would have been different. It was too late when the defeated and exiled Emperor underwent a multistage intervention performed by Sir Henry Thompson in England in January 1873, in an attempt to remove his vesical stone. He died before the third session and the autopsy revealed bilateral marked pyonephrosis and a large residual stone fragment in the bladder measuring 5×3 cm and weighing 22 g which is still preserved in the Hunterian Museum of the Royal College of Surgeons of England [21, 22, 23].

References

1. Shattock JG. A prehistoric or predynastic Egyptian calculus. Trans Pathol Soc Lond. 1905;61:275.
2. Manfredini R, De Giorgi A, Storari A, Fabbian F. Pears and renal stones: possible weapon for prevention? A comprehensive narrative review. Eur Rev Med Pharmacol Sci. 2016;20(3):414–25.
3. Shah J, Whitfield HN. Urolithiasis through the ages. BJU Int. 2002;89(8):801–10.

4. Tefekli A, Cezayirli F. The history of urinary stones: in parallel with civilization. Sci World J. 2013;2013:423964.
5. Herr HW. 'Cutting for the stone': the ancient art of lithotomy. BJU Int. 2008;101(10):1214–6.
6. Abdel-Halim RE, Altwaijiri AS, Elfaqih SR, Mitwalli AH. Extraction of urinary bladder stone as described by Abul-Qasim Khalaf Ibn Abbas Alzahrawi (Albucasis) (325–404 H, 930–1013 AD). A translation of original text and a commentary. Saudi Med J. 2003;24(12):1283–91.
7. Franco P. Traité des Hernies, contenant une ample déclaration de toutes les espèces, et autres excellentes parties de la chirurgie, assavoir: de la pierre, etc. Lyon: 1561.
8. Karamanou M, Mylonas A, Laios C, Poulakou-Rebelakou E. The French contribution to the evolution of the procedure and the instrumentation for lithotripsy. Urology. 2015;85(6):1263–6.
9. Matthews JR. The Paris Academy of Science report on Jean Civiale's statistical research and the 19th century background to evidence-based medicine. Int J Epidemiol. 2001;30(6):1246–9.
10. Bigelow HJ. Lithotrity by a single operation. Am J Med Sci. 1879;75(149):117–34.
11. http://urofrance.org/quisommes-nous/histoire-de-lurologie/histoire-urologie-france/felix-guyon-et-la-naissance-de-lurologie-moderne.html
12. Osborn NK, Baron TH. The history of the "French" gauge. Gastrointest Endosc. 2006;63(3):461–2.
13. Nitze M. Beitrage zur Endosckopie der mannlichen Hamblase*. Arch Klin Chir. 1881;36:661–732.
14. Young HH, McKay RW. Congenital valvular obstruction of the prostatic urethra. Surg Gynecol Obstet. 1929;48:509–12.
15. Goodman TM. Ureteroscopy with pediatric cystoscope in adults. Urology. 1977;9(4):394–7.
16. Lyon ES, Kyker JS, Schoenberg HW. Transurethral ureteroscopy in women: a ready addition to the urological armamentarium. J Urol. 1978;119(1):35–41.
17. Meldrum KK, Mathews R, Gearhart JP. Hugh Hampton Young: a pioneer in pediatric urology. J Urol. 2001;166(4):1415–7.
18. Engel RM. Hugh Hampton Young: father of American urology. J Urol. 2003;169(2):458–64.
19. Bera MK, Maji TK, Bera KP. A tribute to Hugh Hampton Young – the father of modern urology. Indian J Surg. 2007;69(4):169–70.

20. Toledo-Pereyra LH. Hugh Hampton Young-father of modern American urology. J Investig Surg. 2005;18(2):55–7.
21. Moran ME. Famous stone sufferers. In: Moran AE, editor. Urolithiasis. A comprehensive history. New York: Springer; 2014. p. 117–9.
22. Ellis H. A history of bladder stone. J R Soc Med. 1979;72(4):248–51.
23. Androutsos G. Napoleon III's urogenital disease (1808-1873). Prog Urol. 2000;10(1):142–52.

Chapter 3
Epidemiology of Urinary Stones

"As our world continues to generate unimaginable amounts of data, more data lead to more correlations, and more correlations can lead to more discoveries."

Hans Rosling (1948–2017) (Grierson Awards of Best Science Documentary in 2011)

There is a global increase in the incidence and prevalence of urinary calculi in developed as well as in developing countries. In addition to the use of more accurate diagnostic tools, many factors play an important role in this increase, including population aging, diet, lifestyle, and global warming of the planet (Fig. 3.1a, b) [1].

There are geographic variations in the overall probability to develop urinary stones; the risk of developing urolithiasis in adults is higher in the Western countries (5–9% in Europe, 12% in Canada, 13–15% in the USA) than in the rest of the world (1–5%), with the exception of some Middle-East countries such as Saudi Arabia where the reported risk is as high as 20.1% [2]. Urolithiasis mostly affects patients of 25–60 years of age [3] (Fig. 3.2).

A cross-sectional analysis of data from the US National Health and Nutrition Examination Survey (NHANES) for the period from 2007 to 2010 revealed an overall prevalence of urinary calculi in the American population of 8.8%, comprising of 10.6% among men and 7.1% among women [4]. This represents a significant increase compared to an earlier study conducted in 1994 which showed only a prevalence of 5.2% [5].

© Springer International Publishing AG 2017
S.A. Al-Mamari, *Urolithiasis in Clinical Practice*,
In Clinical Practice, DOI 10.1007/978-3-319-62437-2_3

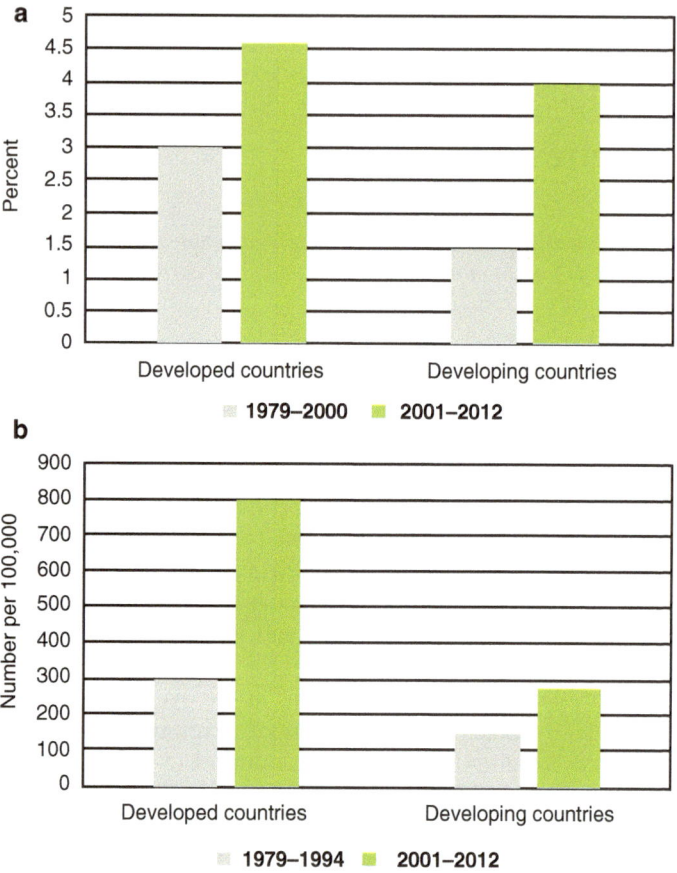

FIGURE 3.1 (**a**) Increase in urolithiasis prevalence in the developed and developing worlds over time. Reproduced and modified from Atalab et al. [1], with permission from the IJKD. (**b**) Increase in urolithiasis incidence in the developed and developing worlds over time (per 100,000 population). Reproduced and modified from Atalab et al. [1], with permission from the IJKD

Strong associations were found with obesity and diabetes and approximately 1 in 11 people in the United States is likely to be affected during his lifespan [4]. In the USA, urolithiasis is mostly encountered in the South-Eastern

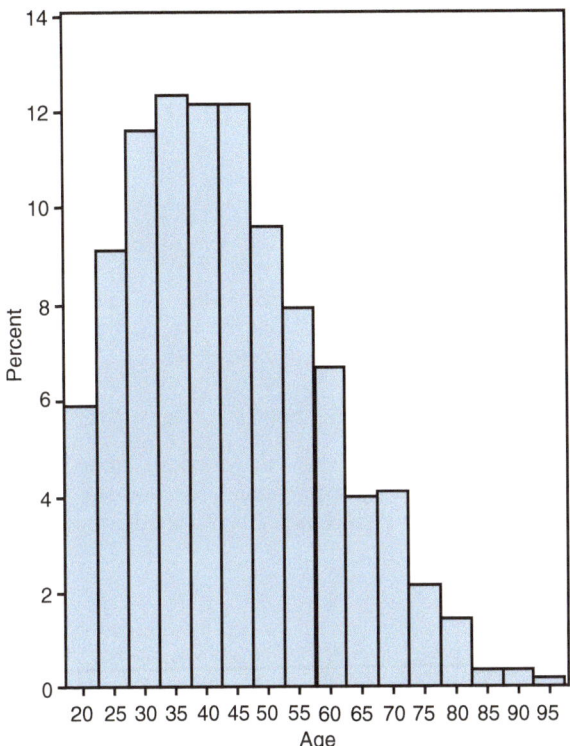

FIGURE 3.2 Age distribution of 1590 valid incident stone formers in Olmsted County, Minnesota, 1984–2003. From Krambeck AE et al. [3]. With permission from Elsevier

region, within the so-called "North-American stone belt" which includes the states of Virginia, North Carolina, Georgia, Tennessee, and Kentucky [2] (Fig. 3.3).

The same trends have been observed in European countries, Japan, and China. A so-called "African-Asian stone belt" was also described and includes North African, Middle East, and Asian countries (Fig. 3.4) [1, 2].

In contrast, very scarce reports exist from the Russian Siberian region, Sub-Saharan Africa, and Latin America (with the exception of the Northeast region of Brazil) (Fig. 3.5) [6].

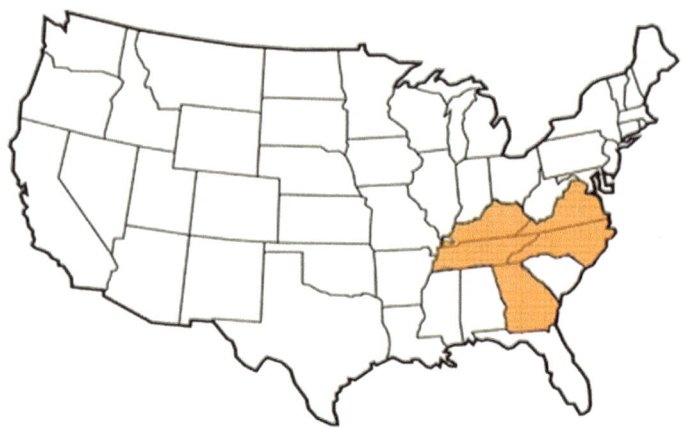

FIGURE 3.3 The so-called "North-American stone belt". From López M, Hoppe B. [2], with permission from the International Pediatric Nephrology Association (IPNA) and Springer

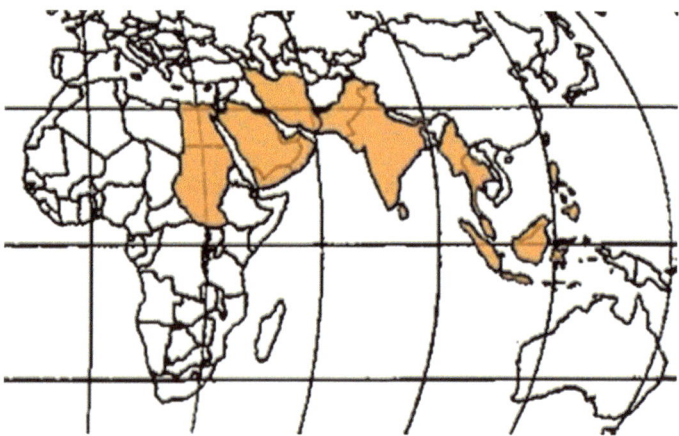

FIGURE 3.4 The so-called African-Asian stone belt. From López M and Hoppe B. [2], with permission from the International Pediatric Nephrology Association (IPNA) and Springer

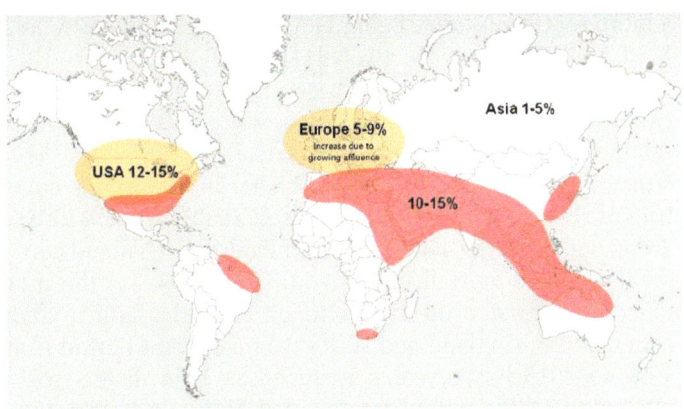

FIGURE 3.5 The so-called stone belt (*red*) extends all the way around the world and is characterized by urinary stone prevalence of 10–15%. From Fisang C et al. [6]. With permission from the Authors and Deutsches Ärzteblatt

The prevalence and incidence of stone disease in the USA are strongly associated with race or ethnicity, being higher among white population compared to Hispanics, Blacks, and Asians in decreasing order. However the prevalence has doubled in African Americans aged 60–74 years from the years 70s through the 90s. In all races, the disease burden is higher in men than in women [5]. The Male to Female ratio in the world varies from 2.5:1 in Japan to 1.15:1 in Iran [7].

Stone disease incidence has also shown an increase in the paediatric population in many countries. In the United States, The Rochester Epidemiology Project study has estimated this increase to be 4% per calendar-year throughout a 25-year period (1984–2008) [8] and there was a significant increase in the percentage of patients having calcium phosphate stones during the same period (18.5–27%) while the percentage of calcium oxalate has declined (60–47%) [9].

After a first stone episode, an old study has estimated the natural cumulative recurrence rate of urolithiasis to be 14%, 35%, and 52% at 1, 5, and 10 years respectively [10]. However the recurrence progression pattern was found to be slower in a more recent research, being 11%, 20%, 31%, and 39% at 2, 5, 10, and 15 years respectively [11]

Worth of note, urinary stone disease still kills in the twenty-first century. Worldwide there were 19,000 urolithiasis-related deaths reported in 2010 versus 18,400 in 1990 [12]. Not surprisingly this mortality is higher in developing countries as shown by the Global Diseases HealthGrove, with São Tomé and Príncipe, Honduras, Armenia, and Thailand carrying the highest mortality rate in 2013 [13]. However this mortality does exist even in developed countries and a study conducted in England and Wales over a 15-year period from 1999 to 2013 has revealed as much as 1954 deaths solely attributed to the complications of urolithiasis (mean 130.3 deaths/year), with a female to male ratio of 1.5:1 [14].

References

1. Atalab S, Pourmand G, El Howairis MF, et al. National profiles of urinary calculi: a comparison between developing and developed worlds. Iran J Kidney Dis. 2016;10(2):51–61.
2. López M, Hoppe B. History, epidemiology and regional diversities of urolithiasis. Pediatr Nephrol. 2010;25:49–59.
3. Krambeck AE, Lieske JC, Li X, et al. Effect of age on the clinical presentation of incident symptomatic urolithiasis in the general population. J Urol. 2013;189(1):158–64.
4. Scales CD Jr, Smith AC, Hanley JM, Saigal CS. Prevalence of kidney calculi in the United States. Urologic Diseases in America Project. Eur Urol. 2012;62:160–5.
5. Stamatelou KK, Francis ME, Jones CA, Nyberg LM, Curhan GC. Time trends in reported prevalence of kidney stones in the United States: 1976–1994. Kidney Int. 2003;63:1817–23.
6. Fisang C, Anding R, Müller SC, et al. Urolithiasis—an interdisciplinary diagnostic, therapeutic and secondary preventive challenge. Dtsch Arztebl Int. 2015;112(6):83–91.
7. Romero V, Akpinar H, Assimos DG. Kidney stones: a global picture of prevalence, incidence, and associated risk factors. Rev Urol. 2010;12(2–3):e86–96.
8. Dwyer ME, Krambeck AE, Bergstralh EJ, Milliner DS, Lieske JC, Rule AD. Temporal trends in incidence of kidney calculi

among children: a 25-year population based study. J Urol. 2012;188:247–52.

9. Wood KD, Stanasel IS, Koslov DS, Mufarrij PW, McLorie GA, Assimos DG. Changing stone composition profile of children with nephrolithiasis. Urology. 2013;82:210–3.

10. Uribarri J, Oh MS, Carroll HJ. The first kidney stone. Ann Intern Med. 1989;111(12):1006–9.

11. Rule AD, Lieske JC, Li X, Melton LJ, Krambeck AE, Bergstralh EJ. The ROKS Nomogram for Predicting a Second Symptomatic Stone Episode. Journal of the American Society of Nephrology. 2014;25(12):2878–86.

12. Lozano R, Naghavi M, Foreman K, et al. Global and regional mortality from 235 causes of death for 20 age groups in 1990 and 2010: a systematic analysis for the Global Burden of Disease Study 2010. Lancet. 2012;380(9859):2095–128.

13. http://global-diseases.healthgrove.com/l/203/Urolithiasis. Sources: Global Health Data Exchange (ghdx.healthdata.org) and The World Bank (data.worldbank.org).

14. Kum F, Mahmalji W, Hale J, et al. Do stones still kill? An analysis of death from stone disease 1999-2013 in England and Wales. BJU Int. 2016;118(1):140–4.

Chapter 4
Stone Composition

"The truth of the story lies in the details."

> *Paul Auster (1947–) (Prince of Asturias Award*
> *for Literature in 2006)*

The determination of the exact stone composition is necessary when one aims to understand its pathophysiology and to provide the optimal treatment to the patient. Contrary to a general belief, stone analysis is recommended in all first-time formers and not only in those with recurrent history of urolithiasis [1].

4.1 Stone Components

A comprehensive table of urinary stones composition with detailed chemical and mineral names as well as chemical formulas is presented below (Table 4.1) [2].

Many of the mineral names are eponymous given after famous Scientists or Explorers [3, 4]:

– **Whewellite** (calcium oxalate monohydrate) (Fig. 4.1a–c) is named after the English Professor William Whewell (1794–1866) who published an extensive research on mineralogy, geology, and many other fields.
– **Wheddelite** (calcium oxalate dihydrate) (Fig. 4.2a, b) is named after the Antarctic Weddell Sea, itself named after the British sailor and navigator James Weddell (1787–1834). As a mnemonic to differentiate between Wheddelite and Whewellite, just remember that there are

© Springer International Publishing AG 2017
S.A. Al-Mamari, *Urolithiasis in Clinical Practice*,
In Clinical Practice, DOI 10.1007/978-3-319-62437-2_4

TABLE 4.1 Stone composition

Chemical name	Mineral name	Chemical formula
Calcium oxalate monohydrate	Whewellite	$CaC_2O_4 \cdot H_2O$
Calcium oxalate dihydrate	Wheddelite	$CaC_2O_4 \cdot 2H_2O$
Basic calcium phosphate	Apatite	$Ca_{10}(PO_4)_6 \cdot (OH)_2$
Calcium hydroxyl phosphate	Carbonite apatite	$Ca_5(PO_3)_3(OH)$
b-tricalcium phosphate	Whitlockite	$Ca_3(PO_4)_2$
Carbonate apatite phosphate	Dahllite	$Ca_5(PO_4)_3OH$
Calcium hydrogen phosphate	Brushite	$CaHPO_4 \cdot 2H_2O$
Calcium carbonate	Aragonite	$CaCO3$
Octacalcium phosphate		$Ca_8H2(PO_4)_6 \cdot 5H_2O$
Uric acid	Uricite	$C_5H_4N_4O_3$
Uric acid dihydrate	Uricite	$C_5H_4O_3\text{-}2H_2O$
Ammonium urate		$NH_4C_5H_3N_4O_3$
Sodium acid urate monohydrate		$NaC_5H_3N_4O_3 \cdot H_2O$
Magnesium ammonium phosphate	Struvite	$MgNH_4PO_4 \cdot 6H_2O$
Magnesium acid phosphate trihydrate	Newberyite	$MgHPO_4 \cdot 3H_2O$
Magnesium ammonium phosphate monohydrate	Dittmarite	$MgNH_4(PO_4) \cdot 1H_2O$
Cystine		$[SCH_2CH(NH_2)COOH]_2$

TABLE 4.1 (continued)

Chemical name	Mineral name	Chemical formula
Gypsum	Calcium sulphate dihydrate	$CaSO_4 \cdot 2H_2O$
	Zinc phosphate tetrahydrate	$Zn_3(PO_4)_2 \cdot 4H_2O$
Xanthine		
2,8-Dihydroxyadenine		
Proteins		
Cholesterol		
Calcite		
Potassium urate		
Trimagnesium phosphate		
Melamine		
Matrix		
Drug stones	• Active compounds crystallising in urine • Substances impairing urine composition	
Foreign body calculi		

From Turk C et al. [2], reproduced and modified with Permission. © European Association of Urology 2015

two "d" in Whe**dd**elite corresponding to the two "d" in "**d**ihy**d**rate".

– **Struvite** (Magnesium ammonium phosphate) (Fig. 4.3) is named after the Russian Diplomat and naturalist Heinrich Christian Gottfried von Struve (1772–1851) who lived in Germany.

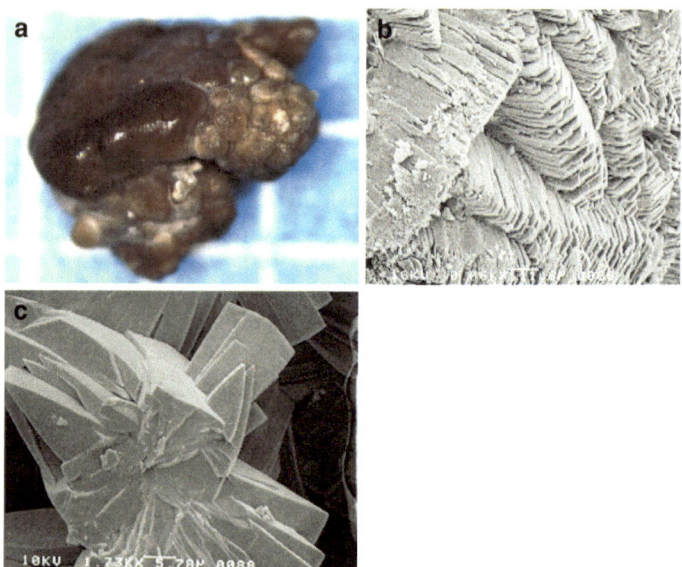

FIGURE 4.1 Calcium oxalate monohydrate stones. (**a**) Gross appearance. (**b**) and (**c**) electron micrographs. Courtesy of Louis C Herring & Co Lab, Orlando, Florida, USA

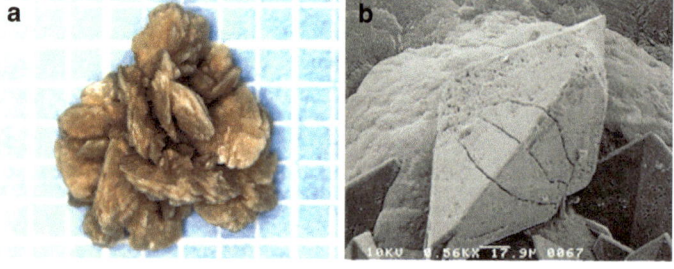

FIGURE 4.2 Calcium oxalate dihydrate stone. (**a**) Gross appearance. (**b**) Electron micrograph. Courtesy of Louis C Herring & Co Lab, Orlando, Florida, USA

FIGURE 4.3 A struvite stone.
Courtesy of Louis C
Herring & Co Lab,
Orlando, Florida, USA

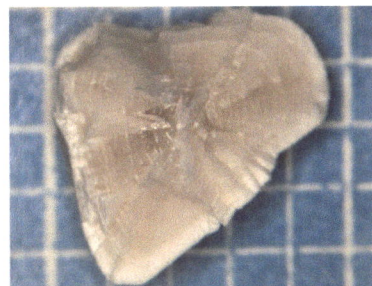

FIGURE 4.4 A brushite
stone. Courtesy of Louis C
Herring & Co Lab,
Orlando, Florida, USA

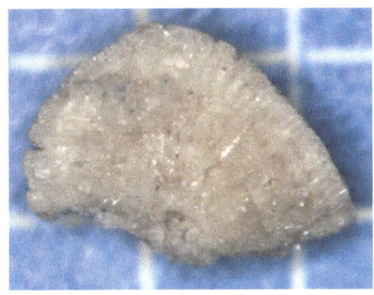

– **Newberyite** (Magnesium acid phosphate trihydrate) is
  named after the Australian geologist and mineralogist
  James Cosmo Newbery (1843–1895).
– **Brushite** (Calcium hydrogen phosphate) (Fig. 4.4) is
  named in honor of the American mineralogist George
  Jarvis Brush (1831–1912).
– **Whitlockite** (b-tricalcium phosphate) is named after the
  American mineralogist Herbert Percy Whitlock
  (1868–1948).
– **Dittmarite** (Magnesium ammonium phosphate mono-
  hydrate) is named after the German-Born Professor of
  Chemistry William Dittmar (1833–1892) who lived in
  Britain.
– **Hannayite**: Very rare, this mineral composition was
  named after the Scottish chemist James Ballantyne
  Hannay (1855–1931).

FIGURE 4.5 (**a**) Apatite crystal in Mexico (By Reno Chris, Public domain). (**b**) Electron micrograph of apatite stone. Courtesy of Louis C Herring & Co Lab, Orlando, Florida, USA

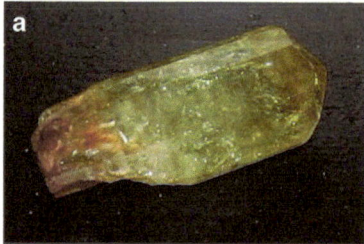

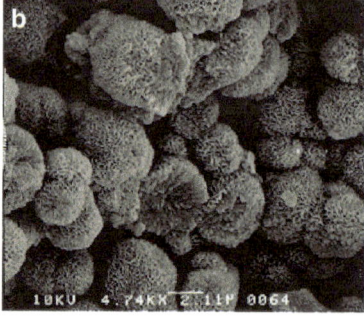

The name **Apatite** however was coined by the German geologist Abraham Gottlob Werner in 1786. It derives from the Greek verb "απατείν" (apatein), which means to deceive or to be misleading because this mineral is often mistaken for quartz or nepheline, or other more valuable minerals such as the gems peridot and beryl [3, 4] (Fig. 4.5a, b).

In contrast, other stones exclusively form in living humans or animals and do not have geological equivalents in the nature. These include Uric acid (Fig. 4.6a, b), Cystine (Fig. 4.7a, b), cholesterol, drugs, proteins, Xanthine, 2,8-dihydroxyadenine stones, etc.

4.2   Stone Subtypes and Associated Common Causes

Within the main stone morphological types, several subtypes have been described in relation to the causes. There are for example five subtypes of Whewellite (type I), three subtypes

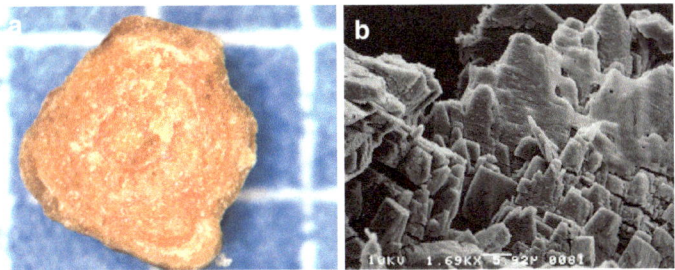

FIGURE 4.6 Uric acid stone. (**a**) Gross appearance of a cut section. (**b**) Electron micrograph. Courtesy of Louis C Herring & Co Lab, Orlando, Florida, USA

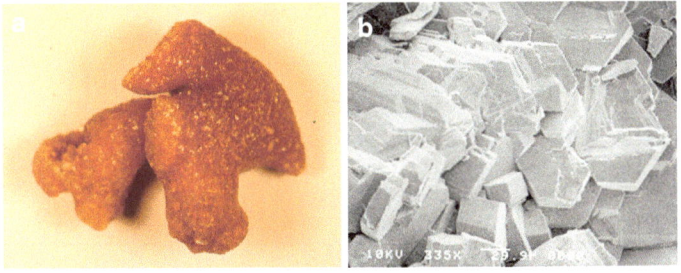

FIGURE 4.7 (**a, b**) Cystine stone. (**a**) Gross appearance. (**b**) Electron micrograph. Courtesy of Louis C Herring & Co Lab, Orlando, Florida, USA

of Wheddelite (type II), and five subtypes of urate stones (type III), and associations frequently exist between the subtypes [5] (Table 4.2 and Figs. 4.8, 4.9, and 4.10).

4.3   Methods to Determine the Stone Composition

No standard technique exists to determine the composition of a stone. Instead there are dozens of methods which should be performed meticulously, combining structural with morphological techniques, in order to reach to the best information [9]. The currently available means for stone analysis are:

TABLE 4.2 Main relations observed between stone type, main component, and etiology

Morphological type	Subtype	Main components	Common causes
I	Ia	Whewellite	Dietary hyperoxaluria
	Ib	Whewellite	Stasis, low diuresis
	Ic	Whewellite	Primary hyperoxaluria type I
	Id	Whewellite	Malformative uropathy, stasis and confined multiple stones
	Ie	Whewellite	Enteric hyperoxaluria
II	IIa	Weddellite	Hypercalciuria
	IIb	Weddellite ± whewellite	Hypercalciuria ± hyperoxaluria ± hypocitraturia
	IIc	Weddellite	Hypercalciuria, stasis and confined multiple stones
III	IIIa	Uric acids	Low urine pH and stasis
	IIIb	Uric acids	Metabolic syndrome, diabetes
	IIIc	Various urates	Hyperuricosuria and alkaline urine, UTI
	IIId	Ammonium urate	Hyperuricosuria and diarrhea

IV	IVa1	Carbapatite	Hypercalciuria, UTI
	IVa2	Carbapatite	Distal renal tubular acidosis
	IVb	Carbapatite	UTI, hypercalciuria. Etiology depends on minor components identified in the stone
	IVc	Struvite	UTI by urease-splitting bacteria
	IVd	Brushite	Hypercalciuria, PHPT, phosphate leak
V	Va	Cystine	Cystinuria
	Vb	Cystine	Cystinuria + inadequate therapy
VI	VIa	Proteins	Chronic pyelonephritis
	VIb	Proteins	Proteinuria, drugs, clots
	VIc	Proteins	ESRF and excessive calcium + vitamin D supplementation

(continued)

TABLE 4.2 (continued)

Morphological type	Subtype	Main components	Common causes
Main associations			
Ia or Ib + IIa or IIb		Whewellite + weddellite	Intermittent hyperoxaluria and hypercalciuria (dietary origin)
Ia + IVa1		Whewellite + carbapatite	Randall's plaque, medullary sponge kidney
IIa or IIb + IVa1		Weddellite + carbapatite	Absorptive or resorptive hypercalciuria
Ia or Ib + IIa or IIb + IVa or IVb		Whewellite + weddellite + carbapatite	Hyperoxaluria + hypercalciuria, medullary sponge kidney
Ia + IIIb		Whewellite + uric acid	Hyperoxaluria + metabolic syndrome

UTI Urinary tract infection, *PHPT* Primary hyperparathyroidism, *ESRF* End-stage renal failure. From Cloutier J et al. [5]. Creative Commons Attribution License

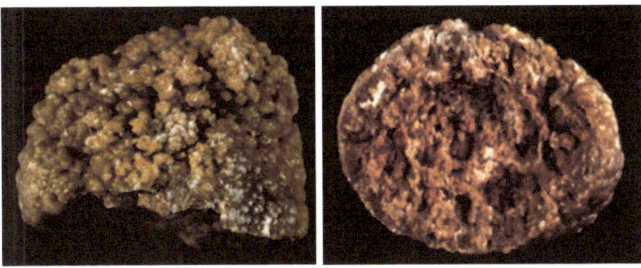

FIGURE 4.8 COM stones subtype Ie. *Left*: surface, *right*: section. From Cloutier J et al. [5] Creative Commons Attribution License

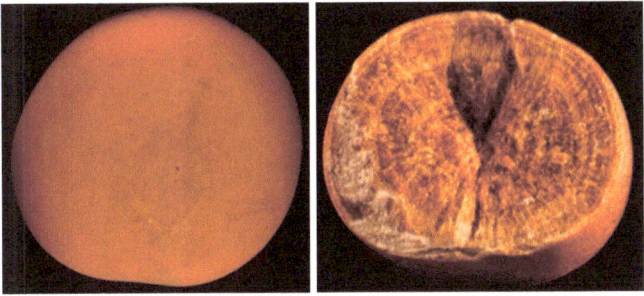

FIGURE 4.9 Uric acid stone subtype IIIa. *Left*: surface, *right*: section. From Cloutier J et al. [5]. Creative Commons Attribution License

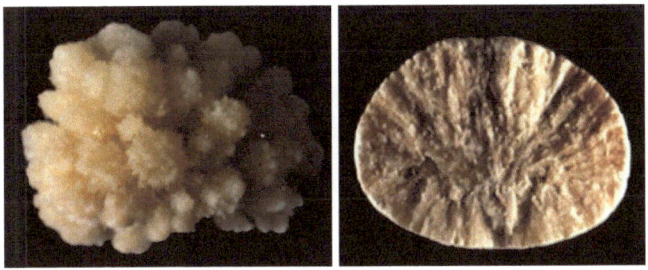

FIGURE 4.10 Brushite stones type IVd (*left* surface; *right* section). From Cloutier J et al. [5]. Creative Commons Attribution License.

Note: Brushite is considered the precursor phase of hydroxyapatite (calcium phosphate). Therefore brushite stones will form if brushite does not convert to hydroxyapatite [6, 7]. However unlike hydroxyapatite, brushite stones are hard and particularly resistant to extracorporeal shock wave lithotripsy [7, 8]

- wet chemical analysis,
- thermogravimetry,
- optic polarizing microscopy,
- scanning electron microscopy (SEM),
- and various methods of spectroscopy:

  - Fourier Transform Infrared spectroscopy (FTIR): examines molecular structure
  - X-Ray Powder Diffraction: determines the crystalline structure
  - Elementary Distribution Analysis

The wet chemical analysis was the most commonly used method to determine stone composition in the 80^s–90^s, but there has been a considerable decline in its use nowadays. It is even considered obsolete because of a very high proportion of errors (6.5–94%) with both the pure substances and binary mixtures [1, 10]. **The EAU experts give a preference to the use of FTIR or X-ray Powder Diffraction, and also to optic polarizing microscopy if available** [1]. However a recent French study has reemphasized on the limitations of all the above methods when used separately, achieving accuracy only when the stone is made of a single specific component such as uric acid, cystine, 2,8-dihydroxyadenine (DHA), struvite, ammonium hydrogen urate or a drug [11]. These tests are not reliable for common calcium nephrolithiasis, because the mere identification of the presence of calcium oxalate (CaOx) and/or calcium phosphate (CaP) is not sufficient to determine the stone aetiology since these constituents may be derived from various causes.

Moreover qualitative differences between the core and the shell of the stone are known since long and have been reported in 29.5% of stones [12]. This could be explained by the fact that the nucleation process is probably initiated by a mechanism different from the factors responsible for the subsequent stone growth [5] (Figs. 4.11 and 4.12).

Therefore, for accurate determination of the stone composition, it is advised to perform a comprehensive

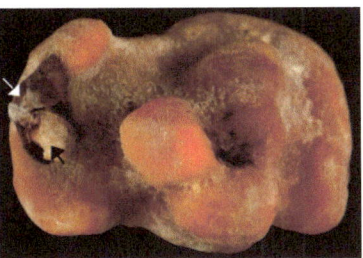

FIGURE 4.11 Uric acid kidney stone in a man aged 58 years old. The patient had a BMI above 30 kg/m^2 and suffered a type 2 diabetes mellitus and hypertension. Uric acid was the consequence of metabolic syndrome and diabetes. However, stone analysis provided evidence that uric acid was secondly deposited on a whewellite stone (*white arrow*) and that the first step of stone formation was a carbapatite Randall's plaque (*black arrow*), suggesting the stone was initiated for a long time. From Cloutier J et al. [5] Creative Commons Attribution License

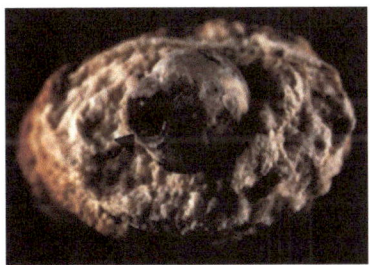

FIGURE 4.12 Section of a stone presumably related to urinary tract infection. In fact, while the peripheral layers are made of a mixture of carbapatite and struvite as a consequence of chronic UTI, the core of the stone is made of pure whewellite, suggesting that metabolic factors are first involved in the stone process. Of note, the morphology of the initial whewellite stone shows a papillary imprint (*arrow*) which is highly suggestive of heterogeneous nucleation from a Randall's plaque (not visible). From Cloutier J et al. [5] Creative Commons Attribution License

morpho-constitutional analysis of urinary stones by combining a careful morphological examination of the surface and the section of stones with detailed FTIR analysis of the nature, location, crystalline phases and a respective proportion of stone constituents [11].

A novel urine based assay using nanoscale flow cytometry of fluorescently labelled bisphosphonate probes (Alendronate-fluorescein/Alendronate-Cy5) was introduced recently; its combination with petrographic thin sections was proposed as an alternative means for determining stone composition [13].

Beside laboratory studies, Dual CT-scan can be used to predict kidney stone composition with a reported 82% accuracy [14] (see Chap 9: Investigations of Urinary Lithiasis), but this has shown limitations in predicting struvite stones [15].

It is also important to note that stone composition may change with repeat sample from the same person, and this has been shown to occur in as much as 21% of patients subjected to multiple stone analyses [16]. Subsequently it is recommended to perform a repeat stone analysis in patients having recurrent stones after receiving drug therapy, in those with early recurrence after a complete stone clearance, as well as in those with late recurrence after a long stone-free period [1].

Moreover the stone composition can be discordant in 25% of bilateral synchronous stones [17].

4.4   Statistics in Stone Composition

The reported stone compositions vary slightly from one study to another and hereafter are some of the most recent and relevant studies.

The largest stone composition study was probably conducted in Mayo Clinic in 2014 and included 43,545 patients [18]. **This study has shown an overall predominance of calcium oxalate stones representing 67.3% of all the stones, followed by apatite, uric acid, struvite, and brushite calculi** accounting for **16.1, 8.3, 3, and 0.9% respectively. Cystine stones were seen in 0.35% only.** It also showed that the calcium oxalate type was preponderant at all ages, starting with 40% in children, and then rising gradually to reach 75% between 50 and 60 years before progressively declining to around 40% by the age of 90. **Interestingly it revealed that the gap between calcium oxalate and apatite stones is smaller in women (58 and 25% respectively), compared with men (74 and 9.6% respectively).** It was also noted in this study that at the age of 50, the apatite and uric acid curves cross over with the uric acid composition surpassing that of the apatite from that age onwards.

A different study has observed a nearly similar trend among Olmsted County residents (Minnesota) (Fig. 4.13) [19].

More recently another comprehensive retrospective study from Mayo Clinic including 2961 first-time symptomatic kidney stone formers revealed similar stone compositions as above. These are described as follows: majority calcium oxalate (76%), majority hydroxyapatite (18%) (i.e. calcium

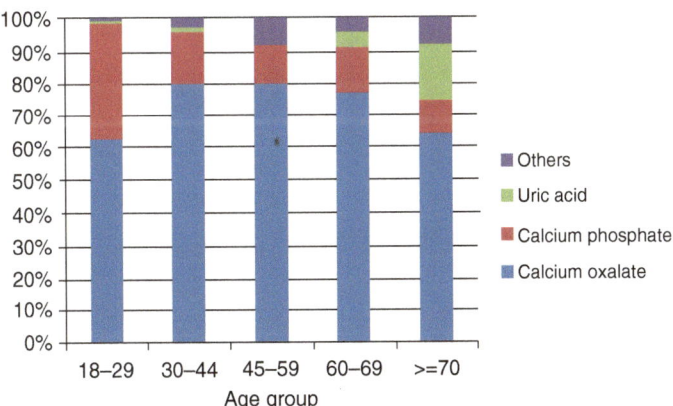

FIGURE 4.13 Stone composition as function of age among Olmsted County, Minnesota residents. From Krambeck AE et al. [19], with permission from Elsevier

stones made up a total of approximately 94% of cases), any uric acid (4.8%), any struvite (0.9%), and any brushite (0.9%) [20].

Stone composition during pregnancy showed predominating calcium phosphate (hydroxyapatite) (65–74%) over calcium oxalate stones (26% of cases), probably because of physiological elevation in maternal urinary calcium excretion and pH [21, 22].

4.5   Geographic Variations of Stone Composition

There are no statistical differences in stone composition within developed countries where the following values have been found: Calcium oxalate/calcium phosphate (81–92%), uric acid stone (5.5–16%), struvite (5.1–7%) [23–26].

There are however small differences observed in developing countries attributable to dietary, socio-economic, and environmental factors, and the following patterns have been reported notably showing a higher proportion of infective stones: calcium oxalate(59.5–87.3%), uric acid (1–19%), phosphate calculi (3–16.7%), struvite (1.4–14.6%) [26].

In the Arabian Peninsula, a Saudi study confirmed that calcium-based stones formed the great majority (84.6%), followed by uric acids (12.8%) [27], while an Omani study characteristically showed a higher rate of cystine stone (4%) than the reported values in the literature [28].

4.6   Changes in Community Stone Composition Over Time

Several investigators have addressed the variations of stone composition in the same community over time. A study in the American state of Massachusetts evaluating a 20-year period (1990–2010) and including over 11,000 stone analyses, found that the percentage of stones from women (i.e. female/male ratio) increased from 29.8 to 39.1%. Furthermore the percentage of uric acid-predominant stones in females increased from 7.6 to 10.2%, while the struvite stones decrease from 7.8 to 3.0% [29]. In the male population, there was no significant change in majority uric acid stones (from 11.7 to 10.8%), while the percentages of apatite, struvite (2.8 to 3.7%), and cystine stones (0.1 to 0.6%) increased significantly. Another study found that the stone composition in Australia has remained relatively static over the past 30 years with regard to the percentage of uric acid (16–17%) and calcium oxalate stones (64–68%), despite modifications in diet and body habitus [25]. There was however a decreased trend in struvite stones (14–7%).

References

1. Türk C, Petřík A, Sarica K, et al. EAU guidelines on diagnosis and conservative management of urolithiasis. Eur Urol. 2016;69(3):468–74.
2. Türk C, Knoll T, Petřík A, et al. EAU guidelines on urolithiasis. © European Association of Urology; 2015. p. 9. http://uroweb.org/wp-content/uploads/22-Urolithiasis_LR_full.pdf
3. Master VA, Meng MV, Stoller ML. Stone nomenclature and history of instrumentation for urinary stone disease. In: Stoller ML, Meng MV, editors. Urinary stone disease: the practical guide to medical and surgical management. Totowa: Humana Press; 2007. p. 3–26.
4. Moran ME. What's in a name? In: Moran AE, editor. Urolithiasis. A comprehensive history. New York: Springer; 2014. p. 168–71.
5. Cloutier J, Villa L, Traxer O, Daudon M. Kidney stone analysis: "give me your stone, I will tell who you are". World J Urol. 2015;33(2):157–69.
6. Pak CY, Eanes ED, Ruskin B. Spontaneous precipitation of brushite in urine: evidence that brushite is the nidus of renal stones originating as calcium phosphate. Proc Natl Acad Sci U S A. 1971;68(7):1456–60.
7. Krambeck AE, Handa SE, Evan AP, Lingeman JE. Profile of the brushite stone former. J Urol. 2010;184(4):1367–71.
8. Klee LW, Brito CG, Lingeman JE. The clinical implications of brushite calculi. J Urol. 1991;145(4):715–8.

9. Basiri A, Taheri M, Taheri F. What is the state of the stone analysis techniques in urolithiasis? Urol J. 2012;9:445.

10. Hesse A, Kruse R, Geilenkeuser WJ, et al. Quality control in urinary stone analysis: results of 44 ring trials (1980-2001). Clin Chem Lab Med. 2005;43(3):298–303.

11. Daudon M, Dessombz A, Frochot V, et al. Comprehensive morpho-constitutional analysis of urinary stones improves etiological diagnosis and therapeutic strategy of nephrolithiasis. C R Chim. 2016;19(11–12):1470–91.

12. Schubert G, Brien G, Bick C. Separate examinations on core and shell of urinary calculi. Urol Int. 1983;38(2):65–9.

13. Gavin CT, Ali SN, Tailly T, et al. Novel methods of determining urinary calculi composition: petrographic thin sectioning of calculi and nanoscale flow cytometry urinalysis. Sci Rep. 2016;6:19328.

14. Hidas G, Eliahou R, Duvdevani M, et al. Determination of renal stone composition with dual-energy CT: in vivo analysis and comparison with x-ray diffraction. Radiology. 2010;257(2):394–401.

15. Marchini GS, Gebreselassie S, Liu X, et al. Absolute Hounsfield unit measurement on noncontrast computed tomography cannot accurately predict struvite stone composition. J Endourol. 2013;27:162.

16. Lee TT, Elkoushy MA, Andonian S. Are stone analysis results different with repeated sampling? Can Urol Assoc J. 2014;8(5–6):E317–22.

17. Kadlec AO, Fridirici ZC, Acosta-Miranda AM, et al. Bilateral urinary calculi with discordant stone composition. World J Urol. 2014;32:281.

18. Lieske JC, Rule AD, Krambeck AE. Stone composition as a function of age and sex. Clin J Am Soc Nephrol. 2014;9(12):2141–6.

19. Krambeck AE, Lieske JC, Li X, et al. Effect of age on the clinical presentation of incident symptomatic urolithiasis in the general population. J Urol. 2013;189(1):158–64.

20. Singh P, Enders FT, Vaughan LE, et al. Stone composition among first-time symptomatic kidney stone formers in the community. Mayo Clin Proc. 2015;90(10):1356–65.

21. Ross AE, Handa S, Lingeman JE, Matlaga BR. Kidney stones during pregnancy: an investigation into stone composition. Urol Res. 2008;36(2):99–102.

22. Meria P, Hadjadj H, Jungers P, et al. Stone formation and pregnancy: pathophysiological insights gained from morphoconstitutional stone analysis. J Urol. 2010;183:1412–8.

23. Parks JH, Worcester EM, Coe FL, Evan AP, Lingeman JE. Clinical implications of abundant calcium phosphate in routinely analyzed kidney calculi. Kidney Int. 2004;66:777–85.

24. Yasui T, Iguchi M, Suzuki S, Kohri K. Prevalence and epidemiological characteristics of urolithiasis in Japan: national trends between 1965 and 2005. Urology. 2008;71:209–13.

25. Lee MC, Bariol SV. Changes in upper urinary tract stone composition in Australia over the past 30 years. BJU Int. 2013;112(Suppl 2):65–8.

26. Atalab S, Pourmand G, El Howairis Mel F, et al. National profiles of urinary calculi: a comparison between developing and developed worlds. Iran J Kidney Dis. 2016;10(2):51–61.

27. Alkhunaizi AM. Urinary stones in Eastern Saudi Arabia. Urol Ann. 2016;8(1):6–9.

28. Al-Marhoon MS, Bayoumi R, Al-Farsi Y, et al. Urinary stone composition in Oman: with high incidence of cystinuria. Urolithiasis. 2015;43(3):207–11.

29. Moses R, Pais VM Jr, Ursiny M, et al. Changes in stone composition over two decades: evaluation of over 10,000 stone analyses. Urolithiasis. 2015;43(2):135–9.

Chapter 5
Lithogenesis

"If you can't explain it simply, you don't understand it well enough"

Albert Einstein (1879–1955) (Nobel Prize in Physics in 1921, Time Person of the Century in 1999)

5.1 Mechanisms of Stone Formation

The physiopathological mechanism of stone formation is a very complex, progressive, and incompletely understood process which includes precipitation, nucleation, crystal growth, aggregation, and concretion of various modulators in urine (Fig. 5.1) [1].

The hypothesis of stone formation is based on 3 mechanisms [2–4]:

- The concentration and the solubility of the precipitating substances in urine
- The presence of promoters of crystallization:
    - Calcium,
    - oxalate,
    - urate and
    - phosphate ions.
- The absence or insufficiency of inhibitors of crystallization:
    - small ions
    - molecules such as magnesium, citrate and pyrophosphate

© Springer International Publishing AG 2017
S.A. Al-Mamari, *Urolithiasis in Clinical Practice*,
In Clinical Practice, DOI 10.1007/978-3-319-62437-2_5

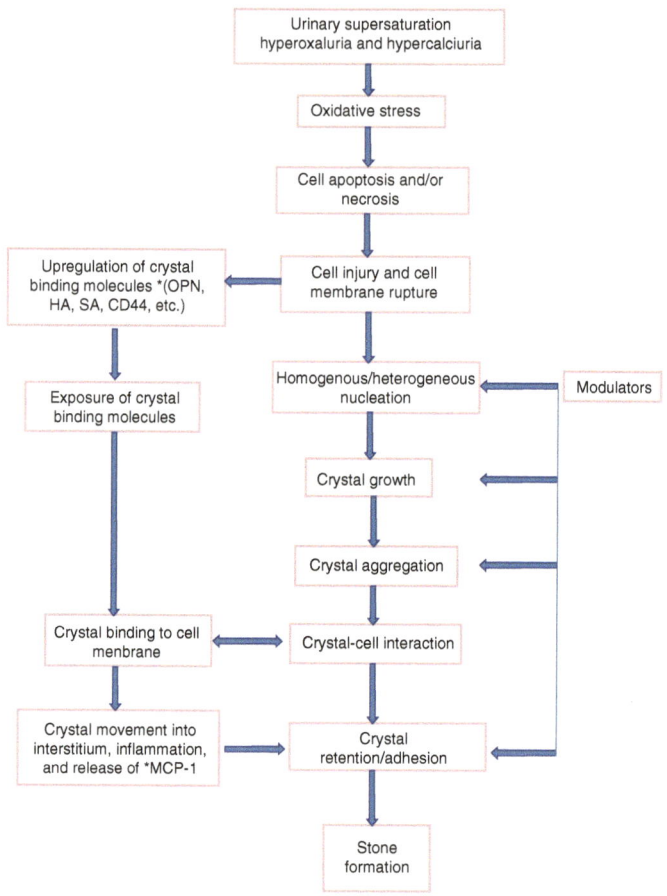

FIGURE 5.1 Schematic representation of various cellular and extracellular events during stone formation. *OPN osteopontin, HA hyaluronic acid, SA sialic acid, MCP-1 monocyte chemoattractant protein-1. From Aggarwal KP et al. [1]. Creative Commons Attribution License

- macromolecules such as osteopontin [5, 6], bikunin [7], matrix GLA protein, Tamm-Horsfall protein, the urinary fragment 1 of prothrombin, diphosphonate, glycosaminoglycans [3, 8].

Inhibitors can further be divided into two sub-groups according to their effect:

– effect on crystal growth: citrate, pyrophosphate and magnesium
– effect on crystal aggregation: glycosaminoglycans, pyrophosphate, and citrate [9].

A "culprit" generally advocated in triggering urinary crystallization and precipitation is a circumstantial poor hydration state of the individual, as seen during hot seasons [10–12].

An easy way to summarize the process of lithogenesis can be proposed as follows:

Hypersaturated urine with a particular solute (either low urine volume or increased excretion of the solute) → crystals formation → progressive growing and aggregation → stone.

Despite being correct, this simplistic explanation does not tell us how and where exactly crystallization starts in the renal parenchyma. The following are findings and advocated theories attempting to lighten this shadowed area.

5.2 Randall's Plaques

In 1937, Alexander Randall stated that crystalline growth starts from plaques of calcium phosphate in the interstitium within renal papillae at the bottom of the renal calyces [13] (Figs. 5.2, 1–6). These plaques have been named after him since then. Although Randall's plaques have not been observed in few conditions, this theory has not yet been contradicted, and contemporary authors are attempting to give more precision on the origin of the plaques. When analysing intra-operative biopsies of kidneys from idiopathic calcium-stone formers, some authors found that the plaques arose from the basement membrane of the thin loop of Henle before spreading through the interstitium to beneath the urothelium. In addition there was no plaque development observed in patients with stones due to obesity-related bypass procedures, who form instead intratubular hydroxyapatite

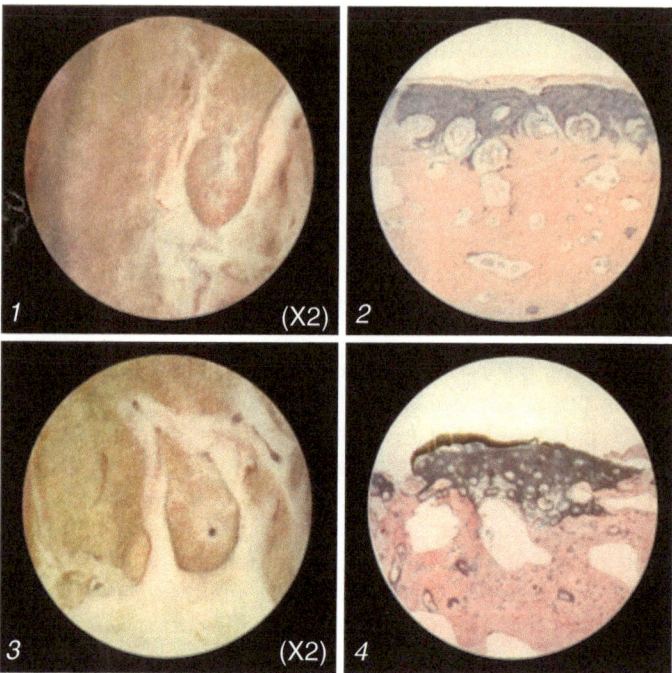

FIGURE 5.2 (*1*) Drawing of a typical subsurface calcium plaque in the wall of a renal papilla. (*2*) Detailed drawing of high magnification of a subsurface calcium deposit on the renal papilla. Note the shrunken tubules at the base of the plaque, their loss of normal epithelium, and the absence of any reaction suggesting infection. (*3*) Colored photograph of a renal papilla, showing the subsurface calcium deposit, and in its center a tiny black secondary deposit. This is the earliest evidence of secondary deposit which forms stone. (*4*). Colored photomicrograph of *3*, showing the calcium plaque which has lost its covering mucosa, and on which is a secondary deposit of brown material, taken to be the earliest evidence of renal calculus formation. No evidence of infection. (*5*) Colored photograph showing calcium deposits in two papillae, and a stone attached and growing on the calcium deposit in the third papilla. Another stone of similar character found in this kidney has been analyzed and proven to be composed of calcium phosphate. (*6*) Colored photomicrograph of *5*, showing the papillary stone attached to its calcium plaque. The differential staining shows the stone composed of calcium phosphate. The plaque with some phosphate staining; counterstains for calcium of different composition. No evidence of infection. From Randall [13]. With permission from Wolters Kluwer Health, Inc

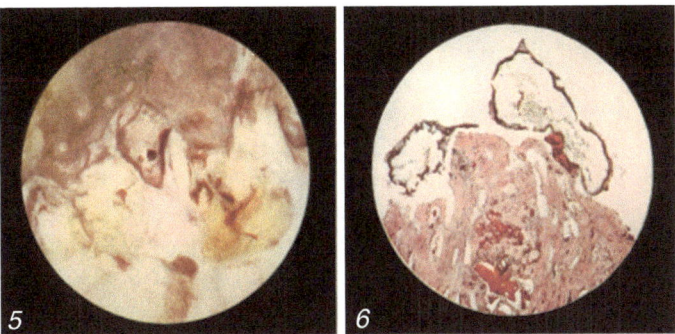

FIGURE 5.2 (continued)

crystals in collecting ducts [14]. Other authors pointed out a deeper origin of the plaques within the papilla in an intimate association with the collecting tubules and vasa recta [15].

5.3 The Free or Fixed Particle Theory

Are the stones developing from an aggregation of free crystals in the tubular lumen or from coated crystals on the tubular wall? An attempt to answer to this crucial question can be summarized in the following points:

(a) In 1978 B. Finlayson and F. Reid excluded the possibility of stone formation in the renal tubules and renal pelvis developing from unattached (free) particles, and stated on the likelihood of this mechanism occurring for bladder stones only [16].

(b) In 1994, DJ Kok and SR Khan demonstrated that during the normal transit time through the kidney, large free crystalline particles can be formed in long loop of Henle and be retained at the end of the collecting ducts, becoming the nidus of a stone [17, 18].

(c) Both mechanisms (free and fixed particles) seem to be accepted nowadays, and four distinct pathways in lithogenesis have been proposed based on endourological findings [19]:

- growth over white (Randall's) interstitial hydroxyapatite plaque, especially for calcium oxalate stones in hypercalciuric patients (Fig. 5.3a, b). Nowadays, thanks to the electron microscopy, a better and more detailed histological definition of the Randall's plaque is proposed by contemporary researchers (Fig. 5.4a–g).
- growth over Bellini duct plugs: this mechanism is possible for all stone types, but has not yet been proven independently to trigger stone formation. Some investigators have proposed a unified theory of plaque and plug formation for renal stones [20].
- formation of micro-liths within inner medullary collecting ducts (IMCD) (Fig. 5.5a, b).

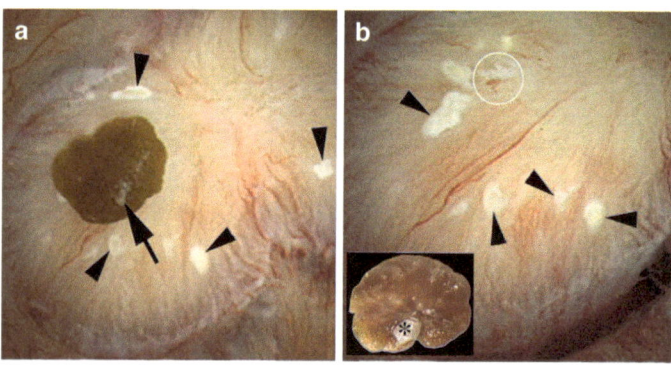

FIGURE 5.3 Attached stone to site of Randall's plaque in an idiopathic calcium oxalate stone former. (**a**) Endoscopic view of a calcium oxalate stone (*arrow*) attached to the tip of a papilla. Several sites of interstitial (Randall's) plaque (*arrowheads*) are seen around the attached stone. Note the normal appearance of the papilla. (**b**) The same papilla seen after the stone was removed. The papillary surface of that same stone is seen by light microscopy as an inset at the bottom left of this panel. **A small site of whitish mineral (marked by *asterisk*) is clearly visible and was identified as hydroxyapatite while the rest of the stone is calcium oxalate.** From Evan AP et al. [19], with permission from Springer-Verlag

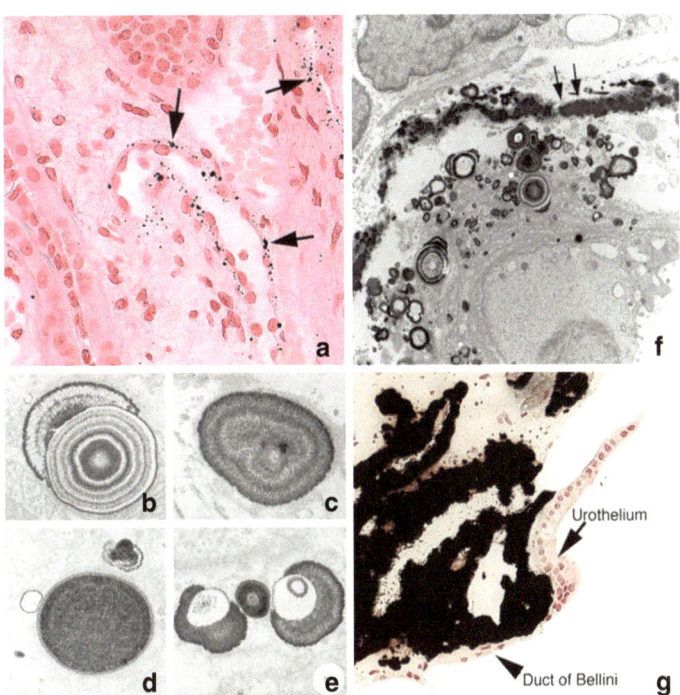

FIGURE 5.4 Histologic images showing initial sites of Randall's plaque and its progression. (**a**) Light microscopy revealing the initial sites of interstitial deposits (*arrows*) to be in the basement membranes of the thin loops of Henle at the papilla tip. (**b–e**) Transmission electron microscopy showing that the sites of interstitial deposits are made up of numerous micro-spherulites of alternating lamina of matrix with and without crystals. The individual deposits are as small as 50 nm and grow into multi-layered spheres of alternating light and electron dense rings with the light regions representing crystals and the electron dense sites matrix material. (**f**) Extensive accumulation of crystalline deposits occurring around the loops of Henle (*double arrows*). (**g**) Spread into the nearby interstitial space extending to the urothelial lining of the urinary space. Disruption of the urothelial layer exposes the site of interstitial deposits to the urine which can trigger overgrowth of mineral and thus stone formation. From Evan AP et al. [19], with permission from Springer-Verlag

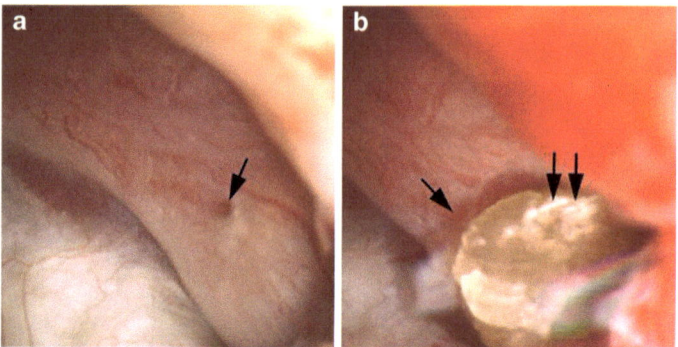

FIGURE 5.5 Endoscopic unroofing of an IMCD ductal stone in cystinuric stone former. (**a**) Micro-liths of cystine are present at the distal ends of IMCD and are easily seen at the time of percutaneous nephrolithotomy to lie under the urothelium at a site marked by a dark shadow (*arrow*) on a dilated duct. (**b**) When the IMCD is unroofed with a laser, an unattached, round tiny 'stone' is exposed (*double arrow*) within dilated IMCD and easily flows out of the IMCD lumen. (IMCD: inner medullary collecting ducts). From Evan AP et al. [19], with permission from Springer-Verlag

  – formation in free solution within the calyces or renal collecting system (Fig. 5.6a, b): No attachment site for the stone is seen on renoscopy. This has been observed for all cystine stones, but also for some CaOx stones in Primary Hyperoxaluria type I (PH1) and obesity bypass, most brushite and hydroxyapatite stones.

5.4   Further Hypothesis

A new theory has recently been raised stipulating that Randall's plaque at the papillary tip doesn't form until a threshold of proximal mineralization is reached. More precisely it was found that mineral density measurements vary between 330 mg/cm^3 and 270 mg/cm^3 respectively in proximal intratubular and in distal interstitial deposits supporting that proximal mineralisation triggers distal Randall's plaque formation [21].

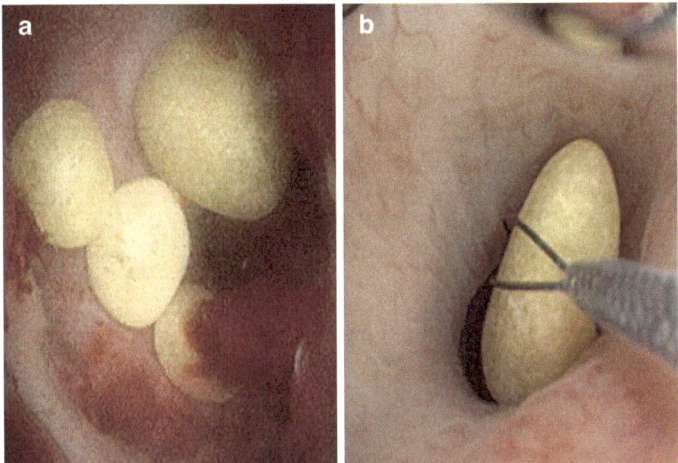

FIGURE 5.6 (**a**) Stones from cystinuric patients have consistent characteristics of a stone formed in 'free solution'. (**b**) The cystine stones look like 'Easter eggs' in that they are completely smooth, oval in shape, have a homogenous yellow coloration and are freely floating in a renal calyx. They are easily grasped and removed. From Evan AP et al. [19], with permission from Springer-Verlag

References

1. Aggarwal KP, Narula S, Kakkar M, Tandon C. Nephrolithiasis: molecular mechanism of renal stone formation and the critical role played by modulators. Biomed Res Int. 2013;2013:292953.
2. Daudon M, Frochot V. Crystalluria. Clin Chem Lab Med. 2015;53(Suppl 2):s1479–87.
3. Fleisch H. Inhibitors and promoters of stone formation. Kidney Int. 1978;13(5):361–71.
4. Robertson WG. Pathophysiology of stone formation. Urol Int. 1986;41(5):329–33.
5. Wesson JA, Johnson RJ, Mazzali M, et al. Osteopontin is a critical inhibitor of calcium oxalate crystal formation and retention in renal tubules. J Am Soc Nephrol. 2003;14(1):139–47.
6. Li X, Liu K, Pan Y, et al. Roles of osteopontin gene polymorphism (rs1126616), osteopontin levels in urine and serum, and the risk of urolithiasis: a meta-analysis. Biomed Res Int. 2015;2015:315043.

7. Atmani F, Mizon J, Khan SR. Inter-alpha-inhibitor: a protein family involved in the inhibition of calcium oxalate crystallization. Scanning Microsc. 1996;10(2):425–33; discussion 433–4.

8. Ryall RL, Harnett RM, Marshall VR. The effect of urine pyrophosphate, citrate, magnesium and glycosaminoglycans on the growth and aggregation of calcium oxalate crystals in vitro. Clin Chim Acta. 1981;112:349–56.

9. Fleisch H. Mechanisms of stone formation: role of promoters and inhibitors. Scand J Urol Nephrol Suppl. 1980;53:53–66.

10. Lieske JC, Rule AD, Krambeck AE. Stone composition as a function of age and sex. Clin J Am Soc Nephrol. 2014;9(12):2141–6.

11. Alkhunaizi AM. Urinary stones in Eastern Saudi Arabia. Urol Ann. 2016;8(1):6–9.

12. Fukuhara H, Ichiyahagi O, Kakizaki H, et al. Clinical relevance of seasonal changes in the prevalence of ureterolithiasis in the diagnosis of renal colic. Urolithiasis. 2016;44(6):529–37.

13. Randall A. The origin and growth of renal calculi. Ann Surg. 1937;105(6):1009–27.

14. Evan AP, Lingeman JE, Coe FL, et al. Randall's plaque of patients with nephrolithiasis begins in basement membranes of thin loops of Henle. J Clin Invest. 2003;111(5):607–16.

15. Stoller ML, Low RK, Shami GS, et al. High resolution radiography of cadaveric kidneys: unraveling the mystery of Randall's plaque formation. J Urol. 1996;156(4):1263–6.

16. Finlayson B, Reid F. The expectation of free and fixed particles in urinary stone disease. Invest Urol. 1978;15(6):442–8.

17. Kok DJ, Khan SR. Calcium oxalate nephrolithiasis, a free or fixed particle disease. Kidney Int. 1994;46(3):847–54.

18. Gambaro G, Trinchieri A. Recent advances in managing and understanding nephrolithiasis/nephrocalcinosis. F1000Res. 2016;5. pii: F1000 Faculty Rev-695.

19. Evan AP, Worcester EM, Coe FL, et al. Mechanisms of human kidney stone formation. Urolithiasis. 2015;43(Suppl 1):19–32.

20. Khan SR, Canales BK. Unified theory on the pathogenesis of Randall's plaques and plugs. Urolithiasis. 2015;43(Suppl 1): 109–23.

21. Hsi RS, Ramaswamy K, Ho SP, Stoller ML. The origins of urinary stone disease: upstream mineral formations initiate downstream Randall's plaque. BJU Int. 2017;119(1):177–84.

Chapter 6
Etiology of Urolithiasis

"Shallow men believe in luck or in circumstance. Strong men believe in cause and effect."

Ralph Waldo Emerson (1803–1882)

Kidney stone disease is a complex disorder associated with a multitude of possible causes, among which metabolic and genetic components occupy an important position, being represented by hyperoxaluria, hypercalciuria, hypocitraturia, hyperuricemia, renal tubular acidosis, hypophosphatemia, cystinuria, etc. Other causes include: urinary infections, impaired drainage (i.e. obstruction), post-bariatric surgery, foreign bodies, drugs, etc. In many cases these factors are intermingling, necessitating a comprehensive clinical evaluation of the patient.

The primary cause and contributory factors of urolithiasis can only be determined after a thorough history, physical examination and paraclinical investigations including: 24-h urine analysis, urinary microscopy and culture, stone analysis, shape, radiodensity/radiopacity, size, number, and location, determination of any associated dysmetabolism, and imaging of the kidney and urinary tract anatomy.

It should always be remembered that a complete clinical description is invaluable as a first step in the route to the etiological definition of a stone. Herein several parameters help to describe the urinary lithiasis:

- Symptomatic or asymptomatic, i.e. fortuitously discovered during investigations for other pathologies,
- Radiopaque or radiolucent,

© Springer International Publishing AG 2017   57
S.A. Al-Mamari, *Urolithiasis in Clinical Practice*,
In Clinical Practice, DOI 10.1007/978-3-319-62437-2_6

- obstructing or non-obstructing,
- anatomical locations: renal (pelvis, upper, mid, lower calyceal, or diverticular), ureteric (upper, mid, or lower), vesical (in the bladder lumen or in a diverticulum), or urethral (posterior or anterior urethra, or urethral diverticulum)
- size: small (<5 mm), intermediate (5–19 mm), or large (>20 mm).
- number: solitary or multiple
- shape: roundish, irregular, stellar, spiky, staghorn
- Laterality: unilateral or bilateral
- First time seen, recurrent, or residual after treatment of the primary stone
- Associated with an obvious cause: dysmetabolism, urinary infection, anatomical or functional abnormality, i.e. retention or impaired drainage,
- Family history

The trainee or the practitioner in Urology is expected to complete this description as meticulously as possible, as a clue to reach to the aetiology and a guide in the initiation of the correct management.

In the present section we will systematically discuss the possible causes of urinary stones.

6.1   Genetic Predispositions

A distinction has been made between the common polygenic and rare monogenic forms of urolithiasis [1–3].

The polygenic forms are well exemplified by the idiopathic calcium oxalate urolithiasis, a common entity affecting the majority of stone formers and associated with many metabolic disorders [3]: hypercalciuria, hyperoxaluria, hypocitraturia, hyperphosphaturia, hyperuricosuria, etc. For sake of clarity these disorders will be addressed separately below under the paragraph "Dysmetabolism".

The monogenic forms account only for 2 and 10% of adult and pediatric kidney formers respectively [2]. However they are characterized by a more severe clinical pattern and their propensity to progress to renal impairment. They include rare entities such as cystinuria, primary hyperoxaluria, Dent's disease, adenine phosphoribosyltransferase (APRT) deficiency, hypoxanthine-guanine phosphoribosyl-transferase (HPRT) deficiency and familial hypomagnesemia with hypercalciuria and nephrocalcinosis (FHHNC) [3].

6.1.1 Dysmetabolism

It is of paramount importance to undertake a metabolic evaluation following initial diagnosis of urolithiasis. This will allow for more specific prescription, either of pharmacological or non-pharmacological interventions, aiming at preventing recurrent stone formation [4].

Eighty-five percent of children presenting with urinary stones were shown to have a positive family history of urolithiasis and 93.2% of them had a metabolic abnormality with hypercalciuria being the most common finding [5]. Consequently hereditary metabolic causes should be suspected in children presenting with a urinary stone particularly at a younger age.

Analyses of 24-h urine composition performed in the Harvard Medical School (Boston) comparing first-time and recurrent stone-formers in the adult population showed similar urine abnormalities in both groups. Overall metabolic abnormalities were encountered in 83.1% and 88.8% respectively, and the rates of various abnormalities did not show any significant difference between the two groups (Table 6.1) [6].

Comparable results were found in another study performed in Pakistan where metabolic abnormalities were found in as much as 90.5% of adults presenting with either multiple or recurrent urinary stones. Again hyperoxaluria, hypercalciuria and hypocitraturia were the most encountered disorders, and 78.5% of the patients had multiple abnormalities. The only notable difference is the higher rate of hyperoxaluria reported in the latter study, **being the most frequent abnormality with 64.5%** (Table 6.2) [7]. These differences can

TABLE 6.1 Univariate analysis of urine abnormalities in first-time and recurrent stone-formers

	First-time stone-former	Recurrent stone-former	P value
Hypercalciuria	28 (39.4%)	104 (43.3%)	.56
Hyperoxaluria	23 (32.4%)	80 (33.3%)	.88
Hyperuricosuria	32 (45.0%)	108 (45.0%)	.99
Hypocitraturia	21 (29.5%)	56 (23.3%)	.29
Any abnormality	59 (83.1%)	213 (88.8%)	.22

From Eisner BH et al. [6], with permission from Elsevier

TABLE 6.2 Frequency of metabolic abnormalities

Metabolic abnormality	Frequency	%age
Hyperoxaluria (oxalate >45 mg/day)	129	64.5
Hypercalciuria (>250 mg/day for women and >300 mg/day for men)	87	43.5
Hypocitraturia (citrate levels <320 mg/day)	81	40.5
Hypernatriuria (sodium level >220 mmol/day)	59	29.5
Hyperuricosuria (>600 mg/day in women and >750 mg/day in men)	43	21.5
Hypomagnesuria (magnesium level <3 mg/day)	27	13.5
Hyperphosphaturia (phosphate level >1.3 g/day)	23	11.5
Hypercalcemia (calcium above the normal range i.e. 8.4–10.2 mg/dL):	93	46.5
Hyperuricemia: (normal range 2.5–8 mg/dL for males and 1.5–6.0 mg/dL for females)	59	29.5

From Ahmad I et al. [7]. Creative Commons Attribution License

probably be explained by genetic and dietary variations as suggested by the following two studies which are characterized by very low hyperoxaluria rates.

It was found among 3040 kidney stone formers in Argentina that biochemical abnormalities were present in 91.5% of patients. The abnormalities consisted of idiopathic hypercalciuria in 56.88%, hyperuricosuria in 21.08%, unduly acidic urine in 10.95%, hypocitraturia in 10.55%, hypomagnesuria in 7.9%, primary hyperparathyroidism on 3.01%, **hyperoxaluria in 2.6%**, and cystinuria in 0.32% of patients [8].

The most frequent metabolic abnormality in Thai population with recurrent idiopathic calcium stones has been reported to be hypocitraturia accounting for 69.6% of cases, while **hyperoxaluria was the lowest reported in the literature with only 1.3%** [9].

Notwithstanding these variations, all these studies and many others underscore the need for a metabolic evaluation of patients presenting with urolithiasis.

6.1.1.1   Hypercalciuria

Many studies have reported hypercalciuria to be the most common metabolic abnormality associated with urolithiasis [6, 8]. It is defined as the urinary excretion of more than 0.1 mmol/kg/24 h of calcium (or more than 4 mg calcium/kg/day) in an individual on normal diet. Due to the sexual difference, this definition can be globally adjusted as more than 300 mg calcium per day in men and more than 250 mg calcium per day in women.

Two categories of hypercalciuria have been described:

• Idiopathic: This is the most frequent one, being observed in about 50% of patients with calcium oxalate/apatite nephrolithiasis [10]. There is no detectable cause and the patient does not exhibit hypercalcemia.

Pak et al. described three types of idiopathic hypercalciuria, absorptive, resorptive, and renal [11], which consist of the following mechanisms respectively: increased intestinal absorption of calcium, increased bone resorption, and defective reabsorption of calcium by the renal tubule [12]. Absorptive hypercalciuria has three sub-types: Sub-type I is dietary independent, sub-type II is dietary dependent, and sub-type III is secondary to a phosphate renal leak which triggers a secondarily increased parathyroid hormone level and vitamin D production.

- Secondary: Has underlying causes which include parathyroidism, Renal tubular acidosis, Paget disease, paraneoplastic syndromes, malignancies (multiple myeloma, lymphoma, leukemia, skeletal metastasis), sarcoidosis, granulomatous disease, Addison disease, milk alkali syndrome, sarcoidosis, iatrogenic (glucocorticoid, Vit D intoxication, loop diuretics), prolonged immobilization (quadriplegia or paraplegia).

6.1.1.2 Hypocitraturia

Hypocitraturia occurs in 20–60% of urolithiasis cases and is defined as a daily citrate excretion inferior to 320 mg (1.67 mmol) in adults [13]. Citrate acts by forming complexes with calcium in the renal tubules, thereby increasing the solubility of the latter, and also by binding the surface of calcium oxalate monohydrate crystals preventing their agglomeration and growth as well as their adhesion to renal epithelial cells [14, 15]. The most commonly encountered form of hypocitraturia is idiopathic. Secondary hypocitraturia was shown to be predominantly of dietary origin (high-protein low alkali diet) [16], but is also seen in association with renal tubular acidosis (RTA), hypokalemia, intestinal malabsorption, genetic abnormalities (Vit D receptor gene polymorphism), and drugs (Acetazolamide, Topiramate, Angiotensin-converting enzyme inhibitors, etc.) [13].

6.1.1.3   Hyperuricosuria

(a) Etiologic factors contributing to hyperuricosuria and uric acid (UA) nephrolithiasis [17, 18]:

- Metabolic syndrome (MS)[1]: This is regarded as **the most common cause of uric acid (UA) stone formation**. These patients have the so-called "gouty diathesis" (latent gout) but with no identifiable secondary cause of the UA stones. It is rare to encounter recurrent UA stone formers with no sign of MS.
- Primary gout: These patients have **hyperuricemia** defined as serum UA level >7 mg/dL in men and >6 mg/dL in women. Nearly only 15–20% of patients with uric acid stones have a history of gout, and a small proportion of hyperuricemic patients (about 10–20%) develop kidney stones. These stones are produced by **precipitating insoluble purine metabolism when urinary pH is low,** namely 2- or 8-dihydroxyadenine, adenine, xanthine, and uric acid.
- Chronic diarrhoea and inflammatory bowel diseases (including ulcerative colitis and Crohn's disease). The suspected triggering factor is the loss of bicarbonate in the stool which results into systemic metabolic acidosis and lowering of the urinary pH.
- Myeloproliferative disorders, large solid tumours, haemolytic anaemias: The high cell turnover in these diseases lead to a release of nucleic acids overproduction of UA, and this phenomenon is also triggered by tumour lysis with chemotherapy.
- Rare Mendelian disorders: Association with medullary cystic kidney disease and familial juvenile hyperuricemic nephropathy

---

[1]The metabolic syndrome is a constellation comprising of metabolic disorders, including hypertension, central obesity, dyslipidemia, atherosclerosis and hyperglycemia.

- Low-carbohydrate high-protein diets (i.e. high-purine diet).
- Ileostomy (uric acid stones may comprise 2/3 of all stones in these patients)
- Type 2 diabetes mellitus and obesity as independent factors [19–21].

(b) Uric acid metabolism:
Purine metabolism in mammals → UA as end-product → catabolized by uricase[2] to allantoin (more soluble) → excretion into the urine.

(c) Mechanism of uric acid stone formation: The urinary excretion of UA in humans generally exceeds 600 mg/day. This produces a concentration of 200–300 mg/L for a normal 24-h urine output of 2–3 L. Since the limited urinary uric acid solubility is 96 mg/L, there appears to be an obvious risk for UA precipitation. **Nonetheless low urine pH appears to play the major role in this mechanism** as spectrophotometric data indicate that uric acid is a weak organic acid with an ionization constant (pKa) of 5.35 at 37° [22].

Precipitating factors in the UA stone formation can be summarized by the following tripod: Acidic urine, hyperuricosuria, and low urine volume [23]. **Out of these, unduly acidic urine is the most important and obligatory factor and is universally and always encountered in all UA stone formers** [18]. At pH levels below the pKa, uric acid is predominantly found in a nonionized form which is less soluble than the urate ion. At a urinary pH of less than 5.5, uric acid is poorly soluble, and solubility increases when the pH is above 6.5. **Therefore any urine pH ≤ 5.5 will lead to precipitation of the UA, increasing the risk of nephrolithiasis** [17]. In addition to the role of urinary pH, the fact that uric acid concentration which is often superior to the higher solubility limit doesn't always precipitate could probably be due to the presence of urinary inhibitors and/or the lack of promoters of crystallization. Some of these factors have been studied in vitro [24] but are yet to be identified in vivo [17].

---

[2]Humans and higher primates lack uricase, therefore serum and urine uric acid concentrations are high.

6.1.1.4 Renal Tubular Acidosis

RTA is subdivided into two major types: type 1 or distal where there is inability of the distal nephron to excrete the daily load of endogenous acid and type 2 or proximal where there is impairment of bicarbonate resorption by the proximal nephron. The daily retention of acid in distal RTA triggers hypercalciuria which explains the high frequency of nephrocalcinosis and nephrolithiasis (Fig. 6.1), as opposed to proximal RTA where urinary stones seldom occur [25].

6.1.2 Cystinuria

This entity is one of the most challenging stone diseases and perhaps the most extensively researched topic in the urolithiasis-related genetics. It deserves the grim title of "Cancer of lithology".

The estimated global prevalence of cystinuria is 1 per 7000 population, but there are important geographical variations even among European countries where the rates in UK and Sweden are 1:2000 and 1:100,000 respectively, while Australia

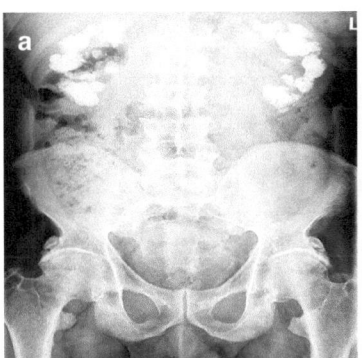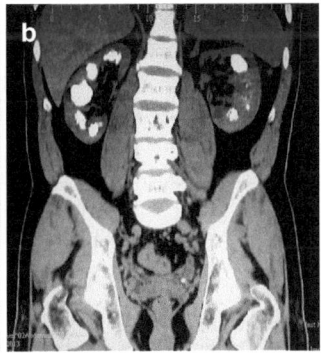

FIGURE 6.1 (**a, b**) KUB Radiograph and coronal CT-scan showing nephrocalcinosis in a 48-year old man with type 1 RTA and impaired renal function. Note the predominance of calculi in the periphery (renal parenchyma) rather than in the collecting system (Courtesy Salim Al Busaidy, Urology, The Royal Hospital, Muscat, Oman)

and Japan have intermediate values with 1:4000 and 1:18,000 respectively [26]. The prevalence is equal in both sexes.

This disease was first described clinically by Sir Archibald Garrod in 1908 [27] but had already been mentioned by Lassaigne in dogs in 1823 [28]. It is an inherited autosomal recessive disorder characterized by the formation of cystine calculi in the kidneys. The primum movens is the mutation in the SLC3A1 gene on chromosome 2 (which contains 10 exons and encodes rBAT), or the SLC7A9 gene on chromosome 19 (which contains 13 exons and encodes bo+AT), or in both genes. This mutation prevents reabsorption of dibasic amino acids by the proximal nephronic tubes as well as by the intestinal microvillosities [29–32]. The dibasic amino acids are Cystine, Ornithine, Lysine, and Arginine, and are better remembered by the mnemonic COLA or COAL.

This chapter is an ever-growing topic as new gene mutations are frequently being discovered almost every year, and around 160 different mutations in the SLC3A1 gene and 116 in the SLC7A9 gene have been reported to date [33–39]. Similar mutations are also observed in the canine model [40].

It has been proposed to genetically classify cystinuria into type A, type B, and type AB, where type A comprises of mutations in both alleles of SLC3A1, type B comprises mutations of both alleles of SLC7A9, and type AB is caused by 1 mutation in SLC3A1 and 1 mutation in SLC7A9 [41]. **Contrary to hyperoxaluria which can develop a systemic form, the only manifestation of cystinuria is urolithiasis.**

The amino-acid Cystine derives from the combination of two cysteine molecules via a disulfide bond (Fig. 6.2a, b).

Clinically three urinary phenotypes have been described for this aminoaciduria:

Type I: This is the most common form. There is normal aminoaciduria in heterozygotes (<200 mg/day), and high excretion if homozygotes (400 mg/day).

Type II: a significant hyperexcretion of cystine and other dibasic aminoacids is seen in homozygotes, but less in heterozygotes (200–400 mg/day) who may still form stones.

FIGURE 6.2 (**a**) Cysteine molecule. From https://en.wikipedia.org/wiki/Cysteine#/media/File:L-Cystein_-_L-Cysteine.svg (Public domain). (**b**) A molecule of cystine. From https://en.wikipedia.org/wiki/Cystine#/media/File:Cystine-skeletal.png (Public domain)

Type III: the intestinal absorption of cystine and dibasic acids is only mildly diminished and cystinuria values are intermediate between types I and II [26, 32, 42].

The final diagnosis of Cystinuria is made by the stone analysis which reveals **the characteristic hexagonal-shaped cystine crystal (see chapter "Investigations of Urinary Lithiasis")**. However a positive family history of cystinuria, hypercystinuria in a 24-h urine analysis (>400 mg/day), or a positive borohydride-cyanonitrosylferrate (sodium cyanide-nitroprusside) test or Brand's test can be sufficient for the diagnosis [43–46].

The sodium Cyanide-nitroprusside test is a rapid, simple and qualitative assay which detects cystinuria of more than 75 mg/L (normal excretion is 30 mg/day or 0.13 mmol/day). Cyanide breaks the di-sulphide bond of cystine, converting it to cysteine which then binds to Nitroprusside producing a purple hue in 2–10 min [46]. When positive, it is better followed by a quantitative study of a 24-h urine sample. The limitation of these colorimetric methods is their inability to differentiate between cystine, cysteine, homocystine and homocysteine, as well as the interference of sulfa-containing drugs such as the thiols.

A novel test, called ***positive cystine capacity*** is now commercially available in the USA; it directly measures the ability of a patient's urine to solubilize or precipitate cystine and avoid the difficulty in the interpretation for patients using thiols. It enables accurate assessment of the drug effect and the eventual need for dosage adjustment [47, 48].

6.1.3   Hyperoxaluria (HO)

Hyperoxaluria may be primary or secondary.

Primary hyperoxaluria (PHO) is a very rare autosomal recessive disorder. A French survey conducted over 20 years ago and addressing PHO type I (the most common and striking type) revealed a prevalence of 1.05/1,000,000, and an average incidence rate of 0.12/1,000,000/year [49]. This entity would fail to dethrone cystinuria from the title of "cancer of lithology" only because of its extreme rarity. However it carries the worst prognosis with a high proportion of patient developing renal failure (64%) and a mortality rate of 19% at a median age of 36 years [49].

The commonest type (type I) (PH1) consists of a deficiency in the activity of the peroxisomal hepatic enzyme **alanine-glyoxylate aminotransferase**, leading to endogenous overproduction of oxalate, and causing urolithiasis, progressive nephrocalcinosis, and end-stage renal disease (ESRD) in children. The equivalent form in adults is generally a mild disorder with occasional urolithiasis, but more severe forms with rapid progression to ESRD have also been documented even in this category of age [50, 51]. Due to consanguineous marriages, Tunisia has perhaps the highest reported PH1 incidence and prevalence as this disease is responsible of 13% of ESRD in the pediatric population, while it accounts for less than 0.7% of ESRD in North America and Europe [52].

Currently three types of PHO have been described with a different enzyme deficiency for each [53] (Table 6.3 and

TABLE 6.3 Classification of hyperoxaluric states

Primary hyperoxaluria: metabolic overproduction

- Type I: alanine: glyoxylate aminotransferase deficiency
- Type II: D-glycerate dehydrogenase deficiency
- Type III: 4-hydroxy-2-oxoglutarate aldolase

Secondary hyperoxaluria

Enteric hyperoxaluria

Extensive intestinal resections with colon intact

- Jejunoileal bypass
- Partial gastrectomy
- Bariatric surgery

Inflammatory bowel disease

- Crohn's disease
- Biliopancreatic disorders (including cystic fibrosis)

Increase of precursors

Ethylene glycol intake

Abuse of vitamin C

Colon decolonisation of oxalate metabolising bacteria

From Lorenzo V et al. [53], with permission from the Authors and Revista Nefrologia

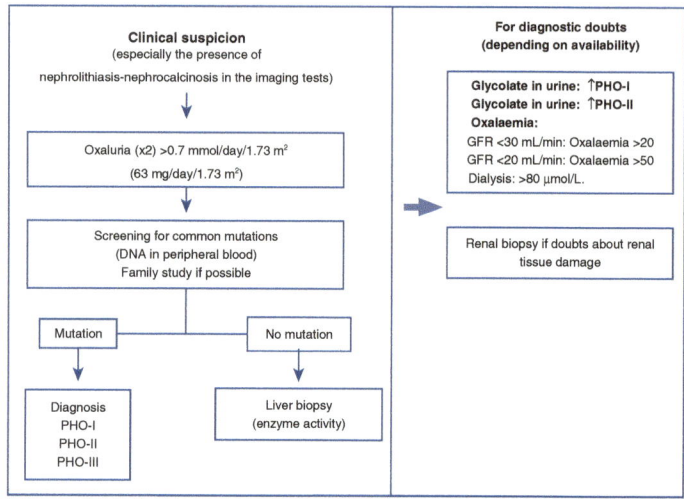

FIGURE 6.3 Primary hyperoxaluria diagnostic algorithm. From Lorenzo V et al. [53], with permission from the Authors and Revista Nefrologia. *GFR* Glomerular filtration rate, *PHO* Primary hyperoxaluria

Fig. 6.3): types I, II, III. The type III was described as recently as the year 2010, leaving the probability for further types still remaining to be discovered. In all types, 24-h oxaluria is in excess of 1 mmol or 80 mg/1.73 m^2 body surface area per day (normal <0.5 mmol or 40 mg/1.73 m^2)[3], and induces **recurrent urolithiasis and progressive nephrocalcinosis**. When kidney damage occurs, it is followed by a systemic deposition of calcium oxalate crystals, known as **systemic oxalosis. Progressive ESRD develops in > 30% of type I PHO;** it can also affect type II, but has never been reported in type III patients [54].

Similar to Cystinuria, there are many genetic variations described in PHO; p.Gly170Arg AGXT mutation was found to be associated with a better outcome in type I [55].

Five different clinical presentations have been described for type 1 PHO [55, 56]:

[3]The normal value of 24-h oxaluria is generally higher in men than in women with respective values of ≤43 mg/day and ≤32 mg/day.

(a) infantile form with early nephrocalcinosis and renal failure (26%),

(b) recurrent urolithiasis and progressive renal failure leading to diagnosis in adolescence or early adulthood (30%),

(c) late-onset form with occasional stone passage leading to diagnosis in adulthood (21%),

(d) diagnosis occurring on post-transplantation recurrence (10%), and

(e) diagnosis made by family screening (13%).

Diagnosis of PHO is suspected when there is a positive family history, supported by the finding of high urinary oxalate levels (normal 10–40 mg per 24 h) or, more accurately by high plasma oxalate levels in combination with chronic kidney disease (Table 6.4) [53].

However the final diagnosis of PHO type I requires to determine the hepatic alanine: glyoxylate amino-transferase activity and to perform genetic studies. If these are inconclusive or not available, liver biopsy should be undertaken [57].

Systemic oxalosis is the most dramatic complication of PHO and is defined as the widespread deposition of high

TABLE 6.4 Clinical parameters in which the diagnosis of primary hyperoxaluria (HPO) must be studied

– Family history of nephrolithiasis

– Infants and children with a first episode of urolithiasis

– Adults with recurring nephrolithiasis associated with early renal failure. Especially in patients with a family history of nephrolithiasis

– Any individual with nephrocalcinosis and renal function deterioration

– Presence of monohydrate calcium oxalate crystals in biological fluids or tissues

– Family members of patients with PHO or suspicion of disease

From Lorenzo V et al. [53], with permission from the Authors and Revista Nefrologia

plasmatic oxalate levels in various organs or systems. This condition is associated with a high mortality rate and should be prevented by an early diagnosis. Unfortunately delay in diagnosis occurs in more than 40% of patients [58].

Contrary to its primary counterpart, secondary hyperoxaluria is caused by an increased dietary ingestion of oxalate or of its precursors (dietary hyperoxaluria), or by alteration in intestinal microflora (enteric hyperoxaluria) (Table 6.3). Dietary oxalate is found in high concentrations in animal as well as in vegetal sources, including chocolate, tea, nut, cocoa, beetroot, nuts, plums, tofu, strawberries, spinach and rhubarb [58]. Enteric hyperoxaluria can be due to malabsorption syndromes (Crohn's disease, ulcerative colitis, celiac disease, cystic fibrosis, post ileal resection or jejuno-ileal bypass, etc.) or to oxalate-degrading bacteria such as the obligate anaerobe bacterium Oxalobacter formigenes, Enterobacter faecalis and lactic acid bacteria [59].

Secondary hyperoxaluria is suspected in the presence of a suggestive dietary or malabsorption history and its diagnosis may be reached through tests aiming at the detection of increased intestinal absorption of oxalate, like stool examination for Oxalobacter formigenes and the $[^{13}C_2]$ oxalate absorption test [58].

Pyridoxine (Vit B6) has been found to be helpful in about 30% of patients with primary hyperoxaluria type 1. Combined Liver-kidney and isolated kidney transplantation are the treatment of choice in primary hyperoxaluria type 1 and type 2 respectively [49, 58]. In ESRD patients, time on dialysis should be short and transplantation be offered as soon as possible to avoid overt systemic oxalosis [54].

6.1.4   Other Monogenic Hereditary Disorders Associated with Nephrolithiasis

(a) Hereditary xanthinuria type I: This rare metabolic disorder was first described in 1954 by Dent and Philpot in a 4-year-old girl [60]. The primum movens is a **genetic deficiency of xanthine oxidase** which triggers a defect of purine metabolism resulting in hypouricemia and hypouricosuria. On the other hand however there are **elevated serum levels of xanthine and hypoxanthine** and a subsequent increased urinary excretion of these oxypurines [61]. Very few cases have been reported in the literature [61–63]. In addition to the hereditary xanthinuria, xanthine stones have also been described in association with Lesch-Nyhan syndrome and conditions where there is profound hyperuricemia such as myeloproliferative disease after treatment with allopurinol [62].

(b) <u>Dent's disease</u>: This rare X-linked recessive renal tubulopathy is caused by mutations in both CLCN5 and OCRL genes, and characterized by **low-molecular-weight-proteinuria in nearly all the patients** (98.4%), followed by hypercalciuria in 85.9% and nephrocalcinosis in 71.9% of patients. Other features are phosphaturic tubulopathy, bone disorders, nephrolithiasis, and chronic kidney disease (CKD) seen in 40.6%, 34.4%, 29.7%, and 14.1% respectively [64].

(c) <u>Hypophosphatemia</u>: This rare entity may be caused by dietary deficiency or intestinal malabsorption of phosphate. Genetic disorders are an important cause of the intestinal phosphate waste; they manifest in infancy and include the autosomal dominant hypophosphatemic rickets, the heterozygous mutations in the main renal sodium-phosphate cotransporter (NPT2a) gene [65], the X-linked dominant hypophosphatemic rickets (XLHR) [66] etc.

(d) <u>Others</u>: Many more genetic causes of hypercalciuric nephrolithiasis have been described [67]. These include the mutation of calcium-sensing receptor (CASR), the adenine phosphoribosyltransferase deficiency (an autosomal recessive disease, also known as 2,8-dihydroxyadeninuria) [68, 69], the polymorphism of klotho gene (G395A gene) [70], the Bartter syndrome type V, the oculo-cerebro-renal syndrome of Lowe, the hereditary hypophosphatemic rickets with hypercalciuria, the familial hypomagnesemia with hypercalciuria and nephrocalcinosis due to paracellin-1 (claudin 16) mutations, etc.

6.2   Urinary Infections

Infective stones account for 3–15% of all urinary stones, the proportion being higher in developing countries. They are mostly composed of struvite which consists of Magnesium Ammonium Phosphate (MAP), and smaller proportions of carbonate apatite and monoammonium urate seen with urease-producing bacteria also referred to as Urea-splitting organisms such as *Proteus*, *Staphylococcus*, *Klebsiella* and some *Pseudomonas* [71]. These organisms are notoriously known to split urea into ammonia and carbon dioxide, resulting in an alkaline urinary pH; the formation of struvite and carbonate apatite crystals subsequently lead to struvite calculi [72].

In contrast to the uropathogenic Escherichia coli which readily forms intracellular bacterial communities, Proteus mirabilis generally fails to establish an intracellular niche and rather forms extracellular clusters in the bladder lumen. These clusters produce foci of mineral deposition and consequently lead to the development of urinary stones. A recent study has identified two virulence factors required for the development of these extracellular clusters: urease and mannose-resistant Proteus-like fimbriae [73].

An experimental murine model study has revealed the interaction between enterobacteriaceae infection and urolithiasis, showing the increased risk of pyelonephritis in the presence of calcium oxalate deposits, and the secondary triggering of further calcium deposit [74].

It is important to note that stones associated with infection are not necessarily composed of struvite, nor are they always associated with urea-splitting bacteria. Secondarily infected non-struvite stones were detected in approximately 20% of a prospective cohort study of 125 PCNL patients, and neurogenic bladder appeared to predispose patients to either struvite or secondarily infected stones with hypocitraturia playing a contributing role. The most commonly-cultured Gram-negative organisms in this study were *Escherichia coli* and *Proteus mirabilis* while the most prevalent Gram-positive organisms were *Enterococcus* spp. *and Staphylococcus* [75].

6.3 Impaired Drainage

Often combined with infection, urinary stasis may potentially be found at all anatomical levels of the urinary tract. Hereafter the various urinary tract malformations and structural defects are reviewed from proximal to distal:

1. Horseshoe kidney (HSK): This is the most common congenital genito-urinary abnormality with a reported incidence of 1/400 to 1/600 births [76]. Stone formation occurs in 1–2:5 patients with HSK due to impaired urinary drainage and infections [76–79].
2. Calyceal mouth stenosis, calyceal and parapelvic diverticulum (Fig. 6.4a–d)
3. Pelviureteric junction (PUJ) obstruction. Also referred to as ureteropelvic (UPJ) obstruction, this is the most common cause of congenital abnormality of the ureter being observed in about 1 in 2000 children, with a M:F ratio of 3:1, and is bilateral in 20–25% [80]. **There is an estimated 70-fold increased risk of secondary renal stone associated with PUJ and recurrent renal lithiasis was observed in 68% of children who present with PUJ and concurrent renal stone** [81].
4. Ureteral duplicity or bifidity [82] and retrocaval ureter [83, 84, 85] (Fig. 6.5).
5. Ureteral diverticulosis [86] (Fig. 6.6a, b). There is not yet evidence that stones form de novo within ureteral diverticulosis. More probably the stones are formed in the kidney and are trapped within the diverticula during their descent.
6. Megaureter [82, 87] (Fig. 6.7a, b)

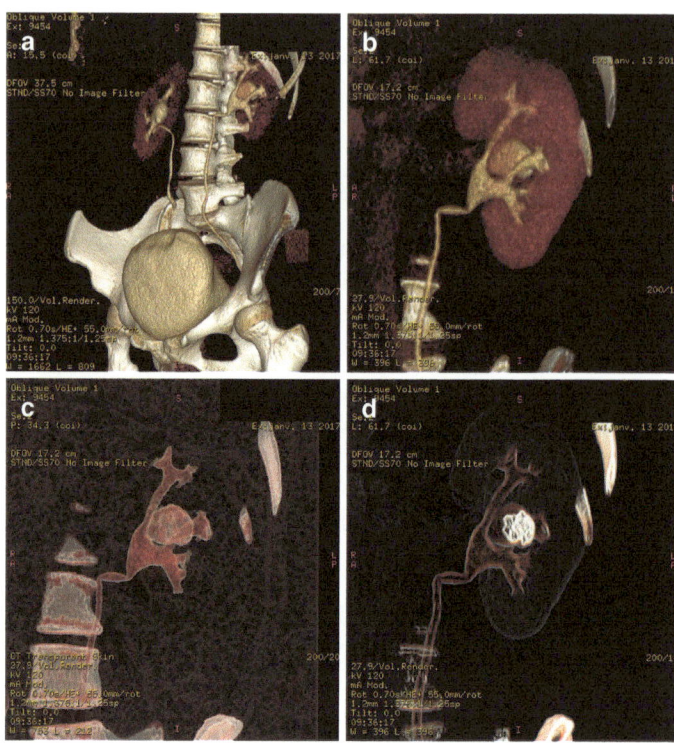

FIGURE 6.4 (**a–d**) 3-D reconstruction of oblique views CT-scan showing multiple calculi within a left renal parapelvic-diverticulum in a 38-year-old woman. Courtesy of Sébastien Novellas. Diagnostic Medical Imaging and Interventional Radiology, Arnault-Tzanck Institute, Saint-Laurent-du-Var, France

7. Vesico-ureteral reflux (VUR): Children with VUR are prone to develop UTI and urinary stasis. They also have a high frequency of hypercalciuria and hyperuricosuria which greatly contribute to the increased association of microlithiasis or stone formation. The frequency of urinary stones and microlithiasis was found to be as higher as 29.6% in a study of 108 children with VUR [88].
8. Ureterocele in children [82] as well as in adults [89].

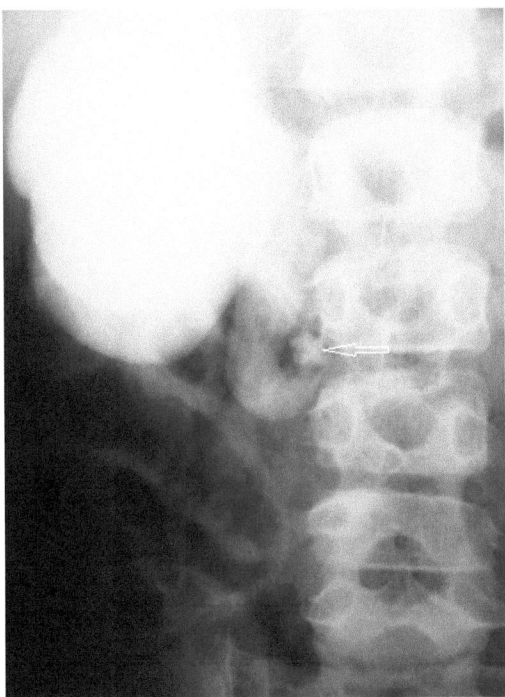

FIGURE 6.5 Intravenous pyelogram showing low-looping fish hook appearance of dilated upper ureter with a radioopaque shadow at the tip suggesting stone (*arrow*). From Kanojia RP et al. [84], with permission from Springer

9. Ileal conduit and continent reservoir: The incidence of urolithiasis in ileal conduit varies from 4.9 to 15.3% [90, 91]. Metabolic disturbances including chronic acidosis and increased excretion of calcium, phosphate and magnesium have been proposed to explain this high incidence, and it was suggested that the risk of urolithiasis may be greater in continent reservoir such as Koch or Indiana pouch [92]. Urinary infection is an important contributing factor of stone formation in these patients.

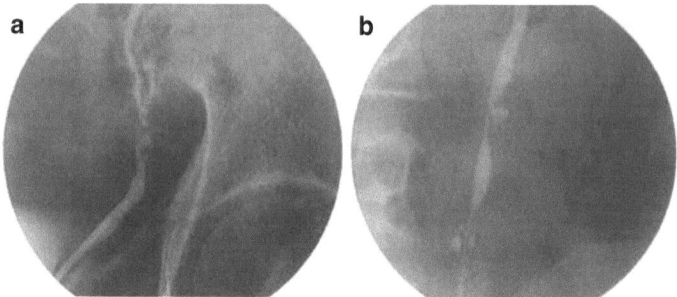

FIGURE 6.6 Retrograde urography images showing multiple left lower (**a**) and upper (**b**) ureteric diverticula. This was performed for a left upper ureteric stone that was found to be in one of the diverticulum. Reproduced from Teo JK et al. [86], with permission from Singapore Medical Journal

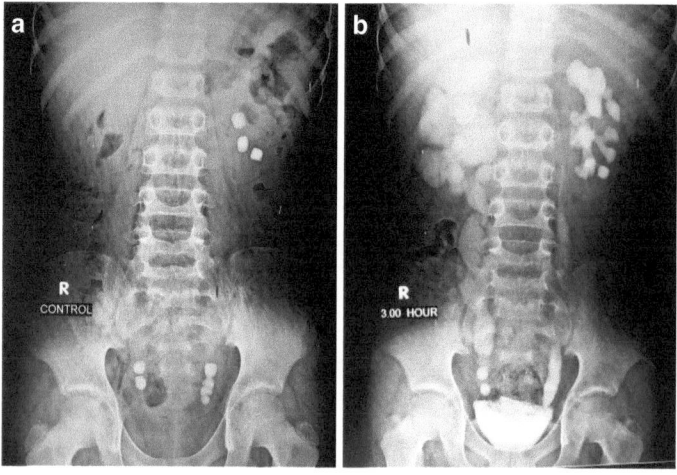

FIGURE 6.7 (**a**) X-ray kidneys, ureters and bladder showing multiple mobile left renal calculi and bilateral ureteral calculi. From Kumar A et al. [87] with permission from BMJ Publishing Group Ltd. (**b**) Intravenous urography showing bilateral dilated ureters and pelvi-calyceal systems. From Kumar A et al. [87] with permission from BMJ Publishing Group Ltd

10. Bladder diverticulum: Bladder diverticula can be congenital or secondary. The congenital form often occur in male children, with an incidence of about 1.7%, and the secondary is mostly described in elderly males (>60 years), with an incidence of 1–6%, in association with a concomitant prostatic hyperplasia [93]. Factors triggering the stone formation are: intradiverticular urine retention, urinary salt deposition, infection and chronic inflammatory stimuli.

11. Vesico-urachal diverticulum: This an extremely rare entity with only a handful of cases reported in the literature (Fig. 6.8) [94].

    However this pathological entity may be underreported, since our recently increased awareness during the preparation of this chapter led us to discover an asymptomatic stone contained in a urachal remnant in a patient investigated in our institution for a left renal calculus (Fig. 6.9a, b).

12. Atonic or augmented bladder: In paediatric augmented bladders, stone formation rates vary with series, from 10% to near half of the cases over a 10-year follow-up [95] and recurrence was observed to occur in almost half of the patients within 5 years [96]. The use of abdominal stoma was shown to expose patients to reservoir calculi more significantly than the use of the native urethra [97]. Stone formation appeared to be predominantly caused by mucus retention within the augmented bladder, and routine bladder irrigation as well as the use of mucolytic agents can significantly reduce the rate of stone formation. Stones have also been reported after closure of bladder exstrophy [98].

13. Neuropathic bladders (e.g. secondary to spinal cord injury): the stone formation here is due to the combination of urinary infection and impaired drainage.

14. Supra-trigonal location of vesico-vaginal fistula (VVF): This is an extremely rare cause of urolithiasis that combines urinary infection and urinary stasis. Obstetrical trauma is the leading cause of VVF in sub-saharian African

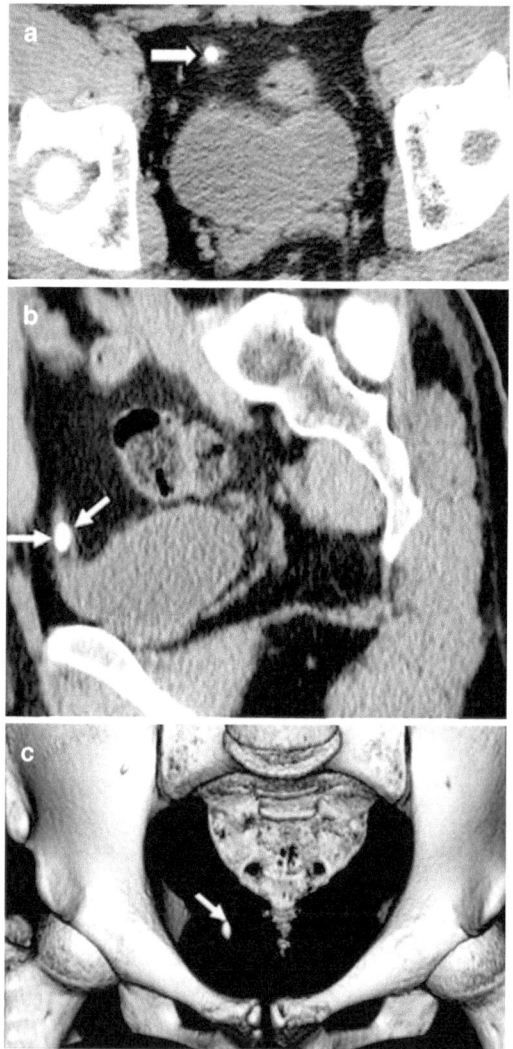

FIGURE 6.8 Stone in a vesico-urachal diverticulum. (**a**) Axial, (**b**) sagittal reformatted, and (**c**) 3-dimensional computed tomographic images showing a tubular structure, containing a hyperdense stone on the anterosuperior aspect of the urinary bladder, slightly on the right side. Reprinted from Atalar MH et al. [94] Copyright © Pol J Radiol, 2016. With permission from the Polish Journal of Radiology and the Authors

FIGURE 6.9 (**a**, **b**) X ray KUB and NCCT showing an incidental calculus seen in a urachal remnant (c). Note also the presence of a small left renal stone (Courtesy Qais Al Hooti, Urology, the Royal Hospital, Muscat, Oman)

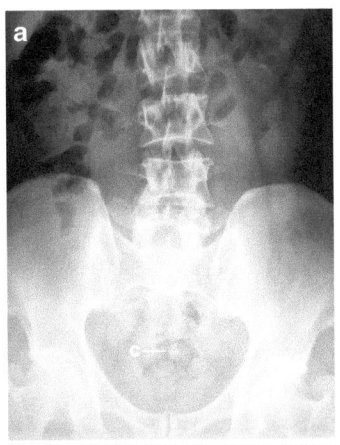

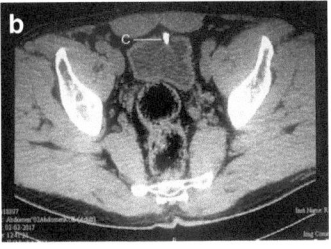

countries. Cases of neglected VVF have been reported in Nigeria and India where the condition resulted in the formation of a giant dumb-bell calculus filling the vagina and the urinary bladder (Fig. 6.10) [99, 100].

15. Bladder outlet obstruction, especially in prostatic hypertrophy (Fig. 6.11), bladder neck stenosis, and urethral stricture with or without urethral diverticulum. In children urinary stone formation can be secondary to posterior urethral valves [82]. Urethral stones generally migrate from the bladder, are small in size, and are more commonly found in men. However literature has reported on larger stone sizes [101], on exceptional female occurrence within a urethral diverticulum [102] (Fig. 6.12) or without underlying genitourinary anatomical abnormalities [103], and even on infantile cases [104, 105].

   Urinary bladder stones associated with obstructive BPH may also assume a characteristic stellar morphology.

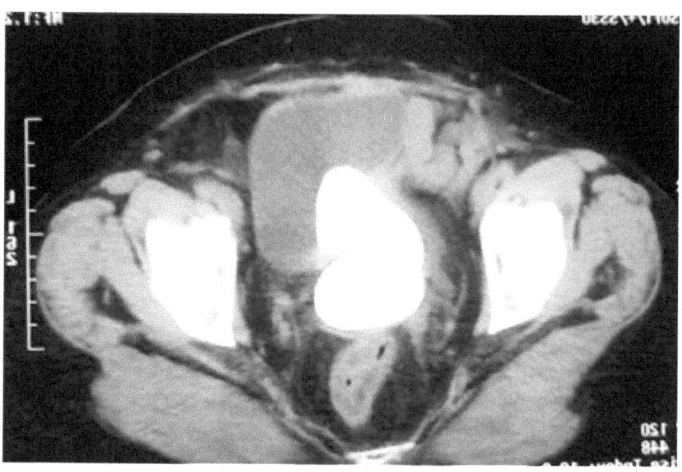

FIGURE 6.10 CT scan showing a 7 × 4.6 cm dumbbell shaped vesico-vaginal calculus with vesico-vaginal fistula. From Sawant A et al. [100], with permission from the Journal of Clinical and Diagnostic Research, Roop Nagar, Delhi, India

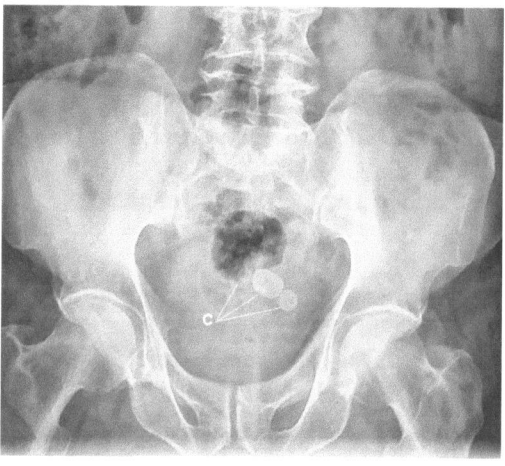

FIGURE 6.11 Supine pelvis X-ray showing three oval-shaped calculi (c) in an 86-year old man presenting with benign prostatic hypertrophy and chronic retention of urine (Courtesy Salim Al-Busaidy, Urology, The Royal Hospital, Muscat, Oman)

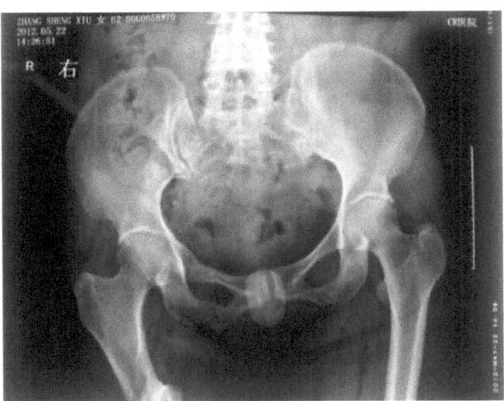

FIGURE 6.12 Radiograph showing giant calculus in a urethral diverticulum in a 60-year-old woman. From Dong Z et al. [102]. With permission from Wolters Kluwer

Because of their dense central core and radiating spicules, they were likened to children toy jacks. These so-called jackstones were first described by Everidge in 1927 [106] and are mostly made of calcium oxalate dihydrate [107] (Fig. 6.13a, b).

Jackstones have exceptionally been reported also in the kidney where they may be made of calcium oxalate monohydrate [108] (Fig. 6.14a–d).

16. Obstructive ejaculatory duct calculi. This is an extremely rare cause of obstructive azoospermia or low-volume oligospermia [109]. It has been reported in a patient with myelomeningocele and neurogenic bladder who underwent bladder augmentation but was incompliant with regular emptying [110]. The open bladder neck and spastic external sphincter in this scenario gave rise to formation of struvite stone in the prostatic urethra and ejaculatory ducts.

17. Prostatic calculi: These are a common finding on X-ray pelvis being seen in up to 40% of men presenting with prostatic enlargement with bladder outflow obstruction. Prostatic stones are asymptomatic per se, but they can rarely be an

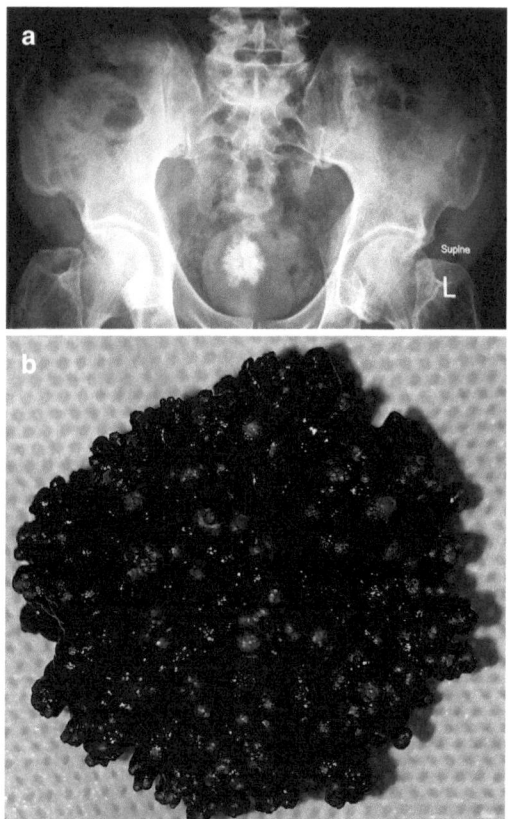

FIGURE 6.13 (**a**) Plain X Ray KUB showing a large jackstone in the urinary bladder (Courtesy Qais Al Hooti, Urology, The Royal Hospital. Muscat, Oman). (**b**) The same stone seen on (**a**) after its retrieval by cystolithotomy (courtesy Qais Al Hooti, Urology, The Royal Hospital, Muscat, Oman)

independent cause of pain or voiding difficulty when they reach very large sizes [111–114]. Prostatic calculi have been described as primary or endogenous, i.e. formed in acini from prostatic fluid, or as secondary or exogenous, i.e. formed in the prostatic duct. Some investigators consider

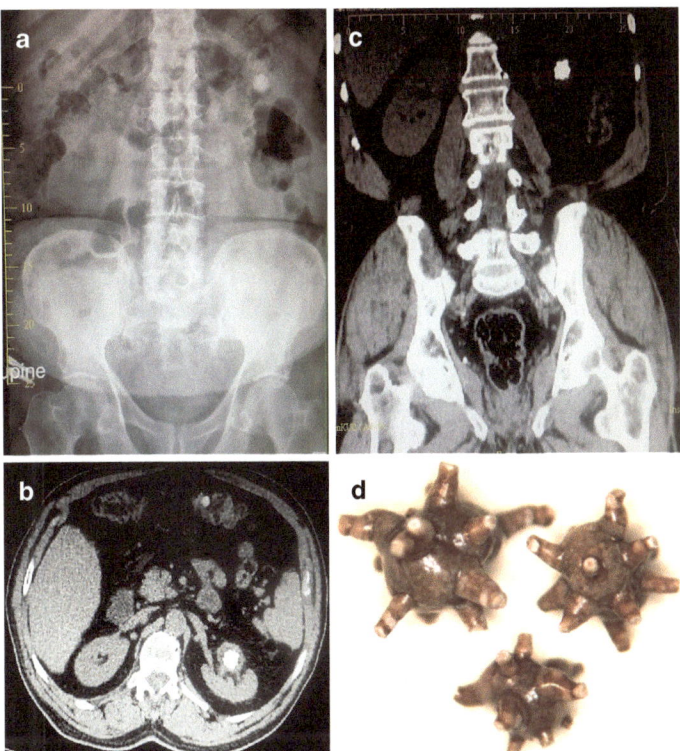

FIGURE 6.14 (**a–c**) X-ray KUB, axial and coronal CT scans showing a jackstone in the extrarenal pelvis of a malrotated left kidney (courtesy Qais Al Hooti, Urology, The Royal Hospital, Muscat, Oman). (**d**) Multiple renal Jackstones made of Calcium oxalate monohydrate. Courtesy of Louis C Herring & Co Lab, Orlando, Florida, USA

prostatic stones merely as calcified forms of corpora amylacea, and studies have shown that they are caused by
acute and/or chronic infections [115, 116].

18. External meatal stenosis: This is a common clinical finding which may cause voiding difficulty and eventually an
impaction of a urethral stone in the fossa navicularis.

19. Urethrocele: This is a rather rare finding associated with a stone and potentially causing recurrent UTI and urinary retention [117, 118].

20. Phimosis: Preputial calculi have been reported in association with phimosis and consequent impaired drainage. They seem to develop through inspissated smegma mixing with lime salts and infected stagnant urine, but migrated upper urinary tract stones can also get trapped in the preputial sac [119–121]. They affect mostly elderly men with poor hygiene in the developing world [119]; however they have also been reported in young adults [120] (Figs. 6.15 and 6.16a, b) and even in children [121] (Fig. 6.17a–d). Either multiple or solitary, these stones are completely removed after a dorsal slit or a circumcision which eliminates the risk of recurrence.

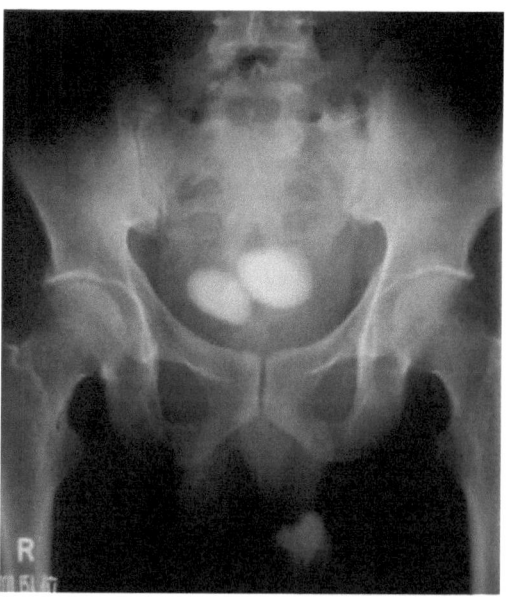

FIGURE 6.15 Plain X ray KUB of a 32-year old man showing multiple preputial calculi and two bladder stones. From Nagata D et al. [120] with permission from John Wiley and Sons

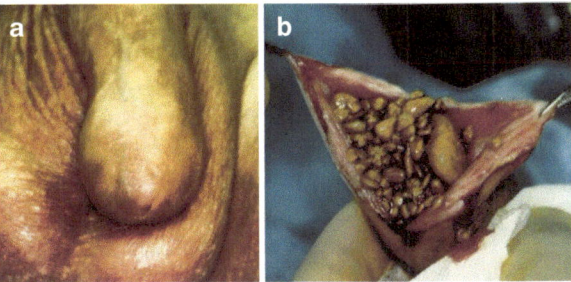

FIGURE 6.16 Same patient seen in Fig. 6.15. (**a**) Gross appearance of the penis with preputial calculi. (**b**) Brown calculi seen in the preputial cavity after dorsal incision. These were made of magnesium ammonium phosphate, calcium phosphate and calcium carbonate. From Nagata D et al. [120], reproduced with permission from John Wiley and Sons

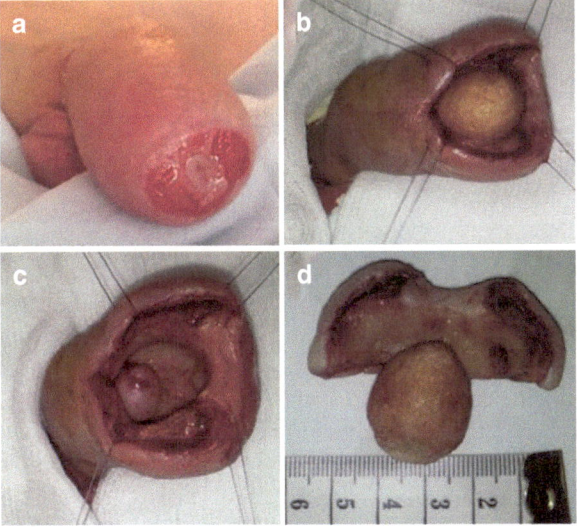

FIGURE 6.17 (**a**) Penis of a 5-year-old child showing severe swelling from the tip upto nearly the penoscrotal junction; there is also a tight phimotic ring with ulceration on its circumference; (**b–d**) removal of a thick preputial sac molded on a 3 × 2 cm oval calculus with the glans imprint on it. From Spataru RI et al. [121], reproduced with permission from Springer

6.4   Post Bariatric Surgery

A comparative study in Mayo Clinic based on a treated population of 759 patients and a control group of equal size has
shown a significant increase in the rate of new urinary stones
in the operated group compared to the control group with
11.1% and 4.3% respectively [122]. One should not overlook
the magnitude of this problem when considering that the
number of bariatric surgeries has tremendously increased in
the developed countries during the last two decades. In the
USA alone, bariatric procedures have reached a peak of
136,000 in the year 2004 [122]. Three mechanisms have been
found to explain the high incidence of calcium oxalate stones
after malabsorptive bariatric surgery [123]: hyperoxaluria,
low urine volume, and hypocitraturia.

6.5   Foreign Bodies

Any foreign body left in contact with the urothelium is a
potential nucleus or nidus around which stones may form:
The most commonly encountered are:

1. Stitch: This has become rare in the modern era. It was common when slowly-absorbable suturing materials were used
   to repair a calyceal violation during partial nephrectomy,
   or to close a pyelo-nephrolithotomy, a dismembered pyeloplasty, to perform a ureteric anastomosis or closure, and
   uretero-vesical anastomosis. It can also be seen after gynaecological procedures when synthetic materials are used
   for the surgical treatment of a prolapsed uterus and come
   inadvertently in contact with the bladder urothelium [124].
2. Long standing indwelling urethral catheter or catheter balloon fragments. The presence of an indwelling catheter is a
   well-known predisposing factor to urinary infection and
   this is an additional factor exposing to stone formation.
3. Forgotten ureteral DJ stent.
4. Migrated intra-uterine contraceptive device (IUCD):
   Many articles in the medical literature have reported on a

migrated IUCD eroding the uterine and bladder walls, protruding into the vesical lumen and inducing a secondary calculus formation around it [125, 126] (Fig. 6.18a–c).

There is an extreme case of forgotten IUCD in an elderly woman for 39 years resulting in an enormous vesi-

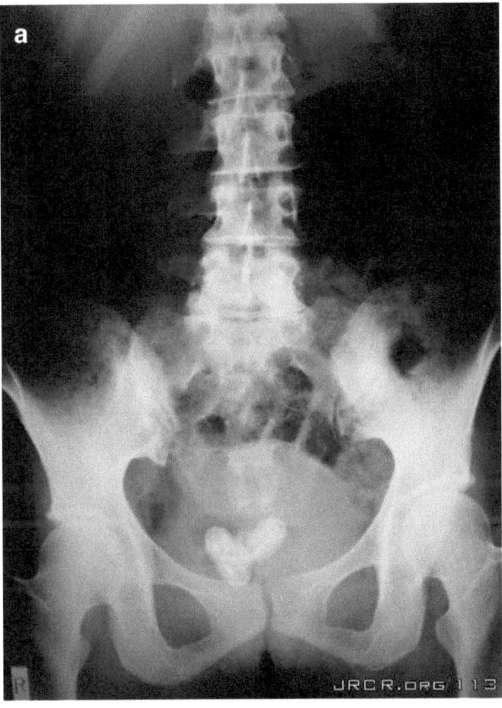

FIGURE 6.18 (**a**) Pelvis X-ray of a 52-year old woman with vesical calculi encrusted around a Copper-T intrauterine contraceptive device which migrated into the urinary bladder. From Amin U and Mahmood R [125], reproduced with permission from the Editors, Journal of Radiology Case Reports. (**b, c**) 52-year old woman with vesical calculi encrusted around a Copper-T intrauterine contraceptive device which migrated to the urinary bladder. Intraoperative view. From Amin U and Mahmood R [125], reproduced with permission from the Editors, Journal of Radiology Case Reports

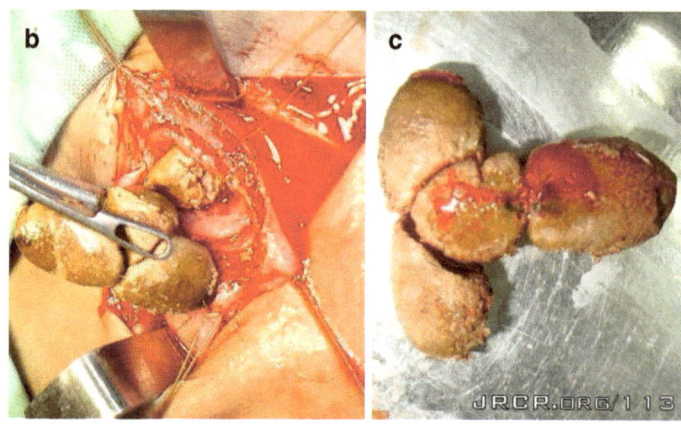

FIGURE 6.18 (continued)

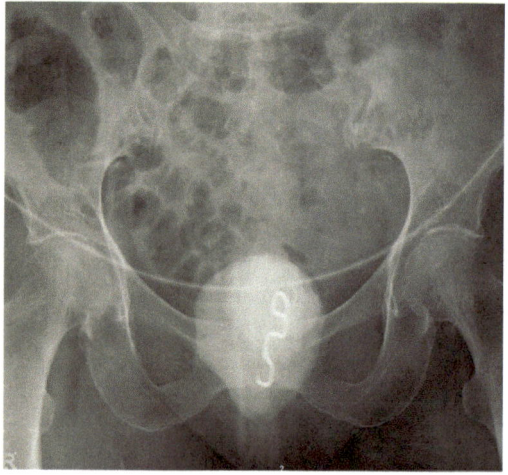

FIGURE 6.19 Plain pelvic x-ray revealing a massive calculus around a foreign body (Lippes loop). From Karsmakers R [127], reproduced with permission from BMJ Publishing Group ltd

cal stone, a vesico-vaginal fistula with urinary incontinence, recurrent urinary tract infections, and advanced chronic kidney disease [127] (Fig. 6.19).

5. Migrated coil used to treat pseudoaneurysm in a segmental branch of right renal artery [128].
6. Mesh used for herniorraphy after erosion through the bladder [129].

6.6   Drugs

The proportion of drug-related stones varies from 0.1% in recent publications [130] to 1% in older studies [131].

Some authors have proposed to divide lithogenic drugs into two groups [132]:

- poorly soluble drugs with high urine excretion favoring crystallisation in the urine: In this group the drug component is identified in the stone analysis. It includes Triamterene (Dyrenium) (the leading cause of drug-related stones in the 1970s) and the anti-HIV infection drugs, namely Protease inhibitors and sulfadiazine (most frequent cause from the 1990s).
- drugs inducing urinary calculi as a consequence of their metabolic effects: calcium/vitamin D supplementation, laxatives, Furosemide, carbonic anhydrase inhibitors such as Acetazolamide (Diamox) [133]. A careful history is required to differentiate this etiology from common metabolic calculi.

Historically sulfonamides are known for more than half a century to be associated with renal stones [134]. Cases of sulfonamides lithiasis are still being reported nowadays and some studies suggest the toxic effect of acetylsulfapyridine, a metabolite of Sulfasalazine which is prescribed for psoriasis or ulcerative colitis [135, 136].

Protease inhibitors are another important group of drugs introduced in the 1990s in the combination therapy against HIV infection better known as highly active antiretroviral therapy (HAART). Indinavir is the most commonly encountered member of this group in association with renal stones; crystalluria and renal stone formation have been reported in 20–50% of patients taking this drug [137, 138]

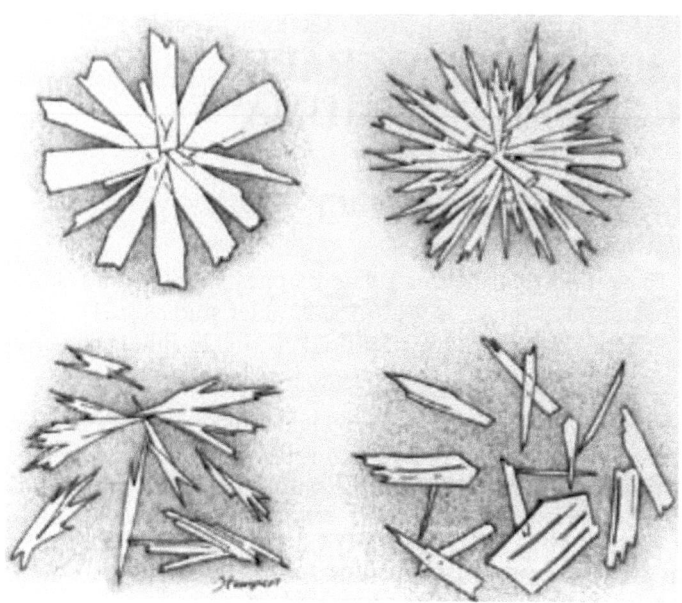

FIGURE 6.20 Urinary indinavir crystals on light microscopy. From Schwartz BF et al. [137], with permission from Elsevier

(Fig. 6.20). However, Atazanavir, Nelfinavir, Amprenavir, Saquinavir, Ritonavir and Darunavir have also been incriminated [139]. Non-protease inhibitors antiretroviral drugs are also involved, including Raltegravir and Efavirenz [139, 140]. Indinavir stones are notoriously known to be radiolucent stones and are also not detectable even on a plain CT-KUB. Ultrasonography is useful for their diagnosis [137] (Table 6.5). Intravenous pyelography may help to detect ureteral stones as filling defects eventually causing obstruction, but the same information can also be obtained with Contrast-Enhanced CT scan.

Many other drugs with a potential for crystallization and renal stone formation have been reported in the medical literature. Here after is their non-exhaustive list: Aminopenicillin (a combination of ampicillin and amoxicillin) [141], Ceftriaxone

TABLE 6.5 Radiographic findings in patients with presumed indinavir calculi

Study	Total no.	No. nondiagnostic	No. suggestive of calculus	No. diagnostic of urinary calculus
Abdominal radiograph	12	7	5	0
IVP	13	5	7	1
Renal ultrasound	11	2	5	4
CT	12	5	7	0

Reproduced and modified from Schwartz BF et al. [137], with permission from Elsevier

[142], Guaifenesin, Dextromethorphan (antitussive and recreational drug), Ephedrine [143, 144], Gelopectose in children [145] Piridoxilate (glyoxylate + pyridoxine) [146], Glafenine (Glifanan®), metabolites of phenazopyridine (Pyridium), N-acetylsulphamethoxazole hydrochloride (Bactrim®) and N-acetylsulphaguanidine (Guanidan®), flumequine (Apurone®) [131], Topiramate (antiepileptic) [147], Triamterene, amorphous silica [148] etc. Even Allopurinol which is used to lower the hyperuricemia can paradoxically crystallise and form urinary calculi as shown in a murine model [149]. A rare case of ethanol gel injection in the prostate to treat lower urinary tract symptoms (LUTS) in an elderly patient with coagulopathy was reported in the literature to cause a soft bladder stone [150]. The stone was formed by prostatic tissue slush following the ethanol-induced necrosis.

6.7   Renal Matrix Stones

Renal matrix stones are also known as fibrinomas, colloid calculi or albumin calculi. These are extremely rare stones with only about 60 cases reported to date, being observed in

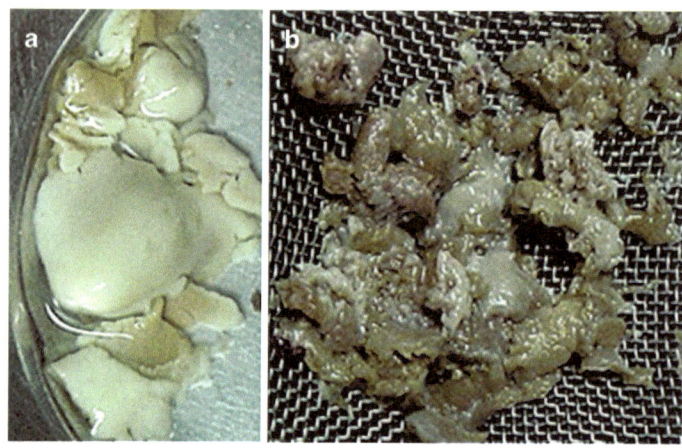

FIGURE 6.21 (**a, b**) Pictures of renal matrix stones. From Shah HN et al. [152], with permission from John Wiley and Sons

females and associated with recurrent urinary infections especially due to Proteus mirabilis or Escherichia coli, history of renal surgery, and chronic kidney failure. They are so-named because their matrix component accounts for about 65% of their dry weight, while this represents only 2.5% of calcium oxalate or urate stones and 9% of cystine stones. This gives them their soft, pliable, and amorphous characteristics [151, 152] (Fig. 6.21a, b).

6.8   Gas-Containing Renal Stones

This is a rare entity with yet unknown pathophysiology. Putative theories state that gas-containing stones may result from a combination of metabolic and infectious factors, and female patients as well as diabetic subjects are reported to be more susceptible [153] (Fig. 6.22a, b).

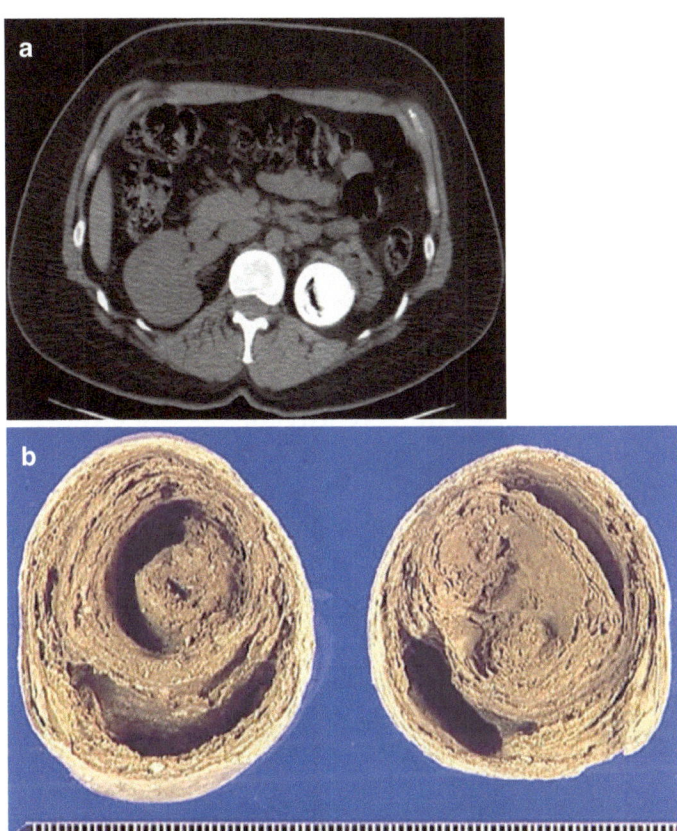

FIGURE 6.22 (**a**) NCCT-scan showing a large gas-containing stone in the left kidney. From Manny TB et al. [153]. With permission from Elsevier. (**b**) Cut section of the stone after its removal. From Manny TB et al. [153]. With permission from Elsevier

6.9   Fetal Origin Hypothesis

Observational studies have shown links between the various medical conditions associated with renal stones (namely hypertension, diabetes mellitus, metabolic syndrome, and osteoporosis) and adverse early-life events, such as low-birth weight. A hypothesis has been formulated recently stating that the stone-associated syndromes have a common programing pathway in early life, suggesting that nephrolithiasis could have developmental origins [154].

6.10   Diseases and Syndromes Associated with Renal Stones

There are frequent associations found between calcium stone formation (derived from alterations in the metabolic regulation of calcium and sodium) and various medical diseases such as hypertension, osteoporosis, and cardiovascular disease, as well as between uric acid stones and the metabolic syndrome (impaired fasting glucose, elevated blood pressure, dyslipidemia, and central obesity) and insulin resistance [155].

Links have also been found between urolithiasis and cardiovascular diseases, namely myocardial infarction, angina, carotid artery atherosclerosis, and stroke [156, 157]. Theories behind this association suggest the role played by vessel walls that buffer the excessive quantity of calcium delivered by a high bone turnover in some renal stone formers. This results in a higher arterial calcification score, an increased arterial stiffness and a reduced bone density [158, 159].

Some of the major syndromes or diseases associated with urolithiasis, namely Cystinuria, primary hyperoxaluria and hyperuricemia (gout) have already been discussed above. Others are:

1. Medullary sponge kidney: First described in 1948 by the Italian Pathologists Cacci R and Ricci V [160], and also referred to by the eponymous Cacci-Ricci disease, medullary sponge kidney is a benign congenital disorder consisting of a malformation of terminal collecting ducts with

secondary ectasis (cysts) and intra-parenchymal stone formation (nephrocalcinosis), mainly composed of calcium phosphate and calcium oxalate. The patients are usually asymptomatic and develop incomplete distal RTA (type 1), hypercalciuria, and hypocitraturia. Recurrent calcium stone formation is found in 12–20% of patients, mainly consisting of CaP and CaOx [161]. The diagnosis is suspected on X-ray KUB and U/S kidneys. The cysts have different sizes, and are generally diffuse and bilateral. This entity may be associated with Caroli's syndrome (a rare congenital non-obstructive multifocal dilatation of the intrahepatic bile ducts) [162].

2. ADPKD: Patients with autosomal dominant polycystic kidney disease (ADPKD) have a renal stone incidence which is approximately 5–10 folds higher than the reported rate in the general population, ranging from 20 to 36% [163, 164]. A Mayo Clinic study revealed a high proportion of uric acid (56.6%) and calcium oxalate (46.6%) as well as hypocitric aciduria, suggesting the contribution of metabolic factors in the high frequency of urolithiasis in ADPKD [165]. However mechanical factors such as intrarenal anatomical obstruction also play an important part because larger polycystic kidneys are more prone to develop stones. A renal volume >500 mL was shown to be an independent significant predictor of nephrolithiasis in patients with ADPKD and normal renal function irrespective of the presence of metabolic disturbances [163].

3. Lesh-Nyhan Syndrome: Congenital disease characterized by motor dysfunction, cognitive and behavioral disturbances, and uric acid overproduction (hyperuricemia). The diagnosis is established by the measurement of hypoxanthine-guanine phosphoribosyltransferase (HPRT) enzyme activity which is less than 1.5% of normal in any tissue sampled from the patient's cell. The *HPRT1* is the only gene known to be associated with Lesch-Nyhan syndrome [165].

4. Hyperparathyroidism: either isolated or as part of Multiple Endocrine Neoplasia (MEN) syndrome type I (or Wermer's syndrome: parathyroid, pancreatic and anterior pituitary tumor). Hyperparathyroidism causes renal stones through hypercalcemia.

5. Intestinal fat malabsorption [166, 167].
6. Cushing disease [168].
7. Chronic inflammatory bowel disease (Crohn's disease and ulcerative colitis) [169, 170].
8. Sarcoidosis: The frequency of nephrolithiasis in sarcoidosis is 20 times more than in the general population [171] and renal stone can be the first manifestation of sarcoidosis in rare cases [171, 172].
9. Milk-alkali syndrome: This entity is caused by the ingestion of large amounts of calcium and absorbable alkali. Hypercalcemia and metabolic alkalosis are the direct result with a remote possibility of renal stones and renal failure. Some authors recommend changing its name to calcium-alkali syndrome which better reflects the etiological origin of the modern version of this disorder. This is now the third most common cause of hospital admission for hypercalcemia after hyperparathyroidism and malignancy hypercalcemia [173, 174].
10. Megacalycosis: A rare pathological entity characterized by dilatation of all renal calyces with normal renal pelvis and ureter and with no identifiable obstructive cause [175].
11. Bartter's syndrome, Dent's disease and X-linked recessive nephrolithiasis [176, 177].
12. Sjögren's syndrome [178].
13. Nail-Patella syndrome (Hood syndrome) [179].

6.11   Other Factors

- The ritual Islamic fasting during the holy Ramadan month is sometimes pointed out but a recent study showed that fasting in Ramadan does not change the number of renal colic visits [180]. Evidence is still lacking to prove that the transient changes caused in the urinary metabolites during day-time fasting increase urinary calculus formation if there is enough nocturnal compensatory water intake.
- Lack of physical activity and smoking [181].
- Long term bed rest and space flight [182].

References

1. Zerwekh JE, Reed-Gitomer BY, Pak CY. Pathogenesis of hyper-calciuric nephrolithiasis. Endocrinol Metab Clin North Am. 2002;31(4):869–84.
2. Jungers P, Joly D, Blanchard A. Inherited monogenic kidney stone diseases: recent diagnostic and therapeutic advances. Nephrol Ther. 2008;4(4):231–55.
3. Monico CG, Milliner DS. Genetic determinants of urolithiasis. Nat Rev Nephrol. 2011;8(3):151–62.
4. Penido MG, de Sousa Tavares M. Pediatric primary urolithia-sis: symptoms, medical management and prevention strategies. World J Nephrol. 2015;4(4):444–54.
5. Amancio L, Fedrizzi M, Bresolin NL, Penido MG. Pediatric uro-lithiasis: experience at a tertiary care pediatric hospital. J Bras Nefrol. 2016;38(1):90–8.
6. Eisner BH, Sheth S, Dretler SP, et al. Abnormalities of 24-hour urine composition in first-time and recurrent stone-formers. Urology. 2012;80(4):776–9.
7. Ahmad I, Pansota MS, Tariq M, Tabassum SA. Frequency of met-abolic abnormalities in urinary stones patients. Pak J Med Sci. 2013;29(6):1363–6.
8. Spivacow FR, del Valle EE, Negri AL, et al. Biochemical diag-nosis in 3040 kidney stone formers in Argentina. Urolithiasis. 2015;43(4):323–30.
9. Stitchantrakul W, Kochakarn W, Ruangraksa C, Domrongkitchaiporn S. Urinary risk factors for recurrent cal-cium stone formation in Thai stone formers. J Med Assoc Thail. 2007;90(4):688–98.
10. Lemann J Jr, Gray RW. Idiopathic hypercalciuria. J Urol. 1989;141(3 Pt 2):715–8.
11. Pak CY, Oata M, Lawrence EC, Snyder W. The hypercalciurias. Causes, parathyroid functions, and diagnostic criteria. J Clin Invest. 1974;54(2):387–400.
12. Audran M, Legrand E. Hypercalciuria. Joint Bone Spine. 2000;67(6):509–15.
13. Zuckerman JM, Assimos DG. Hypocitraturia: pathophysiology and medical management. Rev Urol. 2009;11(3):134–44.
14. Nicar MJ, Hill K, Pak CY. Inhibition by citrate of spontaneous precipitation of calcium oxalate in vitro. J Bone Miner Res. 1987;2(3):215–20.

15. Sheng X, Jung T, Wesson JA, Ward MD. Adhesion at calcium oxalate crystal surfaces and the effect of urinary constituents. Proc Natl Acad Sci U S A. 2005;102(2):267–72.
16. Domrongkitchaiporn S, Stitchantrakul W, Kochakarn W. Causes of hypocitraturia in recurrent calcium stone formers: focusing on urinary potassium excretion. Am J Kidney Dis. 2006;48(4):546–54.
17. Sakhaee K. Epidemiology and clinical pathophysiology of uric acid kidney stones. J Nephrol. 2014;27(3):241–5.
18. Wiederkehr MR, Moe OW. Uric acid nephrolithiasis: a systemic metabolic disorder. Clin Rev Bone Miner Metab. 2011; 9(3–4):207–17.
19. Pak CY, Sakhaee K, Moe O, Preminger GM, Poindexter JR, Peterson RD, Pietrow P, Ekeruo W. Biochemical profile of stone-forming patients with diabetes mellitus. Urology. 2003; 61(3):523–7.
20. Sakhaee K, Adams-Huet B, Moe OW, Pak CY. Pathophysiologic basis for normouricosuric uric acid nephrolithiasis. Kidney Int. 2002;62(3):971–9.
21. Daudon M, Traxer O, Conort P, Lacour B, Jungers P. Type 2 diabetes increases the risk for uric acid stones. J Am Soc Nephrol. 2006;17(7):2026–33.
22. Finlayson B, Smith A. Stability of first dissociable proton of uric acid. J Chem Eng Data. 1974;19(1):94–7.
23. Asplin JR. Uric acid stones. Semin Nephrol. 1996;16(5):412–24.
24. Koka RM, Huang E, Lieske JC. Adhesion of uric acid crystals to the surface of renal epithelial cells. Am J Physiol Renal Physiol. 2000;278(6):F989–98.
25. Narins RG, Goldberg M. Renal tubular acidosis: pathophysiology, diagnosis and treatment. Dis Mon. 1977;23:1–66.
26. Biyani CS, Cartledge JJ. Cystinuria: diagnosis and management. EAU-EBU Updat Ser. 2006;4:175–83.
27. Garrod A. The Croonian lectures on inborn errors of metabolism. Lancet. 1908;172:1–7.
28. Lassaigne J. Observation sur l'existence de l'oxide cystique dans un calcul vesical du chien, et essai analytique sur la composition élémentaire de cette substance particulière. Ann Chim Phys. 1823;23:328–34.
29. Feliubadaló L, Font M, Purroy J, et al. International Cystinuria Consortium. Non-type I cystinuria caused by mutations in SLC7A9, encoding a subunit (bo,+AT) of rBAT. Nat Genet. 1999;23(1):52–7.

30. Chillarón J, Estévez R, Mora C, et al. Obligatory amino acid exchange via systems bo,+-like and y+L-like. A tertiary active transport mechanism for renal reabsorption of cystine and dibasic amino acids. J Biol Chem. 1996;271:17761–70.

31. Calonge MJ, Gasparini P, Chillarón J, et al. Cystinuria caused by mutations in rBAT, a gene involved in the transport of cystine. Nat Genet. 1994;6:420–5.

32. Bisceglia L, Calonge MJ, Totaro A, et al. Localization, by linkage analysis, of the cystinuria type III gene to chromosome 19q13.1. Am J Hum Genet. 1997;60:611–6.

33. Andreassen KH, Pedersen KV, Osther SS, et al. How should patients with cystine stone disease be evaluated and treated in the twenty-first century? Urolithiasis. 2016;44(1):65–76.

34. Oddsson A, Sulem P, Helgason H, et al. Common and rare variants associated with kidney stones and biochemical traits. Nat Commun. 2015;6:7975.

35. Rhodes HL, Yarram-Smith L, Rice SJ, et al. Clinical and genetic analysis of patients with cystinuria in the United Kingdom. Clin J Am Soc Nephrol. 2015;10(7):1235–45.

36. Markazi S, Kheirollahi M, Doosti A, et al. A novel mutation in SLC3A1 gene in patients with cystinuria. Iran J Kidney Dis. 2016;10(1):44–7.

37. Wong KA, Mein R, Wass M, et al. The genetic diversity of cystinuria in a UK population of patients. BJU Int. 2015;116(1):109–16.

38. Di Perna M, Louizou E, Fischetti L, et al. Twenty-four novel mutations identified in a cohort of 85 patients by direct sequencing of the SLC3A1 and SLC7A9 cystinuria genes. Genet Test. 2008;12(3):351–5.

39. Font-Llitjós M, Jiménez-Vidal M, Bisceglia L, et al. New insights into cystinuria: 40 new mutations, genotype-phenotype correlation, and digenic inheritance causing partial phenotype. J Med Genet. 2005;42(1):58–68.

40. Brons AK, Henthorn PS, Raj K, et al. SLC3A1 and SLC7A9 mutations in autosomal recessive or dominant canine cystinuria: a new classification system. J Vet Intern Med. 2013;27(6):1400–8.

41. Dello Strologo L, Pras E, Pontesilli C, et al. Comparison between SLC3A1 and SLC7A9 cystinuria patients and carriers: a need for a new classification. J Am Soc Nephrol. 2002;13:2547–53.

42. Rosenberg L, Durant J, Albrecht I. Genetic heterogeneity in cystinuria: evidence for allelism. Trans Assoc Am Phys. 1966;79:284–96.

43. Middleton JE. A simple, safe nitroprusside test using Ketostix reagent strips for detecting cystine and homocystine in urine. J Clin Pathol. 1970;23(1):90–1.
44. Smith A. Evaluation of the nitroprusside test for the diagnosis of cystinuria. Med J Aust. 1977;2(5):153–5.
45. Finocchiaro R, D'Eufemia P, Celli M, et al. Usefulness of cyanide-nitroprusside test in detecting incomplete recessive heterozygotes for cystinuria: a standardized dilution procedure. Urol Res. 1998;26(6):401–5.
46. Brand E, Harris MM, Biloon S. Cystinuria: excretion of a cystine complex which decomposes in the urine with the liberation of free cystine. J Biol Chem. 1930;86(1):315–31.
47. Coe FL, Clark C, Parks JH, Asplin JR. Solid phase assay of urine cystine supersaturation in the presence of cystine binding drugs. J Urol. 2001;166:688–93.
48. Sumorok N, Goldfarb DS. Update on cystinuria. Curr Opin Nephrol Hypertens. 2013;22(4):427–31.
49. Cochat P, Deloraine A, Rotily M, et al. Epidemiology of primary hyperoxaluria type 1. Société de Néphrologie and the Société de Néphrologie Pédiatrique. Nephrol Dial Transplant. 1995;10(Suppl 8):3–7.
50. El-Reshaid K, Al-Bader D, Madda JP. Primary hyperoxaluria in an adult male: a rare cause of end-stage kidney disease yet potentially fatal if misdiagnosed. Saudi J Kidney Dis Transpl. 2016;27(3):606–9.
51. Lieske JC, Monico CG, Holmes WS, et al. International registry for primary hyperoxaluria. Am J Nephrol. 2005;25:290–6.
52. Leumann E, Hoppe B. The primary hyperoxalurias. J Am Soc Nephrol. 2001;12(9):1986–93.
53. Lorenzo V, Torres A, Salido E. Primary hyperoxaluria. Nefrologia. 2014;34(3):398–412.
54. Hoppe B. An update on primary hyperoxaluria. Nat Rev Nephrol. 2012;8(8):467–75.
55. Harambat J, Fargue S, Acquaviva C, et al. Genotype-phenotype correlation in primary hyperoxaluria type 1: the p.Gly170Arg AGXT mutation is associated with a better outcome. Kidney Int. 2010;77:443–9.
56. Cochat P, Liutkus A, Fargue S, et al. Primary hyperoxaluria type 1: still challenging! Pediatr Nephrol. 2006;21:1075–81.
57. Jellouli M, Ferjani M, Abidi K, et al. Primary hyperoxaluria in infants. Saudi J Kidney Dis Transpl. 2016;27(3):526–32.

58. Bhasin B, Ürekli HM, Atta MG. Primary and secondary hyperoxaluria: understanding the enigma. World J Nephrol. 2015;4(2):235–44.

59. Hoppe B, Leumann E, von Unruh G, et al. Diagnostic and therapeutic approaches in patients with secondary hyperoxaluria. Front Biosci. 2003;8:e437–43.

60. Dent CE, Philpot GR. Xanthinuria, an inborn error (or deviation) of metabolism. Lancet. 1954;263(6804):182–5.

61. Cartier P, Perignon JL. Xanthinuria. Nouv Press Med. 1978;7(16):1381–90.

62. Pais VM Jr, Lowe G, Lallas CD, et al. Xanthine urolithiasis. Urology. 2006;67(5):1084.e9–11.

63. Gargah T, Essid A, Labassi A, et al. Xanthine urolithiasis. Saudi J Kidney Dis Transpl. 2010;21(2):328–31.

64. Anglani F, D'Angelo A, Bertizzolo LM, et al. Nephrolithiasis, kidney failure and bone disorders in Dent disease patients with and without CLCN5 mutations. Springerplus. 2015;4:492.

65. Prié D, Huart V, Bakouh N, et al. Nephrolithiasis and osteoporosis associated with hypophosphatemia caused by mutations in the type 2asodium-phosphate cotransporter. N Engl J Med. 2002;347(13):983–91.

66. Rafaelsen S, Johansson S, Ræder H, Bjerknes R. Hereditary hypophosphatemia in Norway: a retrospective population-based study of genotypes, phenotypes, and treatment complications. Eur J Endocrinol. 2016;174(2):125–36.

67. Stechman MJ, Loh NY, Thakker RV. Genetic causes of hypercalciuric nephrolithiasis. Pediatr Nephrol. 2009;24(12):2321–32.

68. Runolfsdottir HL, Palsson R, Agustsdottir IM, et al. Kidney disease in adenine phosphoribosyltransferase deficiency. Am J Kidney Dis. 2016;67(3):431–8.

69. Edvardsson VO, Palsson R, Sahota A. Adenine phosphoribosyltransferase deficiency. In: Pagon RA, Adam MP, Ardinger HH, et al., editors. GeneReviews®[Internet]. Seattle: University of Washington, Seattle; 1993–2016. 30 Aug 2012 [updated 18 Jun 2015].

70. Gürel A, Üre İ, Temel HE, et al. The impact of klotho gene polymorphisms on urinary tract stone disease. World J Urol. 2016;34(7):1045–50.

71. Frang D, Götz F, Nagy Z, Gimes L, Kocsis B. Study of infective (secondary) renal calculus formation in vitro. Int Urol Nephrol. 1981;13(1):41–9.

72. Bichler KH, Eipper E, Naber K, Braun V, Zimmermann R, Lahme S. Urinary infection stones. Int J Antimicrob Agents. 2002;19(6):488–98.
73. Schaffer JN, Norsworthy AN, Sun TT, Pearson MM. Proteus mirabilis fimbriae- and urease-dependent clusters assemble in an extracellular niche to initiate bladder stone formation. Proc Natl Acad Sci U S A. 2016;113(16):4494–9.
74. Barr-Beare E, Saxena V, Hilt EE, et al. The interaction between enterobacteriaceae and calcium oxalate deposits. PLoS One. 2015;10(10):e0139575.
75. De Cógáin MR, Lieske JC, Vrtiska TJ, et al. Secondary infected non-struvite urolithiasis: a prospective evaluation. Urology. 2014;84(6):1295–300.
76. Weizer AZ, Silverstein AD, Auge BK, Delvecchio FC, Raj G, Albala DM, et al. Determining the incidence of horseshoe kidney from radiographic data at a single institution. J Urol. 2003;170:1722–6.
77. Jira H, Ameur A, Kasmaoui E, et al. Pathologic horseshoe kidney. Report of 13 cases. Ann Urol (Paris). 2002;36(1): 22–5.
78. Benchekroun A, Lachkar A, Soumana A, et al. Pathological horseshoe kidney. 30 case reports. Ann Urol (Paris). 1998;32(5): 279–82.
79. Bennani S, Touijer A, Aboutaieb R, et al. [Pathological horse-shoe kidney. Therapeutic aspects]. Ann Urol (Paris). 1994;28(5): 254–7; discussion 258.
80. Woodward M, Frank D. Postnatal management of antenatal hydronephrosis. BJU Int. 2002;89(2):149–56.
81. Husmann DA, Milliner DS, Segura JW. Ureteropelvic junction obstruction with concurrent renal pelvic calculi in the pediatric patient: a long term follow up. J Urol. 1996;156:741–3.
82. Chahed J, Jouini R, Krichene I, et al. Urinary lithiasis and urinary tract malformations in children: a retrospective study of 34 cases. Afr J Paediatr Surg. 2011;8(2):168–71.
83. Prakash J, Raj A, Sankhwar S, Singh V. Renal calculi with retrocaval ureter: is percutaneous nephrolithotomy sufficient? BMJ Case Rep. 2013;bcr2013008889. https://doi.org/10.1136/bcr-2013-008889.
84. Kanojia RP, Bawa M, Handu AT, et al. Retrocaval ureter with stone in the retrocaval segment of the ureter. Pediatr Surg Int. 2010;26(8):863–5.
85. Bhatia V, Biyani CS. ESWL for stone in a retrocaval ureter: a case report. Int Urol Nephrol. 1994;26(3):263–8.

86. Teo JK, Poh BK, Ng FC. Ureteral diverticulosis. Singapore Med J. 2010;51(9):e161.
87. Kumar A, Goel A, Singh M, Sankwar SN. Urolithiasis in primary obstructive megaureter: a management dilemma. BMJ Case Rep. 2014;30:2014.
88. Madani A, Kermani N, Ataei N, Esfahani ST, Hajizadeh N, Khazaeipour N, et al. Urinary calcium and uric acid excretion in children with vesicoureteral reflux. Pediatr Nephrol. 2012;27:95–9.
89. Chtourou M, Sallami S, Rekik H. Ureterocele in adults complicated with calculi: diagnostic and therapeutic features. Report of 20 cases. Prog Urol. 2002;12(6):1213–20.
90. Hétet JF, Rigaud J, Karam G, et al. Complications of Bricker ileal conduit urinary diversion: analysis of a series of 246 patients. Prog Urol. 2005;15:23–9.
91. Shimko MS, Tollefson MK, Umbreit EC, Farmer SA, Blute ML, Frank I. Long-term complications of conduit urinary diversion. J Urol. 2011;185:562–7.
92. Terai A, Arai Y, Kawakita M, et al. Effect of urinary intestinal diversion on urinary risk factors for urolithiasis. J Urol. 1995;153:37.
93. Gu SP, You ZY, Huang Y, et al. Minimally invasive percutaneous cystostomy with ureteroscopic pneumatic lithotripsy for calculus in bladder diverticula. Exp Ther Med. 2013;5(6):1627–30.
94. Atalar MH, Salk I, Cetin A, Bozbiyik N. A rare case of vesicourachal diverticulum with calculus in a 24-year-old man. Pol J Radiol. 2016;81:301–2.
95. Kronner KM, Casale AJ, Cain MP, et al. Bladder calculi in the pediatric augmented bladder. J Urol. 1998;160(3 Pt 2):1096–8; discussion 1103.
96. Szymanski KM, Misseri R, Whittam B, et al. Cutting for stone in augmented bladders—what is the risk of recurrence and is it impacted by treatment modality? J Urol. 2014;191(5): 1375–80.
97. Hensle TW, Bingham J, Lam J, Shabsigh A. Preventing reservoir calculi after augmentation cystoplasty and continent urinary diversion: the influence of an irrigation protocol. BJU Int. 2004;93(4):585–7.
98. Silver RI, Gros DA, Jeffs RD, Georhart JP. Urolithiasis in the exstrophy-epispadias complex. J Urol. 1997;158:1322–6.
99. Nnabugwu I, Osakue E. Giant dumb-bell calculus complicating vesico-vaginal fistula—a case report. J West Afr Coll Surg. 2011;1(3):91–7.

100. Sawant A, Tamhankar AS, Pawar P, et al. Large dumbbell shaped vesicovaginal calculus managed with holmium laser cystolithotripsy followed by staged repair of vesicovaginal fistula. J Clin Diagn Res. 2016;10(9):PD23–5. Epub 1 Sept 2016.

101. Sigdel G, Aqarwal A, Keshaw BW. A giant urethral calculus. JNMA J Nepal Med Assoc. 2014;52(195):940–2.

102. Dong Z, Wang H, Zuo L, Hou M. Female urethral diverticulum containing a giant calculus: a CARE-compliant case report. Medicine (Baltimore). 2015;94(20):e826.

103. Turo R, Smolski M, Kujawa M, et al. Acute urinary retention in women due to urethral calculi: a rare case. Can Urol Assoc J. 2014;8(1–2):E99–100.

104. Sasaki T, Onishi T, Hoshina A. Urinary retention caused by a urethral cystine stone in a 10-month-old infant. Pediatr Emerg Care. 2013;29(7):831–2.

105. Akhtar J, Ahmed S, Zamir N. Management of impacted urethral stones in children. J Coll Physicians Surg Pak. 2012;22(8):510–3.

106. Everidge J. Jackstone calculi. Proc R Soc Med. 1927;20(5):717–8.

107. Singh KJ, Tiwari A, Goyal A. Jackstone: a rare entity of vesical calculus. Indian J Urol. 2011;27(4):543–4.

108. Grases F, Costa-Bauza A, Prieto RM, et al. Rare calcium oxalate monohydrate calculus attached to the wall of the renal pelvis. Int J Urol. 2011;18(4):323–5.

109. Gordon Z, Monga M. Endoscopic extraction of an ejaculatory duct calculus to treat obstructive azoospermia. J Endourol. 2001;15(9):949–50.

110. Gor RA, Woodhouse CR, Schober JM. Obstructive ejaculatory duct calculi in a patient with bladder augmentation and myelomeningocele. J Pediatr Urol. 2011;7(2):233–5.

111. Koh KB. Symptomatic prostatic calculi—a rare complication after TURP. Med J Malaysia. 1995;50(3):280–1.

112. Goyal NK, Goel A, Sankhwar S. Transurethral holmium-YAG laser lithotripsy for large symptomatic prostatic calculi: initial experience. Urolithiasis. 2013;41(4):355–9.

113. Park B, Choo SH. The burden of prostatic calculi is more important than the presence. Asian J Androl. 2017;19(4):482–5.

114. Najoui M, Qarro A, Ammani A, Alami M. Giant prostatic calculi. Pan Afr Med J. 2013;14:69.

115. Sfanos KS, Wilson BA, De Marzo AM, Isaacs WB. Acute inflammatory proteins constitute the organic matrix of prostatic corpora amylacea and calculi in men with prostate cancer. Proc Natl Acad Sci U S A. 2009;106:3443–8.

116. Dessombz A, Meria P, Bazin D, Daudon M. Prostatic stones: evidence of a specific chemistry related to infection and presence of bacterial imprints. PLoS One. 2012;7:e51691.
117. Penkoff P, Bariol S. Urethral calculus originating from ureterocele and causing urinary retention. ANZ J Surg. 2015;85(11):892–3.
118. Sinha RK, Singh S, Kumar P. Prolapsed ureterocele, with calculi within, causing urinary retention in adult female. BMJ Case Rep. 2014;2014. pii: bcr2013202165.
119. Bhat GS. Preputial calculi: a case report and review of literature. Indian J Surg. 2017;79(1):70–2.
120. Nagata D, Sasaki S, Umemoto Y, Kohri K. Preputial calculi: case report. BJU Int. 1999;83:1076–7.
121. Spataru RI, Iozsa DA, Ivanov M. Preputial calculus in a neurologically-impaired child. Indian Pediatr. 2015;52(2):149–50.
122. Lieske JC, Mehta RA, Milliner DS, et al. Kidney stones are common after bariatric surgery. Kidney Int. 2015;87(4):839–45.
123. Gonzalez RD, Canales BK. Kidney stone risk following modern bariatric surgery. Curr Urol Rep. 2014;15(5):401.
124. Litschgi MS, Benz JJ, Glatthaar E. Bladder stones as a complication of gynecologic surgery. Fortschr Med. 1975;93(32):1627–8.
125. Amin U, Mahmood R. An unusual vesical calculus. J Radiol Case Rep. 2009;3(2):10–3.
126. Rodríguez Collar TL, Gil del Valle Y, Valdés Estévez B, et al. Bladder lithiasis secondary to intrauterine device migration. Case report. Arch Esp Urol. 2008;61(5):640–3.
127. Karsmakers R, Weis-Potters AE, Buijs G, Joustra EB. Chronic kidney disease after vesico-vaginal stone formation around a migrated intrauterine device. BMJ Case Rep. 2010;23:2010.
128. Kumar S, Jayant K, Singh SK, et al. Delayed migration of embolized coil with large renal stone formation: a rare presentation. Case Rep Urol. 2014;2014:687965.
129. Bjurlin MA, Berger AD. Herniorrhaphy mesh as nidus for bladder calculi. Urology. 2011;78(2):329–30.
130. Lieske JC, Rule AD, Krambeck AE. Stone composition as a function of age and sex. Clin J Am Soc Nephrol. 2014;9(12): 2141–6.
131. Daudon M, Protat MF, Réveillaud RJ. Detection and diagnosis of drug-induced lithiasis. Ann Biol Clin (Paris). 1983;41(4): 239–49.
132. Daudon M, Jungers P. Drug-induced renal calculi: epidemiology, prevention and management. Drugs. 2004;64(3):245–75.

133. Barbey F, Nseir G, Ferrier C, et al. Carbonic anhydrase inhibitors and calcium phosphate stones. Nephrologie. 2004;25(5):169–72.
134. Lehr D. Clinical toxicity of sulfonamides. Ann N Y Acad Sci. 1957;69:417–47.
135. De Koninck AS, Groen LA, Maes H, et al. An unusual type of kidney stone. Clin Lab. 2016;62(1–2):235–9.
136. Yanagasawa R, Kamijo T, Nagase Y. A case of drug induced urolithiasis composed of acetyl sulphapyridine associated with ulcerative colitis. Nihon Hinyokika Gakkai Zasshi. 1999; 90(3):462–5.
137. Schwartz BF, Schenkman N, Armenakas NA, Stoller ML. Imaging characteristics of indinavir calculi. J Urol. 1999;161(4):1085–7.
138. Hess B. Drug-induced urolithiasis. Curr Opin Urol. 1998;8(4): 331–4.
139. Izzedine H, Lescure FX, Bonnet F. HIV medication-based urolithiasis. Clin Kidney J. 2014;7(2):121–6.
140. Khalil C, Mohanty MJ, Kaatz G, Abu-Hamdan D. Efavirenz-associated urinary Matrix stone—a rare presentation. Am J Med Sci. 2016;351(2):213–4.
141. Moesch C, Rince M, Raby C, Leroux-Robert C. Aminopenicillin crystalluria: identification by infrared spectrophotometry. Ann Biol Clin (Paris). 1985;43(3):227–31.
142. Chutipongtanate S, Thongboonkerd V. Ceftriaxone crystallization and its potential role in kidney stone formation. Biochem Biophys Res Commun. 2011;406(3):396–402.
143. Small E, Sandefur BJ. Acute renal failure after ingestion of guaifenesin and dextromethorphan. J Emerg Med. 2014;47(1): 26–9.
144. Assimos DG, Langenstroer P, Leinbach RF, et al. Guaifenesin-and ephedrine-induced stones. J Endourol. 1999;13(9):665–7.
145. Augusti M, Mikaelian JC, Monsaint H, et al. A silica urinary calculus secondary to the absorption of gelopectose in a child. Prog Urol. 1993;3(5):812–5.
146. Daudon M, Reveillaud RJ, Normand M, et al. Piridoxilate-induced calcium oxalate calculi: a new drug-induced metabolic nephrolithiasis. J Urol. 1987;138(2):258–61.
147. Fukumoto R, Katayama K, Hayashi T, et al. Two cases of urolithiasis induced by topiramate. Hinyokika Kiyo. 2011;57(3):125–8.
148. Daudon M. Drug-induced urinary calculi in 1999. Prog Urol. 1999;9(6):1023–33.

149. Horiuchi H, Ota M, Kobayashi M, et al. A comparative study on the hypouricemic activity and potency in renal xanthine calculus formation of two xanthine oxidase/xanthine dehydrogenase inhibitors: TEI-6720 and allopurinol in rats. Res Commun Mol Pathol Pharmacol. 1999;104(3):307–19.

150. Ikari O, Leitão VA, D'ancona CA. Intravesical calculus secondary to ethanol gel injection into the prostate. Urology. 2005;65(5):1002.

151. Beltrami P, Ruggera L, Guttilla A, et al. The endourological treatment of renal matrix stones. Urol Int. 2014;93(4):394–8.

152. Shah HN, Kharodawala S, Sodha HS, et al. The management of renal matrix calculi: a single-centre experience over 5 years. BJU Int. 2009;103(6):810–4.

153. Manny TB, Mufarrij PW, Lange JN, et al. Gas-containing renal stones: findings from five consecutive patients. Urology. 2012;80(6):1203–8.

154. Howles SA, Edwards MH, Cooper C, Thakker RV. Kidney stones: a fetal origins hypothesis. J Bone Miner Res. 2013;28(12): 2535–9.

155. Gambaro G, Trinchieri A. Recent advances in managing and understanding nephrolithiasis/nephrocalcinosis. F1000Res. 2016;5. pii: F1000 Faculty Rev-695.

156. Rule AD, Roger VL, Melton LJ 3rd, et al. Kidney stones associate with increased risk for myocardial infarction. J Am Soc Nephrol. 2010;21:1641–4.

157. Alexander RT, Hemmelgarn BR, Wiebe N, et al. Kidney stones and cardiovascular events: a cohort study. Clin J Am Soc Nephrol. 2014;9:506–12.

158. Fabris A, Ferraro PM, Comellato G, et al. The relationship between calcium kidney stones, arterial stiffness and bone density: unraveling the stone-bone-vessel liaison. J Nephrol. 2015;28(5):549–55.

159. Shavit L, Girfoglio D, Vijay V, et al. Vascular calcification and bone mineral density in recurrent kidney stone formers. Clin J Am Soc Nephrol. 2015;10(2):278–85.

160. Cacci R, Ricci V. Sopra una rara e forse ancora non descritta affezione cistica delle piramidi renali ('rene a spugna'). Atti Soc Ital Urol. 1948;5:59–63.

161. Xu H, Zisman AL, Coe FL, Worcester EM. Kidney stones: an update on current pharmacological management and future directions. Expert Opin Pharmacother. 2013;14(4):435–47.

162. Mrowka C, Adam G, Sieberth HG, Matern S. Caroli's syndrome associated with medullary sponge kidney and nephrocalcinosis. Nephrol Dial Transplant. 1996;11(6):1142–5.
163. Nishiura JL, Neves RF, Eloi SR, et al. Evaluation of nephrolithiasis in autosomal dominant polycystic kidney disease patients. Clin J Am Soc Nephrol. 2009;4(4):838–44.
164. Torres VE, Erickson SB, Smith LH, et al. The association of nephrolithiasis and autosomal dominant polycystic kidney disease. Am J Kidney Dis. 1988;11(4):318–25.
165. Nyhan WL, O'Neill JP, Jinnah HA, Harris JC. Lesch-Nyhan syndrome. In: Pagon RA, Adam MP, Ardinger HH, et al., editors. GeneReviews®[Internet]. Seattle: University of Washington, Seattle; 1993–2016. 25 Sept 2000 [updated 15 May 2014].
166. Siener R, Petzold J, Bitterlich N, et al. Determinants of urolithiasis in patients with intestinal fat malabsorption. Urology. 2013;81(1):17–24.
167. Ferraz RR, Tiselius HG, Heilberg IP. Fat malabsorption induced by gastrointestinal lipase inhibitor leads to an increase in urinary oxalate excretion. Kidney Int. 2004;66(2):676–82.
168. Faggiano A, Pivonello R, Melis D, et al. Nephrolithiasis in Cushing's disease: prevalence, etiopathogenesis, and modification after disease cure. J Clin Endocrinol Metab. 2003;88(5):2076–80.
169. Trinchieri A, Lizzano R, Castelnuovo C, et al. Urinary patterns of patients with renal stones associated with chronic inflammatory bowel disease. Arch Ital Urol Androl. 2002;74(2):61–4.
170. McConnell N, Campbell S, Gillanders I, et al. Risk factors for developing renal stones in inflammatory bowel disease. BJU Int. 2002;89(9):835–41.
171. Rizzato G, Fraioli P, Montemurro L. Nephrolithiasis as a presenting feature of chronic sarcoidosis. Thorax. 1995;50(5):555–9.
172. Darabi K, Torres G, Chewaproug D. Nephrolithiasis as primary symptom in sarcoidosis. Scand J Urol Nephrol. 2005;39(2):173–5.
173. Patel AM, Goldfarb S. Got calcium? Welcome to the calcium-alkali syndrome. J Am Soc Nephrol. 2010;21(9):1440–3.
174. Medarov BI. Milk-alkali syndrome. Mayo Clin Proc. 2009;84(3):261–7.
175. Pereira Arias JG, Gurtubay Arrieta I, Escobal Tamayo V, et al. Megacalycosis and lithiasis. Arch Esp Urol. 1995;48(3):310–4.

176. Thakker RV. Pathogenesis of Dent's disease and related syndromes of X-linked nephrolithiasis. Kidney Int. 2000;57(3): 787–93.
177. Thakker RV. Molecular pathology of renal chloride channels in Dent's disease and Bartter's syndrome. Exp Nephrol. 2000;8(6):351–60.
178. Eriksson P, Denneberg T, Eneström S, et al. Urolithiasis and distal renal tubular acidosis preceding primary Sjögren's syndrome: a retrospective study 5-53 years after the presentation of urolithiasis. J Intern Med. 1996;239(6):483–8.
179. Mittal R, Saxena S, Hotchandani RK, et al. Bilateral renal stones associated with nail-patella syndrome. Nephron. 1994;68(4):509.
180. Cevik Y, Corbacioglu SK, Cikrikci G, et al. The effects of Ramadan fasting on the number of renal colic visits to the emergency department. Pak J Med Sci. 2016;32(1):18–21.
181. Soueidan M, Bartlett SJ, Noureldin YA, et al. Leisure time physical activity, smoking and risk of recent symptomatic urolithiasis: survey of stone clinic patients. Can Urol Assoc J. 2015;9(7–8):257–62.
182. Okada A, Ichikawa J, Tozawa K. Kidney stone formation during space flight and long-term bed rest. Clin Calcium. 2011;21(10):1505–10.

Chapter 7
Symptomatology and Signs of Urinary Stones

"In examining disease, we gain wisdom about anatomy and physiology and biology. In examining the person with disease, we gain wisdom about life."

Oliver Sacks (1933–2015)

7.1 Presenting Symptoms

1. Renal colic: The most common presentation. The pain is triggered by tension in the renal capsule, renal collecting system, or ureter, and travels with the sympathetic nerves along the subcostal, iliohypogastric, ilioinguinal, and/or genitofemoral nerves, to be experienced over the T8 to L2 dermatomes [1, 2]. It is characteristically spasmodic and agonizing and starts at the loin area below the rib cage, and radiates to the ipsilateral flank, iliac fossa and inguinal region. Therefore it can sometimes reach the corresponding labium majus in females and hemiscrotum in males as well as the proximal anterior aspect of the thigh due to L1–2 nerve roots pain transmission through the genitofemoral nerve (Fig. 7.1) [1, 2]. There are paroxysmal and intermittent attacks during the same episode, frequently associated with nausea and vomiting. When the stone causes an obstructive uropathy, in addition to pain, the patient may present with fever, and his laboratory parameters will show deranged renal function and increased inflammatory markers. Renal colics mostly occur during

© Springer International Publishing AG 2017
S.A. Al-Mamari, *Urolithiasis in Clinical Practice*,
In Clinical Practice, DOI 10.1007/978-3-319-62437-2_7

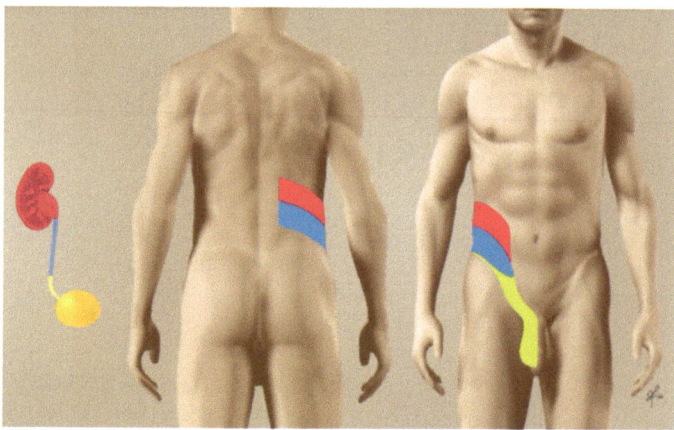

FIGURE 7.1 Location of pain in the flank, right lower quadrant, and groin depends upon the location of pathology in the urinary tract, i.e., a stone making its way to the bladder. *Red* indicates pain originating in the kidney or at the uretero-pelvic junction (UPJ), *blue* shows pain from upper and middle ureteral pathology, and *yellow* indicates pain from the distal ureter or uretero-vesical junction. From Noble MJ [2] with permission from Springer

hot seasons. However the association with lunar phases remains controversial; some authors reported that most cases of renal colics presented around day 15 of the lunar phases and the lowest number was found on days 1 and 30 [3], but these observations were not confirmed by other investigators [4, 5].

2. Haematuria: Frequently associated with the renal colic, haematuria may be microscopic or macroscopic. In relation with urolithiasis confirmed by unenhanced helical Computed Tomography scan (UHCT), the sensitivity, specificity, positive predictive value, and negative predictive value of microscopic haematuria detected on urinalysis are 84%, 48%, 72%, and 65%, respectively [6]. The low specificity is explained by the multiple possible alternative diagnoses associated with haematuria (infections, trauma, foreign body, malignancy, glomerulonephritis, etc.).

3. Urinary retention: this occurs in the presence of a bladder or urethral stone. It is typically a hyperacute and very painful event.
4. Irritative syndrome: It consists of recurrent suprapubic pain associated with frequency and urgency due to trigonal irritation of a vesical stone.
5. Vague loin pain: This ill-defined pain occurs mostly with non-obstructive calyceal or staghorn calculus possibly associated with chronic pyelonephritis.
6. Asymptomatic: Nowadays due to the liberal use of imaging studies of the abdomen (ultrasound and CT-scan), more stones are being discovered serendipitously with or without any clinical bearing.

   A random study of 1590 validated incident symptomatic stone formers among Olmsted County adult residents (Minnesota) has shown that with increasing age, patients were more likely to present with atypical or no pain, but with fever, diarrhea, pyuria, UTI, and bacteremia [7] (Table 7.1). **This atypical presentation in elderly patients represents a clinical challenge requiring a high index of suspicion for a timely diagnosis and intervention**. There was a significant increase of UTI, and the most commonly cultured organism was Escherichia coli seen in 39%, followed by Klebsiella pneumonia, Staphylococcus aureus and Proteus mirabilis encountered in 12%, 6.2%, and 6.2% respectively. The great majority of patients with UTI were females accounting for 82.6%.

   A Turkish review study of 950 patients confirmed the above trend showing relatively less flank pain and more haematuria in patients aged more than 60 years compared to younger subjects [8]. Ureteral stones were more frequent in the younger age while elderly patients had a higher rate of bladder stones accounting for their increased frequency of dysuria and haematuria in this study.

   More rarely, patients may present with odd complaints or signs and the relation with urolithiasis will be difficult to establish at first glance. These include:

• Male infertility with obstructive azoospermia [9],

TABLE 7.1 Presenting symptoms of 1590 incident stone formers

| | Age at diagnosis | | | | | | |
	18–29 Years	30–44 Years	45–59 Years	60–69 Years	70 Years or older	p Value
No. pts	325	589	428	148	100	
No. pain (%):						30.0001
Renal colic	305 (94)	530 (90)	378 (88)	127 (86)	73 (73)	
Atypical	16 (5)	43 (7)	34 (8)	12 (81)	17 (17)	
None	4 (1)	16 (3)	16 (4)	9 (6)	10 (10)	
No. nausea (%)	210 (65)	377 (64)	244 (57)	92 (62)	58 (58)	0.13*
No. emesis (%)	144 (44)	237 (40)	138 (32)	56 (38)	38 (38)	0.014
No. fever greater than 38C or greater than 100.5F (%)	17 (5)	37 (6)	26 (6)	11 (7)	17 (17)	0.0010
No. voiding symptoms (%)	132 (41)	214 (36)	122 (29)	41 (28)	26 (26)	0.0008

No. loose stools or diarrhea (%)	36 (11)	51 (9)	33 (8)	17 (12)	19 (19)	0.0086
No. gross hematuria (%)	63 (19)	129 (22)	88 (21)	33 (22)	20 (20)	0.90
No. microscopic hematuria (%)	220 (68)	367 (62)	275 (64)	92 (62)	64 (64)	0.58
No. UTI with greater than 100,000 cfu/mL (%)	19 (6)	21 (4)	18 (4)	9 (6)	19 (19)	<0.0001
No. pyuria (%)	21 (7)	22 (4)	20 (5)	15 (10)	15 (15)	<0.0001
Spot urine pH:						0.058
No.	26	31	28	16	20	
Mean (SD)	6.39 (0.96)	6.26 (1.08)	6.03 (1.02)	5.75 (0.88)	6.60 (1.09)	

From Krambeck et al. [7] with permission from Elsevier

*Trend test p=0.04

- Hemospermia for ejaculatory duct inspissated material or stones [10],
- Combination of recurrent lower urinary tract infections and painful ejaculation [11].

7.2   Calculating the Probability of Renal Stone Symptoms Recurrence

The Recurrence of Kidney Stone (ROKS) nomogram was developed by Rule et al. based on clinical characteristics of 2239 first-time adult kidney stone formers. It showed that about $\frac{1}{3}$ **of them had recurrent symptomatic episodes**. The pattern of recurrence progression was **11%, 20%, 31%, and 39% at 2, 5, 10, and 15 years respectively** [12]. In this study the following factors were found to be associated with increased risk of recurrent symptomatic episodes: younger age at the first episode, male sex, white race, family history of stones, prior asymptomatic stone on imaging, prior suspected stone episode, gross hematuria, nonobstructing (asymptomatic) stone on imaging, symptomatic renal pelvic or lower-pole stone on imaging, no ureterovesicular junction stone on imaging, and uric acid stone composition [12]. The recurrent pattern of the stones associated with cystinuria, primary hyperoxaluria and other genetic abnormalities should not be forgotten at this point.

References

1. Anderson JK, Kabalin JN, Cadeddu JA. Surgical anatomy of the retroperitoneum, adrenals, kidneys, and ureters. In: Wein AJ, Kavoussi LR, Novick AC, Partin AW, Peters CA, editors. Campbell-Walsh's urology. 9th ed. Philadelphia: Saunders Elsevier; 2007. p. 3–37.
2. Noble MJ. Acute and chronic flank pain. In: Potts MJ, editor. Genitourinary pain and inflammation: diagnosis and management. Humana Press, Totowa, NJ; 2008. p. 19–37.

3. Molaee Govarchin Ghalae H, Zare S, Choopanloo M, Rahimian R. The lunar cycle–effects of full moon on renal colic. Urology Journal. 2009;8:137–40.

4. Arampatzis S, Thalmann GN, Zimmermann H, Exadaktylos AK. Lunar tractive forces and renal stone incidence. Emerg Med Int. 2011. doi: 10.1155/2011/813460.

5. Yang AW, Johnson JD, Fronczak CM, LaGrange CA. Lunar phases and emergency department visits for renal colic due to ureteral calculus. PLoS One. 2016;11(6):e0157589.

6. Luchs JS, Katz DS, Lane MJ, et al. Utility of hematuria testing in patients with suspected renal colic: correlation with unenhanced helical CT results. Urology. 2002;59(6):839–42.

7. Krambeck AE, Lieske JC, Li X, et al. Effect of age on the clinical presentation of incident symptomatic urolithiasis in the general population. J Urol. 2013;189(1):158–64.

8. Dursun M, Ozbek E, Otunctemur A, et al. Clinical presentation of urolithiasis in older and younger population. Arch Ital Urol Androl. 2014;86(4):249–52.

9. Ranjan P, Yadav A, Kapoor R, Singh R. A rare case of obstructive azoospermia due to compression of the seminal vesicle and ejaculatory duct by a large lower ureteric stone. Singap Med J. 2013;54(3):e56–8.

10. Zargooshi J, Nourizad S, Vaziri S, et al. Hemospermia: long-term outcome in 165 patients. Int J Impot Res. 2014;26(3):83–6.

11. Hadidi M, Hadidy A, Alrabadi AF, et al. Bilateral very large calcium oxalate stones in the seminal vesicles: case report and literature review. Urol Res. 2011;39(6):509–13.

12. Rule AD, Lieske JC, Li X, et al. The ROKS nomogram for predicting a second symptomatic stone episode. J Am Soc Nephrol. 2014;25(12):2878–86.

Chapter 8
Complications of Urolithiasis

"Just when you think it can't get any worse, it can."

Nicholas Sparks (1965–)

Many complications may arise from urolithiasis especially if there is a delay in the diagnosis or incomplete treatment. These complications are enumerated hereafter:

1. Obstruction and uremia: generally caused by pelvi-ureteric and ureteral stones, but can also be the consequence of a giant bladder stone as reported in a few studies [1–3].
2. Sepsis: a common consequence of obstruction in presence of UTI.
3. Chronic pyelonephritis [4].
4. Renal failure: acute or chronic.

    (a) Acute renal failure occurs mostly as the result of bilateral obstructing ureteral stones, stone on a solitary kidney, or as the result of sepsis with multiorgan failure.

    (b) Chronic renal failure is the result of chronic pyelonephritis in the setting of recurrent multiple renal stones or staghorn calculus. A study showed that cystinuria in the United Kingdom often presents with staghorn calculi and commonly progresses to chronic kidney disease in as much as 70% of the cases [5]. The grim tendency of primary hyperoxaluria to progress to chronic renal failure has already been discussed in an earlier chapter.

© Springer International Publishing AG 2017
S.A. Al-Mamari, *Urolithiasis in Clinical Practice*,
In Clinical Practice, DOI 10.1007/978-3-319-62437-2_8

5. Xanthogranulomatous pyelonephritis

This is a very rare entity, predominantly affecting adult patients ≥50 years, females (F:M = 2.5:1), and mainly caused by staghorn calculus (51.4%) and obstructing ureteric calculi (22.9%). **Only a minority of patients are diabetic**. The most common clinical presentations appear to be **flank pain, high grade fever > 38 °C, dysuria and weight loss**. The left kidney is more affected than the right one. Laboratory results are consistent with anemia, leukocytosis, and pyuria in the majority of cases. Imaging studies show hydronephrosis, generalized kidney enlargement, or a localized renal mass [6–10]. The diffuse form is more frequent (81%) than the focal one, and extra-renal extension has been described in more than half of the cases [10, 11]. **Nephrectomy is curative with a good outcome** [6–10]. Histologically, the renal parenchyma is destructed and replaced by granulomatous tissue containing lipid-filled macrophages (xanthoma cells) [11]. These macrophages are thus named because of their yellow appearance (Greek "Xanthos": yellow).

6. Hypertension:

ADPKD with renal stones have increased risk to develop HTN than ADPKD without renal stones [12]. Remember the suggested role played by vessel walls in buffering calcium delivered by a high bone turnover in some renal stone formers, resulting in a higher arterial calcification score and an increased arterial stiffness (see section Etiology of Urolithiasis, paragraph 6.10).

7. Emphysematous pyelonephritis (EPN):

This is an uncommon acute, life-threatening, suppurative and necrotizing infection of the renal parenchyma and perirenal tissue, accompanied by gas within the renal parenchyma, collecting system, or perinephric tissue.

From a 48-patient cohort Huang and Tseng proposed in 2000 a clinico-radiological classification of EPN based on the radiological extension of the gas or abscess in a CT-scan [13]:

- Class 1: gas in the collecting system only;
- Class 2: gas in the renal parenchyma without extension to extrarenal space;

- Class 3A: extension of gas or abscess to perinephric space;
- Class 3B: extension of gas or abscess to pararenal space; and
- Class 4: bilateral EPN or solitary kidney with EPN.

The association of EPN with urolithiasis is well documented in the literature [14–17] (Fig. 8.1), **but DM is a nearly constant factor seen in > 90% of cases of EPN** [15]. The female gender is another frequently encountered factor and, for unknown reason, the left kidney is more frequently involved than the right one. The association with urolithiasis varies according to the studies, being 22% in old studies [13, 18] to as higher as 57% in a very recent publication which also showed that EPN in patients with urolithiasis exhibits a less severe course than in patients without urolithiasis [19].

Escherichia coli is the most commonly encountered causative micro-organism present in half of the cases or more [13, 20]. Other possible organisms are Klebsiella pneumonia and Proteus mirabilis. **More than 80% respond to conservative treatment based on an early**

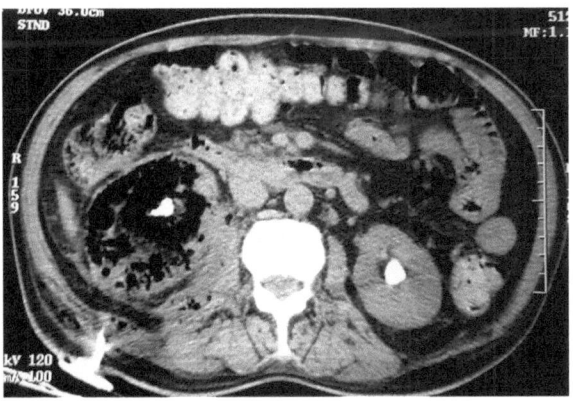

FIGURE 8.1 Noncontrast CT revealing the presence of gas in the right pelvicalyceal system with bilateral intrarenal calculus. From Sridhar et al. [17] with permission from Oxford University Press

broad-spectrum IV antibiotic therapy, renal drainage and a rapid control of blood sugar. Nephrectomy may be required in a minority of cases [21]. The patient is better managed in a high dependency or an intensive care unit and the recommended initial antibiotics are third-generation cephalosporins. However Carbapenems are to be introduced if the progress is not favourable with the former antibiotics, or in debilitated patients who require emergency hemodialysis or develop disseminated intravascular coagulation (DIC); Fluoroquinolone and gentamicin are better avoided [20].

8. Pyonephrosis:
   Pyonephrosis follows infection in a completely obstructed kidney. It may present with acute flank pain associated with sepsis and a palpable and tender kidney, but generally the patient will come with a long standing history of dull ache in the ipsilateral loin associated with a low-grade fever and a progressive unwellness. Pyonephrosis is frequently seen in developing countries due to a delay in the diagnosis of an obstructive uropathy, and was found to be caused by urolithiasis in 73% of cases [22]. However it has also been observed in developed countries in patients with spinal cord injury who develop silent progression of the disease [23].

9. Myocardial Infarction
   Kidney stone formers were found to have an increased risk of myocardial infarction, estimated to reach 31% after a mean follow-up of 9 years, independently of chronic kidney disease and other risk factors [24].

10. Ureteral stricture:
    This is often caused by an aggressive ureteroscopy aiming at removing a stone, and is exceptionally the direct consequence of a longstanding stone causing local inflammatory reaction in the ureteral wall. A recent prospective study showed a stricture rate of 7.8% 3 months after ureteroscopy has been performed for impacted stones [25], however this figure varies with the experience of publishing centers.

11. Fistulization:

    Although uncommon, this complication has been reported in many articles and occurs as a late event of pyonephrosis or xanthogranulomatous pyelonephritis. Renal fistula generally open into the adjacent organs such as the skin (through the psoas muscle), the colon, the peritoneal cavity and the spleen, but rarely it can even open above the diaphragm into the bronchial tree [26–28] (Fig. 8.2a–c).

    An exceptional case of large renal fistula to the posterior abdominal wall has been reported in a patient with spina bifida and paraplegia resulting in spontaneous extrusion of part of a staghorn renal calculus [29].

    Spontaneous bladder rupture and subsequent vesicocutaneous fistula is an extremely rare event scarcely reported in the literature and caused by a giant bladder stone [30, 31].

12. Spontaneous renal pelvis or ureteral rupture

    This is an extremely rare event with only 18 cases reported in the literature, ten of them being caused by an obstructing ureteral stone [32], while malignancy accounted for the majority of the remaining cases.

13. Mechanical dystocia

    This is an extremely rare event caused by enormous bladder stone [33].

14. Epididymoorchitis

    Infection of the epididymis may occur as a complication of an infected urethral stone [34].

15. Urothelial carcinoma

    A cohort including nearly 22,000 Taiwanese patients with urinary stone revealed an increased risk of developing urothelial carcinoma, which was greater in women [35].

16. Penile gangrene

    There is one case of penile gangrene and sepsis reported in the literature directly resulting from impacted multiple urethral stones in a 54-year-old patient in Trinidad and Tobago who did not surprisingly have other co-morbidities [36].

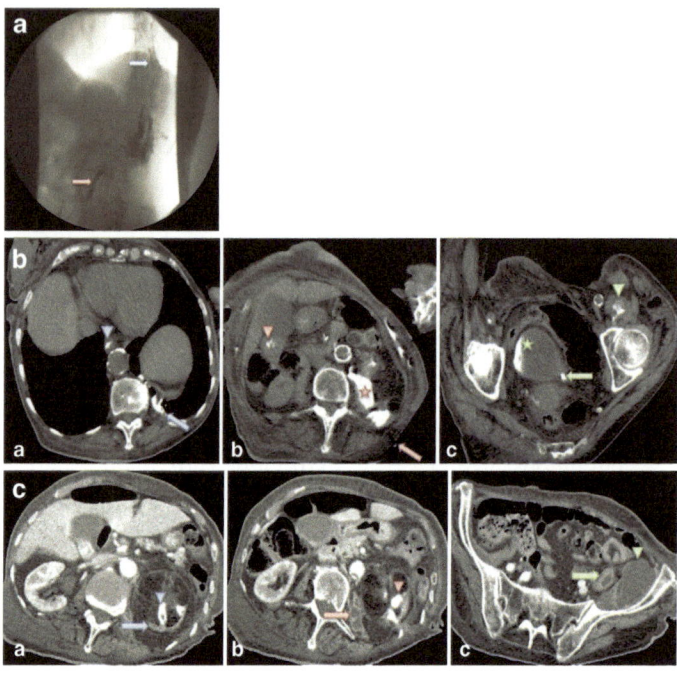

FIGURE 8.2 (**a**) Fistulogram showing nephrocutaneous fistula with contrast leakage cranially (*blue arrow*) and caudally (*red arrow*) from the kidney. From Snoj Z et al. [26]. Creative Commons Attribution License. (**b**) The computer tomographic scan performed immediately after the fistulogram; the patient was positioned on her right flank. (*A*) Contrast in the oesophagus (*blue arrowhead*) and communication with the left lower lobe of the lung (*blue arrow*). (*B*) Cutaneous fistula (*red arrow*), contrast retroperitoneally (*red star*) and in the duodenum (*red arrowhead*). (*C*) Contrast in bladder (*green star*), ureter (*green arrow*) and in the psoas muscle (*green arrowhead*) just proximally to lesser trochanter. From Snoj Z et al. [26]. Creative Commons Attribution License. (**c**) The computer tomographic scan with intravenous contrast. (*A*) Staghorn calculus (*blue arrowhead*) and extremely atrophic parenchyma of the left kidney (*blue arrow*). (*B*) Retroperitoneal abscess (*red arrow*) and staghorn calculus (*red arrowhead*). (*C*) Fistulisation along the psoas muscle (*green arrow*) and large pelvic abscess (*green arrowhead*). From Snoj Z et al. [26]. Creative Commons Attribution License

References

1. Celik O, Suelozgen T, Budak S, Ilbey YO. Post-renal acute renal failure due to a huge bladder stone. Arch Ital Urol Androl. 2014;86(2):146–7.
2. Ofluoglu Y, Aydin HR, Kocaaslan R, et al. A cause of renal dysfunction: a giant bladder stone. Eurasian J Med. 2013; 45(3):211–3. doi:10.5152/eajm.2013.41.
3. Komeya M, Sahoda T, Sugiura S, et al. A huge bladder calculus causing acute renal failure. Urolithiasis. 2013;41(1):85–7.
4. Barr-Beare E, Saxena V, Hilt EE, et al. The interaction between Enterobacteriaceae and calcium oxalate deposits. PLoS One. 2015;10(10):e0139575.
5. Rhodes HL, Yarram-Smith L, Rice SJ, et al. Clinical and genetic analysis of patients with cystinuria in the United Kingdom. Clin J Am Soc Nephrol. 2015;10(7):1235–45.
6. Addison B, Zargar H, Lilic N, et al. Analysis of 35 cases of Xanthogranulomatous pyelonephritis. ANZ J Surg. 2015;85(3):150–3.
7. Datta B, Datta C, Pahari DK. Xanthogranulomatous pyelone-phritis: critical analysis of 18 cases from a rural tertiary care centre of India. J Indian Med Assoc. 2014;112(1):33–5.
8. Kim SW, Yoon BI, Ha US, et al. Xanthogranulomatous pyelo-nephritis: clinical experience with 21 cases. J Infect Chemother. 2013;19(6):1221–4.
9. Siddappa S, Ramprasad K, Muddegowda MK. Xanthogra-nulomatous pyelonephritis: a retrospective review of 16 cases. Korean J Urol. 2011;52(6):421–4.
10. Kim JC. US and CT findings of xanthogranulomatous pyelone-phritis. Clin Imaging. 2001;25(2):118–21.
11. EL Abiad Y, Dehayni Y, Qarro A, Balla B, Ammani A, Alami M. Xantogranulomatous pyelonephritis: the missed diagnosis. Int J Surg Case Rep. 2016;18:21–3.
12. Bajrami V, Idrizi A, Roshi E, Barbullushi M. Association between nephrolithiasis, hypertension and obesity in polycystic kidney disease. Open Access Maced J Med Sci. 2016;4(1):43–6.
13. Huang JJ, Tseng CC. Emphysematous pyelonephritis: clinicora-diological classification, management, prognosis, and pathogen-esis. Arch Intern Med. 2000;160(6):797–805.
14. Goel T, Reddy S, Thomas J. Emphysematous pyelonephritis with calculus: management strategies. Indian J Urol. 2007;23(3): 250–2. Figure 3.

15. Shokeir AA, El-Azab M, Mohsen T, El-Diasty T. Emphysematous pyelonephritis: a 15-year experience with 20 cases. Urology. 1997;49(3):343–6.
16. Kutwin P, Konecki T, Jabłonowski Z. Emphysematous pyelonephritis in a diabetic patient with obstructed kidney. Cent European J Urol. 2014;67(2):196–8.
17. Sridhar S, Rakesh D, Sangumani J. Stones, sugar and air-emphysematous pyelonephritis. QJM. 2015;108(1):73.
18. Somani BK, Nabi G, Thorpe P, et al. ABACUS Research Group. Is percutaneous drainage the new gold standard in the management of emphysematous pyelonephritis? Evidence from a systematic review. J Urol. 2008;179:1844–9.
19. Sanford TH, Myers F, Chi T, Bagga HS, Taylor AG, Stoller ML. Emphysematous pyelonephritis: the impact of urolithiasis on disease severity. Transl Androl Urol. 2016;5(5):774–9.
20. Lu YC, Hong JH, Chiang BJ, et al. Recommended initial antimicrobial therapy for emphysematous pyelonephritis: 51 cases and 14-year-experience of a tertiary referral center. Medicine (Baltimore). 2016;95(21):e3573.
21. Misgar RA, Mubarik I, Wani AI, et al. Emphysematous pyelonephritis: a 10-year experience with 26 cases. Indian J Endocrinol Metab. 2016;20(4):475–80.
22. Sow Y, Fall B, Sarr A, et al. Pyonephrosis: 44 cases in Senegal. Med Trop (Mars). 2011;71(5):495–8.
23. Vaidyanathan S, Singh G, Soni BM, et al. Silent hydronephrosis/pyonephrosis due to upper urinary tract calculi in spinal cord injury patients. Spinal Cord. 2000;38(11):661–8.
24. Rule AD, Roger VL, Melton LJ III, Bergstralh EJ, Li X, Peyser PA, et al. Kidney stones associate with increased risk for myocardial infarction. J Am Soc Nephrol. 2010;21:1641–4.
25. Fam XI, Singam P, Ho CC, et al. Ureteral stricture formation after ureteroscope treatment of impacted calculi: a prospective study. Korean J Urol. 2015;56(1):63–7.
26. Snoj Z, Savic N, Regvat J. Late complication of a renal calculus: fistulisation to the psoas muscle, colon, spleen, peritoneal cavity, skin and bronchi. Int Braz J Urol. 2015;41(4):808–12.
27. Dubey IB, Singh AK, Prasad D, Jain BK. Nephrobronchial fistula complicating neglected nephrolithiasis and Xanthogranulomatous pyelonephritis. Saudi J Kidney Dis Transpl. 2011;22(3):549–51.
28. Calvo Quintero JE, Alcover García J, Gutiérrez del Pozo R, et al. Fistulization in xanthogranulomatous pyelonephritis. Presentation

of 6 clinical cases and review of the literature. Actas Urol Esp. 1989;13(5):363–7.

29. Vaidyanathan S, Hughes PL, Soni BM, et al. Unpredicted spontaneous extrusion of a renal calculus in an adult male with spina bifida and paraplegia: report of a misdiagnosis. Measures to be taken to reduce urological errors in spinal cord injury patients. BMC Urol. 2001;1:3. Epub 2001 Dec 20.

30. Kaur N, Attam A, Gupta A, Amratash. Spontaneous bladder rupture caused by a giant vesical calculus. Int Urol Nephrol. 2006;38(3–4):487–9.

31. Kobori Y, Shigehara K, Amano T, Takemae K. Vesicocutaneous fistula caused by giant bladder calculus. Urol Res. 2007;35(3):161–3.

32. Chen GH, Hsiao PJ, Chang YH, et al. Spontaneous ureteral rupture and review of the literature. Am J Emerg Med. 2014;32(7):772–4.

33. Ait Benkaddour Y, Aboulfalah A, Abbassi H. Bladder stone: uncommon cause of mechanical dystocia. Arch Gynecol Obstet. 2006;274(5):323–4. Epub 2006 Apr 29.

34. Joshi P, Sarda D, Ahmad A, et al. Double dumb-bell calculus in childhood. Afr J Paediatr Surg. 2009;6(2):122–3.

35. Sun LM, Lin CL, Chang YJ, Liang JA, Liu SH, Sung FC, et al. Urinary tract stone raises subsequent risk for urinary tract cancer: a population-based cohort study. BJU Int. 2013;112:1150–5.

36. Ramdass MJ, Naraynsingh V. Multiple urethral stones causing penile gangrene. Case Rep Urol. 2014;2014:182094. doi:10.1155/2014/182094. Epub 2014 May 18.

Chapter 9
Investigations of Urinary Lithiasis

"Supposing is good, but finding out is better."

Mark Twain (1835–1910)

This chapter will review the diagnostic methods that are required to demonstrate the existence of a urinary stone, followed by the investigations needed to detect the eventual cause(s) of stone formation. Finally a brief account will be given on the studies performed to evaluate the aftermath of the urinary stone disease.

9.1   Diagnosis of a Urinary Stone

This is mainly based on the following imaging methods:

9.1.1   Kidney-Ureter-Bladder (KUB) Plain X-ray

X-rays were accidentally discovered by the German Professor Wilhem Conrad Röntgen in his Würzburg (Germany) laboratory in 1895 while working with a cathode-ray tube. He named these rays "X" as he didn't know their exact nature. He observed their ability to cross fleshy or soft anatomical tissues but not dense structures such as bones. Röntgen was granted the first Nobel Prize of Physics in 1901 for this discovery.

© Springer International Publishing AG 2017   131
S.A. Al-Mamari, *Urolithiasis in Clinical Practice*,
In Clinical Practice, DOI 10.1007/978-3-319-62437-2_9

Nowadays the medical use of X-rays has become widespread and can be rapidly performed in every center. However it has a limited sensitivity for urolithiasis; it will not detect any radiolucent stones (20–40%), most borderline radio-opaque stones, and even some radio-opaque stones in the presence of suboptimal bowel preparation. Calcium stones, i.e. calcium oxalate dehydrate and monohydrate as well as calcium phosphate stones, are notably known to be radiopaque. Brushite stones are among the densest stones (Fig. 9.1) [1], while uric acid stones are

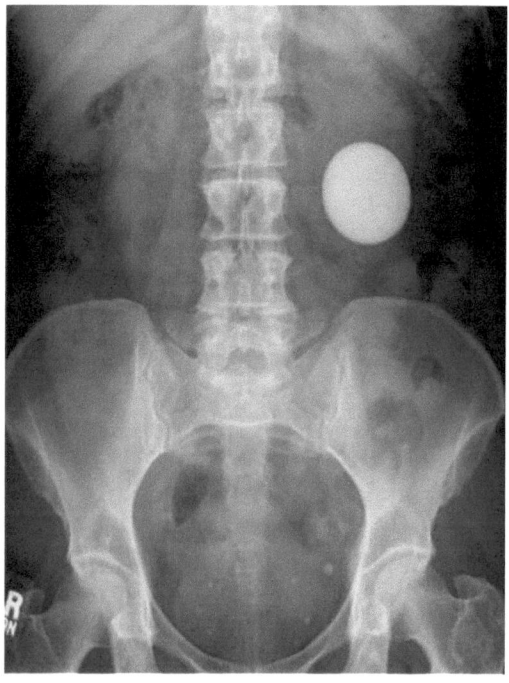

FIGURE 9.1 Large left renal roundish brushite stone. Its radiodensity is well superior to that of the bones. From Krambeck AE et al. [1] with permission from Elsevier

well-known radiolucent entities. Other known radiolucent stones include ammonium urate, xanthine, 2,8-dihydroxyadenine and drug-stones. Magnesium-Ammonium-Phosphate (MAP), apatite and cystine stones have a borderline radiopacity [2].

KUB X-ray is concordant with the gold standard Unenhanced CT-scan in only 50% of patients. It has a very low sensitivity of 18.6%, but an excellent specificity of 95.1%, a good positive predictive value of 84.6%, but a poor negative predictive value of 44.8% [3].

Some predictive factors for stone radiopacity have been proposed using computed tomography parameters. The first factor is **the visibility of the stone in the scout film** which predicts radiopacity of the stone on a KUB X-ray in nearly 100%. For the scout-negative stones, the cut-off of Hounsfield Units (HU) value used to predict radiopacity varies **from > 630 HU to > 772 HU** according to published series. Other predictive factors are a **stone size > 9.7 mm**, a **non-midureteral stone location**, and an **anterior abdominal wall fat thickness ≤ 23.9 mm** [4, 5].

Plain radiograph is also useful as an initial investigation for severe LUTS with fever and haematuria to exclude a stone in the bladder or the prostatic urethra. An impacted stone in the prostatic urethra may appear as a double dumbbell structure especially in children [6]. Cases of giant dumbbell vesicoprostatic calculi have also been diagnosed in the adult population in post-retropubic prostatectomy patients [7] as well as in association with a stricture of the bulbomembranous part of the urethra (Fig. 9.2a, b) [8].

X-ray digital tomosynthesis (DTS) is a refined technology aiming at increasing the sensitivity and accuracy of the standard X-ray imaging. The basic components of D TS are similar to those of a simple digital radiography, but it provides some of the benefits of computed tomography (CT) [7]. It has widely been studied for lung pathology [9, 10]; its application to urolithiasis diagnosis is still limited but has shown encouraging results [11, 12].

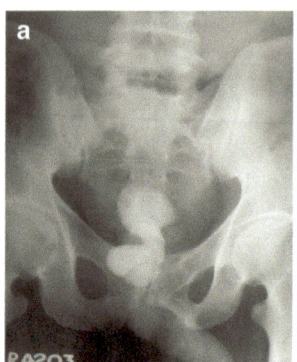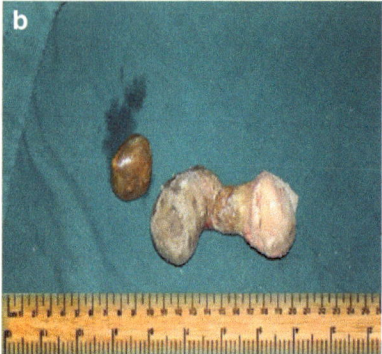

Figure 9.2 (**a**) Erect X-ray KUB of a 38-year-old male patient showing a giant dumb-bell vesico-urethral calculus and a smaller urethral stone distally. These were secondary to a stricture of the bulbo-membranous part of the urethra. From Prabhuswamy VK et al. [8]. Creative Commons Attribution License. (**b**). Picture of the large dumb-bell vesico-urethral calculus and the smaller urethral stone after their removal via transvesical approach. From Prabhuswamy VK et al. [8] Creative Commons Attribution License

9.1.2   Intra-venous Urography or Pyelography (IVU or IVP)

"Intravenous urography is dead. Long live the computerized tomography!", so loudly exclaimed some investigators in 2010 [13]. Since this announcement other authors have prepared the IVU coffin [14]. However IVU is still not yet buried; it has been suggested here and there to be a quicker means than CT-scan in the emergency department [15], to be superior to X-ray KUB in the diagnosis of ureteral indinavir stone [16], or to be more accurate in the diagnosis of retrocaval ureter [17]. Moreover IV-contrast medium injection (not formal departmental IVU) is still used nowadays, though exceptionally, for localization of a radiolucent ureteric stone being treated by Extracorporeal Shock-Waves Lithotripsy (ESWL), when ureteroscopy is not possible or contra-indicated [18]. Nonetheless there are fewer and fewer nostalgic advocates to stand for IVU today in the era of helical CT-scan.

9.1.3   Ultrasonography (U/S) KUB

"Ultra" is a Latin prefix that means "beyond", "greater", or "higher". Ultrasound refers to sound waves whose frequency is **higher** than what can be heard by the human ear. The frequency of audible sounds for humans ranges between 20 and 20,000 Hertz or 20 kiloHertz (kHz). Therefore ultrasounds will be defined as those having a frequency higher that 20 kHz.

The existence of Ultrasounds was demonstrated for the first time by the Italian Physiologist Lazzaro Spallanzani who discovered in 1794 that bats use inaudible sounds for hunting and navigating, introducing the principle of echolocation. Then the Swiss Physicist Jean-Daniel Colladon used an underwater church-bell as an ultrasound transducer in 1841 and discovered that sound travels faster through water than air (indeed, the speed of sound in water is 4.3 times faster than in air, being 1,484 and 343 meters per second respectively). [1]The French brothers Pierre and Jacques Curie discovered the piezoelectricity in 1880. The Physicists Paul Langevin (France), Constantin Chilowsky (Switzerland), and Robert William Boyle (Canadian/British) are credited for the first application of ultrasounds as they succeeded to generate and detect ultrasounds using piezoelectricity in 1916–1917. This launched the use of sonars (acronym for **SO**und **N**avigation **A**nd **R**anging) by submarines during World War I. However it took nearly three more decades until the first application of ultrasound in Medicine was performed for the diagnosis of brain tumors by the Austrian Neuro-Psychiatrist Karl Theodore Dussik in 1942.

Nowadays Ultrasonography is a readily available tool used for medical imaging in almost all emergency departments. It has the capability of detecting a variety of abdominal pathologies, and is very accurate in diagnosing renal and urinary bladder

---

[1]The principle of Piezoelectricity (from the Greek verb "piezein": to press or to squeeze) can be summarized by the production of electricity by pressure application.Indeed when submitted to high pressure, various solid materials such as quartz, ceramics, crystals, etc. accumulate a potential energy that is instantly delivered as an alternating electric current. The simplest example of piezoelectricity nowadays is a gas lighter. "Reverse or inverse piezoelectricity" is the faculty of the same solid materials to become mechanically stressed, i.e. deformed in shape when submitted to electricity.

stones. It is the recommended modality for detecting urinary stones in pregnancy where radiating methods are contra-indicated. Also, to avoid the cumulative deleterious effects of repeated radiation exposure in children during their lives, many guidelines recommend Ultrasonography as the primary imaging technique in children suspected with urolithiasis [2, 19, 20].

However, in addition to its operator-dependency, the limitation of ultrasonography is the low sensitivity for ureteric stones which are often not detectable, but will be suspected because of the symptoms and presence of ipsilateral signs of obstruction when hydro-ureteronephrosis is present. A novel technique, namely the native tissue harmonic imaging ultrasonography has been proposed which aims at improving contrast and spatial resolution although its use is very scarce. When coupled with a KUB X-ray to define ureteral stones, the sensitivity, specificity, and accuracy have been shown to improve to 96%, 91%, and 95% respectively, when compared to plain CT [21]. Another drawback of ultrasonography is its tendency to overestimate the stone size. The stone shadow width was shown to give a more accurate stone size than the direct measurement of the stone itself, and once again harmonic imaging seems to perform better than the other Ultrasound modalities, namely the conventional ray line and the spatial compound, with a one-mm accuracy comparable to CT-scan [22].

9.1.4   Plain Computed-Tomography (CT) Scan KUB

Both the British Engineer Godfrey Hounsfield and the South-African-American Physicist Allan MacLeod Cormack have been recognized as the inventors of the Computed-Tomography (CT) scan in 1972, and shared the Nobel Prize in Physiology/Medicine in 1979.

Etymologically the word tomography derives from the Greek roots "tomos" which means "section" or "slice", and "graphia" which means "image", "writing", "drawing" or "describing". In Medicine, tomography is a **cross-sectional image** of the human body generally using X rays, but the term also applies to ultrasonography, positron emission, or magnetic resonance imaging.

Non-Contrast-enhanced CT-scan (NCCT), also referred to as Unenhanced Helical CT-scan (UHCT), is the standard means to diagnose urolithiasis and is used to assess the accuracy of all other diagnostic methods. It is the imaging modality of choice for the diagnosis of urinary stones, due to its high sensitivity (up to 97%), specificity (≥96%), and accuracy (97%). Furthermore it can detect extra-urinary causes of acute flank pain, and has also the advantage of a faster speed of acquisition [23, 24].

However CT-scan is not always available. Moreover it has a high workload and requires sometimes time-consuming and complex arrangement with the Radiographer and the Radiologist for its performance, especially during night duties and week-ends. In addition, its major drawback is the use of a significant X-ray load; it is contraindicated in pregnant ladies and may be particularly dangerous for children.

The use of low-dose NCCT is an attempt to attenuate the hazardous effects of this imaging means. A low-dose NCCT delivers a radiation exposure of only two-fold greater than that produced by a KUB radiography [2] (Table 9.1). Nonetheless caution is still required when using NCCT to diagnose urolithiasis as radiation exposure may lead to malignancy in 0.5/1000 cases [25], among other deleterious effects. Therefore the old hippocratic golden principle of "Primum non nocere" (first, do no harm) as well as the radiological principle of ALARA (as low as reasonably achievable) should always be borne in mind when prescribing or

TABLE 9.1 Radiation exposure of imaging modalities

Method	Radiation exposure (mSv)
KUB radiography	0.5–1
IVU	1.3–3.5
Regular-dose NCCT	4.5–5
Low-dose NCCT	0.97–1.9
Enhanced CT	25–35

mSv milliSievert. From Türk C [2]. With Permission from Elsevier

TABLE 9.2 Stone density values measured on CT in Hounsfield units (HU)

| | Hounsfield units (HU) | | | |
	Mean ±SD	Minimum	Maximum	Number (%) of stones
CaOxMH	1499 ± 269	840	1940	40 (47)
CaOxDH	1505 ± 221	1050	1800	12 (14)
CaP	1106 ± 220	790	1440	11 (13)
UA	348 ± 67	270	450	9 (10)
Cystine	563 ± 115	320	720	14 (16)

SD Standard deviation, *CT* computed tomography, *CaOxMH* calcium oxalate monohydrate, *CaOxDH* calcium oxalate dihydrate, *CaP* calcium phosphate, *UA* uric acid. From Bulakçı M et al. [28]. With permission from the Turkish Association of Urology

performing this investigation. This warning is not superfluous: NCCT was still the first imaging modality in children with urolithiasis, being performed in 63% of cases in the USA up to the year 2011 despite the recommendations of several guidelines for the use of ultrasounds as the primary imaging technique in the pediatric population! [26, 27].

When interpreting stone characteristics on a CT-scan, the density definition in Hounsfield Units (HU) is important to predict its composition. Table 9.2 shows approximate density values of some common stones [28]. It should be remembered that the densities of air, water, and bone are −1000, 0, and +1000 HU respectively.

Additional information on the composition of the stone may be obtained by a color Doppler Ultrasound study where cystine stones were shown to produce a twinkling artefact contrary to uric acid. Therefore, cystine composition, as opposed to UA composition, should be suspected when the measured density value of the stone is below 780 HU on CT and there is a grade 3 twinkling artefact intensity observed on Doppler U/S [28].

A further advantage of CT-Scan is the accurate evaluation of the stone burden which has a direct bearing in the selection and success of treatment.

The three main methods used to estimate the stone burden are: the cumulative stone diameter, the Ackermann's formula, and the sphere formula. A French study has shown that all the three methods provide good size estimation for stones smaller than 20 mm, but suggested that calculation of volume, i.e. the sphere formula should be preferred for stones greater than 20 mm [29]. However the EAU guidelines favor the Ackermann's formula (an ellipsoidal algebral formula) [2, 30].

An additional advantage of NCCT is its superiority in detecting residual stones after PCNL regardless of the stone size, compared to KUB X-ray and US [31].

Dual-energy computed tomography (DECT) is an advanced technology with the potential to differentiate uric acid from non-uric acid stones with almost 100% accuracy for stones greater than 3 mm in size, and is also very useful in identifying cystine stones [32, 33].

9.2 Investigations of the Cause

After an anamnesis directed towards the predisposing factors (acquired or inherited) and a physical examination, the etiological investigations should be focused on metabolic disturbances and anatomical abnormalities. A few decades ago, it was accepted that extensive metabolic evaluation is unnecessary in patients presenting with a first renal stone episode, because the subsequent use of specific drug therapy in those patients carried specific risks while providing only modest beneficial effects compared to placebo [34].

Nowadays this dogma has been revisited and currently accepted guidelines recommend metabolic testing in recurrent stone formers, but also in high-risk or interested first-time stone formers [19]. Also stone analysis should be performed in all first-time stone formers and repeated in patients with recurrent lithiasis [2].

However the controversy is not yet over since a recent publication proposed to differentiate between uncomplicated and complicated urinary stone patients with the former group accounting for about 75% [35] (Tables 9.3 and 9.4). The

TABLE 9.3 Classification of urinary stone patients as uncomplicated on the basis of their medical history

Findings	Action
First episode Age: adult	Cave: History of "frequent kidney pain" in childhood, but unclear origin
No anatomic abnormalities	Exclusion of for example, horseshoe kidney and outlet stenosis
Probable correlation with lifestyle	For instance, stone formation at or soon after a time of unusual stress and specific compensation reactions
Negative family history of urolithiasis	Cave: Hints of possibly undiscovered stones in family members through statements such as "There was something, but I can't quite remember…"
Single stone	Assessment with suitable imaging procedures

From Fisang et al. [35], with permission from the Authors and Deutsches Ärzteblatt

TABLE 9.4 Classification of urinary stones as high risk

Finding	Action
Age; child or adolescent	Consider assessing siblings for risk of lithogenesis
Brushite, uric acid/urate, infectious stones	Bear other accompanying minerals in mind in diagnosis and treatment
Chronic psychovegetative stress	Establish severity, perhaps with aid of validated stress-assessment systems
Single kidney	
Malformation of the urinary tract	
Disorders of gastrointestinal function	E.g., Crohn disease, ulcerative colitis, sprue, chronic pancreatitis, liver cirrhosis, small bowel resection

TABLE 9.4 (continued)

Finding	Action
High recurrence rate	More than three stones in 3 years. Changes in stone type (principal and subsidiary mineral phase) or composition may indicate alterations in metabolic conditions
Hyperparathyroidism (HPT)	Five forms of HPT, primary to quinary
Nephrocalcinosis	Numerous causes, e.g., following renal tubular acidosis, primary hyperoxaluria, sarcoidosis, HPT, chronic glomerulitis
Positive family history	Consider assessing patient's children for risk of lithogenesis
Primary hyperoxaluria	Two types, autosomal-recessive hereditary disease
Renal tubular acidosis	Test by means of urinary pH curve, blood gas analysis, and ammonium chloride load test
Residual stone fragments	Possibly consider endoscopic means of stone removal, particularly when the concrement is of a type that resists disintegration by ESWL, e.g., brushite, cystine, whewellite
Cystine, 2,8-dihydroxyadenine, xanthine stones	Stone formation genetically determined; lifelong metaphylaxis is mandatory

ESWL extracorporeal shockwave lithotripsy
From Fisang et al. [35], with permission from the Authors and Deutsches Ärzteblatt International

authors propose avoiding extensive metabolic studies for the uncomplicated group but still recommend carrying out general investigations based on the type of stone, including a comprehensive anamnesis of the potential risk factors [36].

9.2.1   Metabolic Abnormalities

The metabolic investigations comprise of a random urine analysis and microscopy, an analysis of the first-voided morning urine, and a 24-h urine examination performed without any specific diet and aiming at defining the following values: pH, total volume, calcium, oxalate, sodium, potassium, creatinine, citrate, etc.

The normal values of 24-h urine examination are presented in the Table 9.5 [36].

It is worth noting that the urinary pH follows a circadian rhythm, being acidic in the morning and tending to be more alkaline in the course of the day, especially after meals. An alkaline pH (>7) is generally associated with CaP and infectious stones while an acidic one (<5.4) favours uric acid, cystine and CaOx stones.

A nomogram using 24-h urine parameters, including urinary sodium, calcium, oxalate and uric acid, in combination with patient's age and BMI (Body Mass Index) was shown to be a significant predictor of stone composition, especially in differentiating uric acid from calcium oxalate stones [37].

In 1975 Pak et al. have proposed a "simple" test to differentiate between the absorptive, the resorptive, and the renal form of hypercalciuria [38]:

A collection of a two-hour urine sample is performed after overnight fast and a four-hour urine sample after a 1-g calcium load per mouth. Then the patients are tested for calcium, cyclic AMP and creatinine.

- In absorptive hypercalciuria, there is normocalcemia, normal fasting urinary calcium (less than 0.11 mg per milligram

TABLE 9.5 Twenty-four-hour urinary constituents and their ratios in normal individuals and stone formers

Parameters	Normal individuals (n = 25)	Stone patients (n = 100)
Volume (mL/24 h)	1650 ± 546	2852 ± 1435
Oxalate (mmol/24 h)	0.39 ± 0.12[a]	0.63 ± 0.35[a]
Calcium (mmol/24 h)	4.75 ± 2.84[b]	7.30 ± 3.99[b]
Magnesium (mmol/24 h)	3.84 ± 0.38	3.65 ± 1.22
Citrate (mmol/24 h)	1.59 ± 0.75	1.46 ± 0.94
Uric acid (mmol/24 h)	1.74 ± 0.93[b]	2.49 ± 1.29[b]
Phosphate (mmol/24 h)	28.33 ± 18.15[b]	21.94 ± 10.67[b]
Creatinine (mmol/24 h)	9.72 ± 2.22	10.54 ± 2.84
Oxalate/Creatinine (mmol/24 h)	0.04 ± 0.02[b]	0.07 ± 0.04[b]
Calcium/Creatinine (mmol/24 h)	0.48 ± 0.26[b]	0.73 ± 0.43[b]
Magnesium/Creatinine (mmol/24 h)	0.40 ± 0.09	0.38 ± 0.19
Citrate/Creatinine (mmol/24 h)	0.18 ± 0.12	0.15 ± 0.12
Uric acid/Creatinine (mmol/24 h)	0.18 ± 0.10	0.26 ± 0.20
Phosphorus/Creatinine (mmol/24 h)	3.00 ± 1.75[b]	2.27 ± 1.30[b]
Magnesium/Calcium (mmol/24 h)	1.16 ± 0.73[c]	0.63 ± 0.37[c]
Citrate/Calcium (mmol/24 h)	0.52 ± 0.41[a]	0.28 ± 0.30[a]

Statistical analysis performed by Student's t test
The data are expressed as Mean ± S.D.
[a]$p < 0.01$
[b]$p < 0.05$
[c]$p < 0.001$
From Kumar R et al. [36], with permission from Springer

of urinary creatinine), and high urinary calcium (≥0.2 mg per milligram of creatinine) after the calcium load.

- In primary hyperparathyroidism (resorptive hypercalciuria), there is hypercalcemia, high fasting urinary calcium, and high urinary cyclic AMP (>4.60 μmoles per gram of creatinine) after calcium load.

- In renal hypercalciuria, there is normocalcemia, high fasting urinary calcium, and high or higher-normal urinary cyclic AMP (>6.86 μmoles per gram of creatinine), normal fasting urinary cyclic AMP.

Urinary cyclic AMP evaluation was formerly an invaluable method to reach to the diagnosis of parathyroidism [39, 40]. It is however seldom assayed nowadays and has been replaced by the measurement of the intact parathormone (PTH) in order to determine primary hyperparathyroidism in the presence of hypercalcemia as per the following protocol [41]: Low-calcium diet 3 days before the calcium load test (CLT) → CLT of 1 gm Ca/50 kg → measurement of intact parathormone and ionized calcium at 0, 1, 2, and 3 h after CLT. PTH is suppressed in patients with normal parathyroid function at 3-h, while those with hyperparathyroidism have a rebound of PTH after a transient decline at 2-h.

9.2.2 Crystalluria

The determination of stone composition has already been discussed earlier. This study implies providing the biochemistry Physician or the laboratory technician with a stone sample after its spontaneous passage or surgical retrieval. Nowadays this procurement is hindered by technological advances that allow endourological treatment with complete intra-corporeal stone disintegration. The same drawback is observed when vaporizing a prostatic adenoma with Laser as no specimen will be available for histopathology.

Nonetheless, microscopic crystals can sometimes be identified in a urine specimen, and this provides possible suggestions as to the stone composition and contributes to the etiological diagnosis [42, 43].

The term "Crystal" is derived from the ancient Greek word "κρύσταλλος" (pronounced "krústallos") which means "clear ice". In the context of urinary stones, it refers to the solid phase of the stone, i.e. the hard component, as opposed to the organic phase or matrix.

Crystalluria is best studied on the whole volume of the first voided urine in the morning because of a good concentration of urine, and determination of the urine pH is essential for their interpretation [42, 43]. When present, a comprehensive examination of crystals should be undertaken for their identification, quantification and size, using a microscope equipped with polarized light or even utilizing infrared spectroscopy for unusual crystals [42, 43]. The main crystals identifiable in urine include calcium oxalate, calcium phosphate, uric acid and urate,[2] struvite, and aminoacids (cystine). Rarer ones are purines (2,8-dihydroxyadenine and xanthine) and drugs-associated [42, 43] (Figs. 9.3, 9.4, 9.5, 9.6, and 9.7).

Furthermore a study has shown the usefulness of follow-up serial crystalluria analyses in determining the future risk of stone recurrence in patients presenting with urolithiasis for the first time. After a prospective evaluation of 205 calcium stone formers for a median duration of 7 years, Michel Daudon et al. found that the presence of crystals in 50% or more of urine samples was associated with stone recurrence in 87% of cases, whereas only 9% of patients with less frequent crystalluria developed stone recurrence [43] (Fig. 9.8).

---

[2]Urate is defined as a salt of uric acid, i.e. a combination of uric acid with another element, usually the sodium, but also calcium and ammonium.

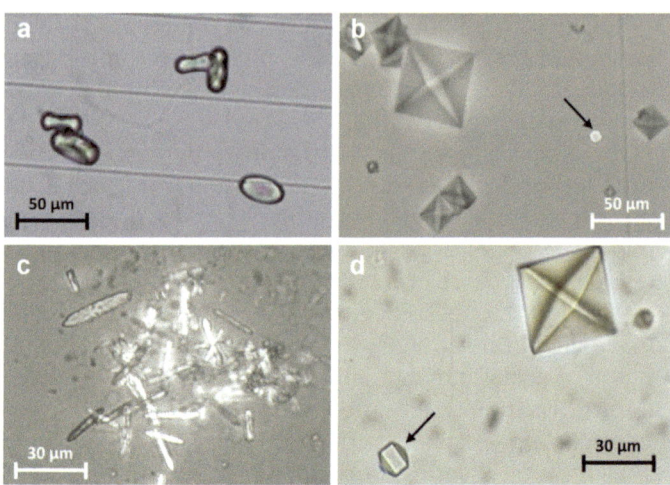

FIGURE 9.3 Calcium oxalate crystals. (**a**) Whewellite crystals with the typical ovoid shape. (**b**) Typical octahedral (bipyramidal) crystals of weddellite and a small red-cell like crystal of whewellite (*arrow*). (**c**) Elongated hexagonal crystals of whewellite as found in the urine of patients after the ingestion of ethylene-glycol. (**d**) Octahedral and dodecahedral (*arrow*) crystals of weddellite. From Daudon M and Frochot V [42], with permission from De Gruyter and the Authors

9.2.3   Anatomical or Structural Abnormalities

Imaging studies are needed to detect any abnormality that may be the direct cause of the stone formation or a contributor to the lithogenesis.

Although U/S is generally used to initiate the diagnosis, CECT is the investigation of choice for a final and accurate definition of abnormalities of the upper urinary tract, including narrow calyx, calyceal diverticulum and PUJ obstruction. When further definition of the upper urinary tract is needed, a retrograde pyelogram (RGP) may be indicated, but this invasive modality is seldom performed alone nowadays.

For bladder stones, uroflowmetry and ultrasonographic determination of the post-voiding residual volume of the bladder are mandatory. Large solitary spiky (Jackstone) or

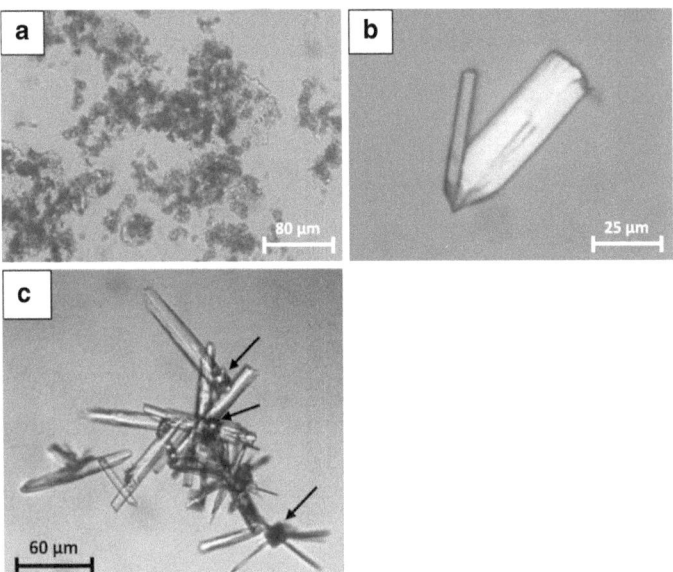

FIGURE 9.4 Calcium phosphate crystals. (**a**) Amorphous granulations of carbonated calcium phosphate. (**b**) Asymmetrical rod-shaped crystals of calcium hydrogen phosphate dihydrate (brushite). (**c**) Crystal aggregate of brushite intermingled with weddellite (*arrows*). From Daudon M and Frochot V [42], with permission from De Gruyter and the Authors

multiple roundish stones are commonly seen in the bladder secondary to bladder outlet obstruction.

When there is history and/or physical signs suggesting neurological causes for the bladder voiding dysfunction, urodynamic studies are indicated.

Note: Bladder stones are generally classified into two categories: Primary and secondary.

– Primary bladder stones may be totally formed de novo inside the bladder or their nuclei may have been formed in the kidneys before they migrate and further grow-up inside the bladder. In both cases they are considered primary because of the absence of local causes such as

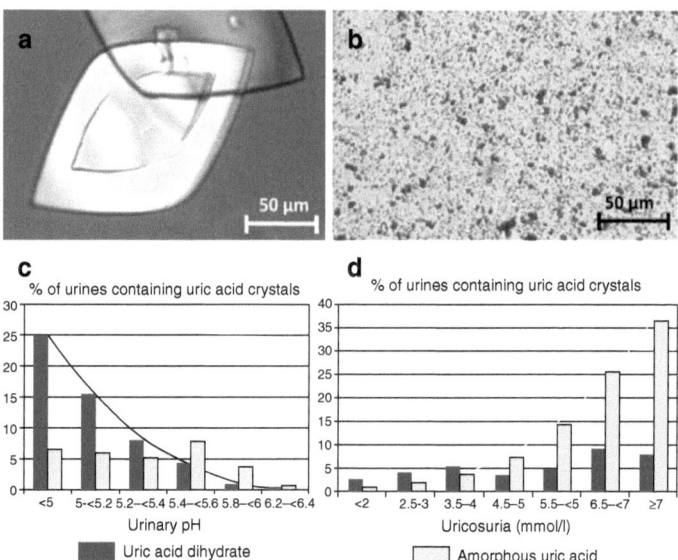

FIGURE 9.5 Uric acid crystals. (**a**) Typical lozenges of uric acid dihydrate crystals. (**b**) Amorphous uric acid granulations. (**c**) Correlation
between uric acid dihydrate crystals and urinary pH. (**d**) Correlation
between amorphous uric acid granulations and uricosuria. From
Daudon M and Frochot V [42], with permission from De Gruyter
and the Authors

obstruction, infection, foreign bodies or neurogenic bladder. These stones are endemic and generally affecting the
pediatric population. They are found in developing African
and Asian countries in association with malnutrition, diarrheal disease, chronic dehydration, and are mostly made of
ammonium acid urate which can be mixed with CaOx and
CaP [44, 45]. This disease in mostly found in children
below 10 years with a peak at 2–4 years and boys are more
commonly affected than girls with a male/female ratio of
12–13:1 [46, 47].
– Secondary vesical calculi are caused by bladder outlet
obstruction or any other local cause including diverticulum,
neurogenic bladder, foreign body, catheterization or trauma.

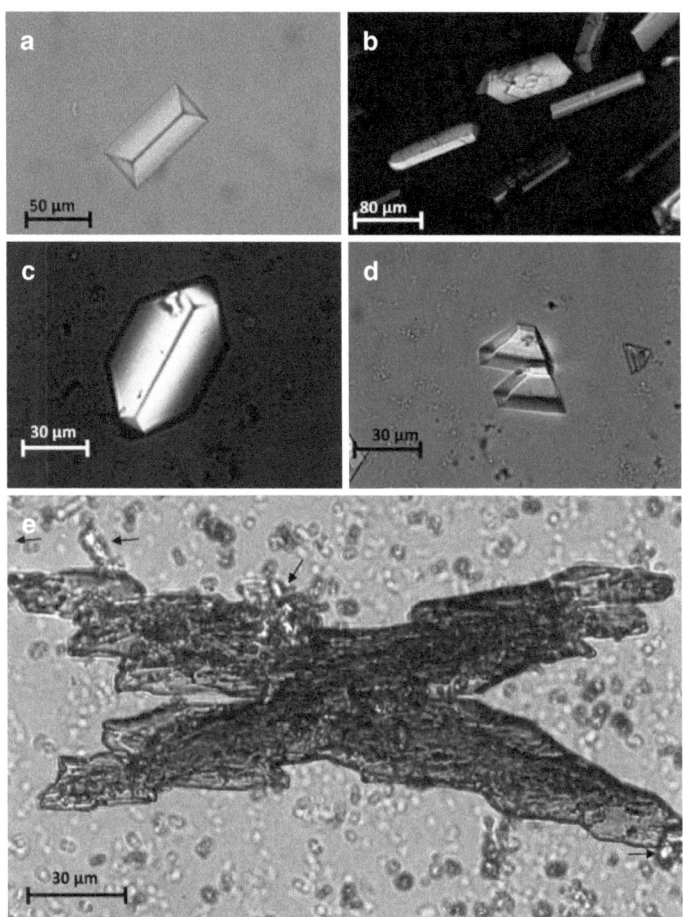

FIGURE 9.6 Struvite crystals as seen under polarized light. (**a**) Coffin-shaped crystal of struvite. (**b**) Rod-shaped and coffin-shaped crystals of struvite. (**c**) A hexagonal crystal of struvite and small agglomerates of amorphous carbonated calcium phosphate grains. (**d**) Trapezoidal crystals of struvite. (**e**) A large X-shaped crystal of struvite with birefringent small aggregates of ammonium hydrogen urate crystals (*black arrows*). From Daudon M and Frochot V [42], with permission from De Gruyter and the Authors

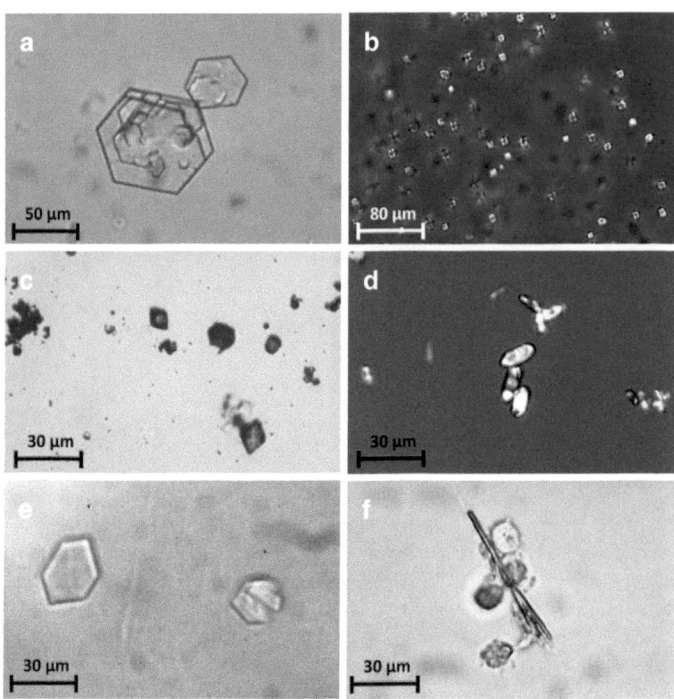

FIGURE   9.7 Uncommon   crystals.   (**a**)   Cystine   crystals.   (**b**) 2,8-dihydroxyadenine crystals as seen by polarized light. (**c**) Diamond-shaped crystal of N-acetylsulfamethoxazole hydrochloride very similar to uric acid dihydrate crystals. (**d**) Oval-shaped crystal of N-acetylsulfamethoxazole hydrochloride very similar to whewellite. (**e**) Hexagonal crystals of N-acetylsulfamethoxazole hydrochloride that may easily be misidentified as cystine crystals. (**f**) Needle-shaped crystals of atazanavir surrounded by leukocytes. From Daudon M and Frochot V [42], with permission from De Gruyter and the Authors

9.3   Investigations of the Aftermath of Urolithiasis

Once the diagnosis of urolithiasis has been ascertained and its cause eventually elucidated as accurately as possible, the Urologist's next aim is to evaluate the local and systemic consequences of the stone disease, either as a single episode or a

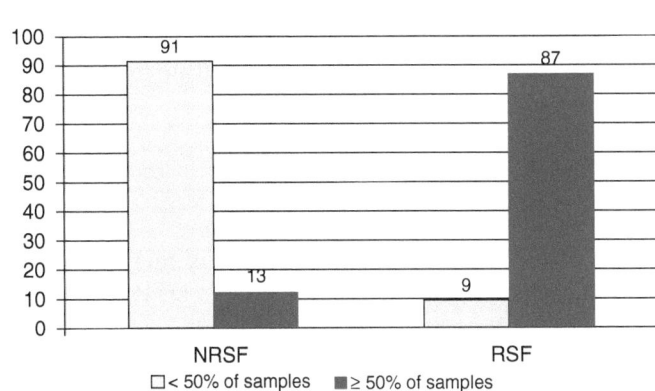

FIGURE 9.8 Percentage of patients with crystalluria. Relation between the occurrence of crystalluria in serial urine samples and the risk of stone recurrence in stone formers. *NRSF* nonrecurrent stone formers, *RSF* recurrent stone formers over a period of 7 years of follow-up. From Daudon M et al. [43], with permission from Elsevier Masson SAS

recurrent phenomenon. The detrimental effects arising from the presence of a stone in the urinary system can be detected by serum renal function tests or by functional and anatomical imaging tests. However it is important to note that functional imaging studies should be reserved only for selected patients in whom there is a strong suspicion of kidney scarring or ureteral stenosis with compromised renal function [48]. The importance of these studies is first medico-legal as they allow one to define the baseline function of the affected kidney before performing any procedure; secondly there is an obvious practical interest as a non-functioning kidney would necessitate a nephrectomy rather than a treatment limited to the stone.

9.3.1 Laboratory

Blood urea and creatinine, and evaluation of the estimated glomerular filtration rate (eGFR): Recurrent kidney stone formers have been shown to have a chronic kidney disease prevalence of 9.3% compared to 1.3 % for a control group [49].

Urine culture is also important to evaluate chronic UTI which correlates with persistent stones.

9.3.2   Isotope Renogram Tests

99mTc-MAG3 (mercaptoacetyltriglycine or mertiatide), 99mTc-DMSA (dimercaptosuccinic acid), 99mTc-DTPA (diethylene-triaminepentacetic acid), 131-iodine labelled OIH (Ortho-iodohippurate), 99mTc-Glucoheptonate, EC (ethylcys-teine) etc.

Radiopharmaceuticals aiming to assess renal function and anatomy are traditionally categorized into three groups [50]:

- Those excreted by glomerular filtration: 99m Tc-DTPA
- Those excreted by tubular secretion: 131I-OIH, 99mTc-MAG3.
- Those retained in the renal tubules for long periods: 99mTc-DMSA.

  – **99mTc-MAG3 is presently the preferred radio-tracer because it is predominantly secreted through renal tubules with only a small amount being filtered through glomeruli due to its considerable protein binding** [51]. Its extraction fraction (the percentage of the agent extracted with each passage through the kidney) is 40–50%. **It provides excellent images of the kidney including scars, and gives also good ureteric visualization in many cases allowing one to diagnose obstruction.** Usual dose: 70–120 MBq (2–3 mCi) [50, 51].
  – 123I-Hippuran (131I-OIH) was the reference standard in the 80s, but the high cost has precluded its distribution nowadays. It is excreted primarily by the renal tubules. Usual dose: 20 MBq (≈0.5 mCi) [51].
  – **99mTc-DTPA has the advantages of cheapness and ease of production. It is cleared by the glomerulus and can therefore be reliably used for GFR measurement.**

However it is a slow agent with a very low extraction fraction of only 20%, making it unsuitable in patients with impaired renal function. The curve forms and diuretic responses of ^{99m}Tc-DTPA are also more difficult to interpret than those of MAG3 and ^{123}I-hippuran. Usual dose: 70–120 MBq (2–3 mCi) [50, 51].

- **^{99m}TC-DMSA is an excellent cortical imaging agent due to its long retention in the renal tubules**. About 40% of the injected dose binds to the renal cortex. It provides therefore high-quality anatomic images which are needed to diagnose pyelonephritis. It is unsuitable for the study of obstruction [50].

9.3.3   Retrograde Pyelography

Helps to define a ureteric stenosis and other anatomical abnormalities in the urinary tract, but should be performed only if there is clinical suspicion and possibility of a concomitant endourological intervention for final treatment or alleviation of the symptoms.

References

1. Krambeck AE, Handa SE, Evan AP, Lingeman JE. Profile of the brushite stone former. J Urol. 2010;184(4):1367–71.
2. Türk C, Petřík A, Sarica K, et al. EAU guidelines on diagnosis and conservative management of urolithiasis. Eur Urol. 2016;69(3):468–74.
3. Chan VO, Buckley O, Persaud T, Torreggiani WC. Urolithiasis: how accurate are plain radiographs? Can Assoc Radiol J. 2008;59(3):131–4.
4. Sfoungaristos S, Gofrit ON, Katz R, et al. A predictive model for stone radiopacity in kidney-ureter-bladder film based on computed tomography parameters. Urology. 2014;84(5):1021–5.
5. Chua ME, Gomez OR, Sapno LD, et al. Use of computed tomography scout film and Hounsfield unit of computed tomography scan in predicting the radio-opacity of urinary calculi

in plain kidney, ureter and bladder radiographs. Urol Ann. 2014;6(3):218–23.

6. Joshi P, Sarda D, Ahmad A, et al. Double dumb-bell calculus in childhood. Afr J Paediatr Surg. 2009;6(2):122–3.

7. Desai KM, Kadow C, Gingell JC. Giant "dumb-bell" vesicopros-tatic calculus. Br J Urol. 1987;59(5):483.

8. Prabhuswamy VK, Tiwari R, Krishnamoorthy R. A giant dumb-bell shaped vesico-prostatic urethral calculus: a case report and review of literature. Case Rep Urol. 2013;2013:167635. doi:10.1155/2013/167635. Epub 2013 May 21.

9. Chou SH, Kicska GA, Pipavath SN, Reddy GP. Digital tomo-synthesis of the chest: current and emerging applications. Radiographics. 2014;34(2):359–72.

10. Gomi T, Nakajima M, Fujiwara H, et al. Comparison between chest digital tomosynthesis and CT as a screening method to detect artificialpulmonary nodules: a phantom study. Br J Radiol. 2012;85(1017):e622–9.

11. Liu S, Guo J, Hu X, et al. Comparative study of X-ray digital DTS imaging and kidney ureter bladder radiography in urinary calculi. Zhonghua Yi Xue Za Zhi. 2015;95(25):2010–3.

12. Tuerdi B, Wang H, Huo Z, et al. Comparative study of X-ray digital tomosynthesis imaging based on intravenous urography and unenhanced multidetector-row computerized tomography in urinary calculi. Zhonghua Yi Xue Za Zhi. 2014;94(15):1157–60.

13. Franco A, Tomás M, Alonso-Burgos A. Intravenous urography is died. Long live the computerized tomography! Actas Urol Esp. 2010;34(9):764–74.

14. Hale Z, Hanna E, Miyake M, Rosser CJ. Imaging the urologic patient: the utility of intravenous pyelogram in the CT scan era. World J Urol. 2014;32(1):137–42.

15. Quirke M, Divilly F, O'Kelly P, et al. Imaging patients with renal colic: a comparative analysis of the impact of non-contrast heli-cal computed tomography versus intravenous pyelography on the speed of patient processing in the Emergency Department. Emerg Med J. 2011;28(3):197–200.

16. Schwartz BF, Schenkman N, Armenakas NA, Stoller ML. Imaging characteristics of indinavir calculi. J Urol. 1999;161(4): 1085–7.

17. Hassan R, Aziz AA, Mohamed SK. Retrocaval ureter: the importance of intravenous urography. Malays J Med Sci. 2011;18(4):84–7.

18. Hiros M, Spahovic H, Selimovic M, Sadovic S. Extracorporeal shock wave lithotripsy and intravenous contrast media application for localization of radiolucent calculi. Med Arh. 2011;65(2):86–8.

19. Kokorowski PJ, Hubert K, Nelson CP. Evaluation of pediatric nephrolithiasis. Indian J Urol. 2010;26(4):531–5.

20. Shah NB, Platt SL. ALARA: is there a cause for alarm? Reducing radiation risks from computed tomography scanning in children. Curr Opin Pediatr. 2008;20(3):243–7.

21. Mitterberger M, Pinggera GM, Pallwein L, et al. Plain abdominal radiography with transabdominal native tissue harmonic imaging ultrasonography vs unenhanced computed tomography in renal colic. BJU Int. 2007;100(4):887–90.

22. Dunmire B, Harper JD, Cunitz BW, et al. Use of the acoustic shadow width to determine kidney stone size with ultrasound. J Urol. 2016;195(1):171–7.

23. Smith RC, Verga M, McCarthy S, Rosenfield AT. Diagnosis of acute flank pain: value of unenhanced helical CT. AJR Am J Roentgenol. 1996;166:97–101.

24. Andrabi Y, Patino M, Das CJ, et al. Advances in CT imaging for urolithiasis. Indian J Urol. 2015;31(3):185–93.

25. Berrington de González A, Mahesh M, Kim KP, et al. Projected cancer risks from computed tomographic scans performed in the United States in 2007. Arch Intern Med. 2009;169(22):2071–7.

26. Tasian GE, Pulido JE, Keren R, et al. Use of and regional variation in initial CT imaging for kidney stones. Pediatrics. 2014;134:909–15.

27. Strohmaier WL. Imaging in pediatric urolithiasis-what's the best choice? Transl Pediatr. 2015;4(1):36–40.

28. Bulakçı M, Tefik T, Akbulut F, et al. The use of non-contrast computed tomography and color Doppler ultrasound in the characterization of urinary stones - preliminary results. Turk J Urol. 2015;41(4):165–70.

29. Merigot de Treigny O, Bou Nasr E, Almont T, et al. The cumulated stone diameter: a limited tool for stone burden estimation. Urology. 2015;86(3):477–81.

30. Ackermann D, Griffith DP, Dunthorn M, Newman RC, Finlayson B. Calculation of stone volume and urinary stone staging with computer assistance. J Endourol. 1989;3:355–9.

31. Gokce MI, Ozden E, Suer E, et al. Comparison of imaging modalities for detection of residual fragments and prediction of stone related events following percutaneous nephrolitotomy. Int Braz J Urol. 2015;41(1):86–90.

32. Primak AN, Fletcher JG, Vrtiska TJ, et al. Noninvasive differentiation of uric acid versus non-uric acid kidney stones using dual-energy CT. Acad Radiol. 2007;14(12):1441–7.
33. Haley WE, Ibrahim e-SH, Qu M, et al. The clinical impact of accurate cystine calculi characterization using dual-energy computed tomography. Case Rep Radiol. 2015;2015:801021.
34. Uribarri J, Oh MS, Carroll HJ. The first kidney stone. Ann Intern Med. 1989;111(12):1006–9.
35. Fisang C, Anding R, Müller SC, et al. Urolithiasis—an interdisciplinary diagnostic, therapeutic and secondary preventive challenge. Dtsch Arztebl Int. 2015;112(6):83–91.
36. Kumar R, Kapoor R, Mittal B, et al. Evaluation of urinary abnormalities in urolithiasis patients: a study from North India. Indian J Clin Biochem. 2003;18(2):209–15.
37. Torricelli FC, De S, Liu X, et al. Can 24-hour urine stone risk profiles predict urinary stone composition? J Endourol. 2014;28(6):735–8.
38. Pak CY, Kaplan R, Bone H, et al. A simple test for the diagnosis of absorptive, resorptive and renal hypercalciurias. N Engl J Med. 1975;292(10):497–500.
39. Broadus AE. Nephrogenous cyclic AMP as a parathyroid function test. Nephron. 1979;23(2–3):136–41.
40. Shaw JW, Oldham SB, Rosoff L, et al. Urinary cyclic AMP analyzed as a function of the serum calcium and parathyroid hormone in the differential diagnosis of hypercalcemia. J Clin Invest. 1977;59(1):14–21.
41. McHenry CR, Rosen IB, Walfish PG, Pollard A. Oral calcium load test: diagnostic and physiologic implications in hyperparathyroidism. Surgery. 1990;108(6):1026–31. Discussion 1032
42. Daudon M, Frochot V. Crystalluria. Clin Chem Lab Med. 2015;53(Suppl 2):s1479–87.
43. Daudon M, Frochot V, Bazin D, Jungers P. Crystalluria analysis improves significantly etiologic diagnosis and therapeutic monitoring of nephrolithiasis. C R Chim. 2016;19(11–12):1514–26.
44. Soliman NA, Rizvi SA. Endemic bladder calculi in children. Pediatr Nephrol. 2016; doi:10.1007/s00467-016-3492-4.
45. Naqvi SAA, Rizvi SAH, Shahjehan S. Analysis of urinary calculi by chemical methods. J Pak Med Assoc. 1984;34:147–53.
46. Thalut K, Rizal A, Brockis JG, et al. The endemic bladder stones of Indonesia—epidemiology and clinical features. Br J Urol. 1976;48(7):617–21.

47. Kamoun A, Daudon M, Abdelmoula J, et al. Urolithiasis in Tunisian children: a study of 120 cases based on stone composition. Pediatr Nephrol. 1999;13(9):920–5. Discussion 926.
48. Assimos D, Krambeck A, Miller NL, et al. Surgical management of stones: American Urological Association/Endourological Society guideline, Part I. J Urol. 2016;196(4):1153–60.
49. Sigurjonsdottir VK, Runolfsdottir HL, Indridason OS, et al. Impact of nephrolithiasis on kidney function. BMC Nephrol. 2015;16:149.
50. Taylor AJ, Nally JV. Clinical applications of renal scintigraphy. Am J Roentgenol. 1995;164:31–41.
51. O'Reilly PH. Consensus Committee of the Society of Radionuclides in Nephrourology. Standardization of the renogram technique for investigating the dilated upper urinary tract and assessing the results of surgery. BJU Int. 2003;91(3):239–43.

Chapter 10
Differential Diagnosis of Urolithiasis

"If you're not confused, you're not paying attention."

Tom Peters (1942–)

The differential diagnosis of urolithiasis includes all the causes of abdominal pain, dysuria, haematuria, and hydroureteronephrosis. They also include all entities susceptible to be mistaken for stones on imaging investigations.

1. Abdominal pain:

    (a) Appendicitis is the most commonly encountered alternative diagnosis competing with urolithiasis in the acute presentation. The pain pattern may help to differentiate the two entities: appendicitis causes a continuous pain in the right iliac fossa at the McBurney's point often with a localized peritonitis (positive rebound sign), whereas urolithiasis causes colicky pain in the corresponding loin and flank, which can radiate to the ipsilateral iliac fossa and external genitalia (hemiscrotum or labium majus). Moreover it is well known in semiology of the acute abdomens that the renal patient is agitated and shouting, while the peritoneal one is prostrated and sick looking.

    (b) Lumbar pain from any etiology is another common differential diagnosis of urolithiasis, either in an acute

© Springer International Publishing AG 2017
S.A. Al-Mamari, *Urolithiasis in Clinical Practice*,
In Clinical Practice, DOI 10.1007/978-3-319-62437-2_10

or chronic presentation. The causes can be osteo-muscular or neurological as seen in lumbar disc prolapse. A very rare case of severe unilateral loin to groin pain due to an acute paravertebral lumbar compartment syndrome has been reported after weightlifting exercises [1].

(c) Other causes of pain that can be confused with urolithiasis are: acute epididymitis, testicular torsion, retroperitoneal fibrosis, acute cholelithiasis, cholecystitis, diverticulitis, pancreatitis, large or hemorrhagic renal cyst, inflammatory bowel disease, papillary necrosis, peptic ulcer, pyonephrosis, cystic fibrosis [2], viral gastro-enteritis, bowel obstruction, Henoch-Schönlein purpura [3], acute renal infarction (e.g. secondary to atrial fibrillation) [4], Fitz-Hugh-Curtis syndrome, and various gynaecological pathologies such as pelvic inflammatory disease, salpingitis, oophoritis, ovarian cyst torsion, ectopic pregnancy, endometriosis. Ureteral endometriosis produces periodic ipsilateral pain, haematuria and hydrouretero nephrosis.

A rare cause of loin pain is the "nutcracker syndrome" also referred to as "left renal vein entrapment". The left renal vein crossing in front of the aorta is compressed anteriorly by the superior mesenteric artery arising from the anterior aspect of the aorta [5]. There is also a so-called "posterior nutcracker" where a retroaortic or circumaortic left renal vein is compressed between the aorta and the vertebral column [6] (Fig. 10.1).

Another extremely rare case of acute loin pain is the obstructive uropathy associated with ureteral herniation. This has been described in elderly patients and the most commonly encountered hernial site is the inguinal canal. However few cases of ureteral herniation through femoral canal and greater sciatic foramen have also been reported [7, 8] (Fig. 10.2a–d).

(d) Munchausen   syndrome: Named   after   Baron Munchausen, a fictitious character created by the German writer Rudolf Erich Raspe (1737–1794), and

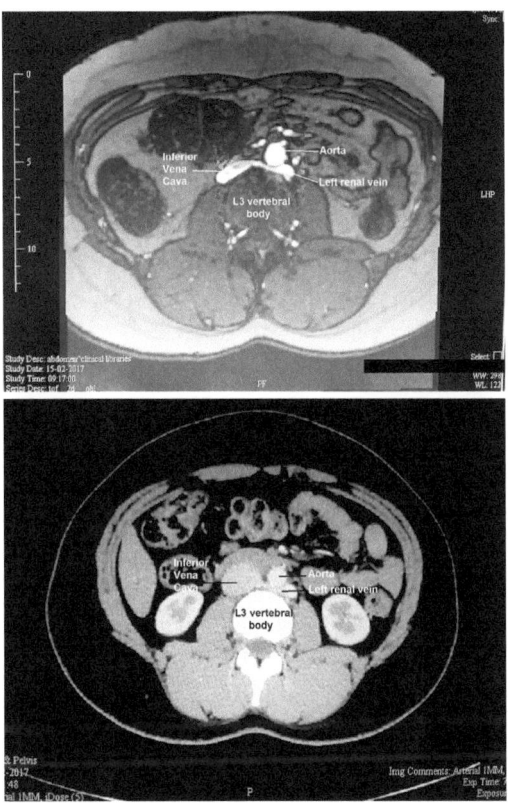

FIGURE 10.1 Axial MRI and CT-scans showing compression of the left renal vein between the aorta and the vertebral column in a 45-year female patient complaining of intermittent left loin pain. Courtesy Dr Salim Al-Busaidy, Urology, the Royal Hospital, Muscat, Oman.

Note: In this case the left renal vein courses in a descending pathway reaching the level of L3 vertebra before it joins the inferior vena cava. This is not uncommon for retrocaval veins [9]

based on a real baron, Karl Friedrich Hieronymous von Münchhausen (1720–1797), nicknamed "the baron of lies" ("Lügenbaron" in German) [10]. This is a syndrome of factitious illness, associated with self-inflicted signs of disease such as haematuria. The individuals

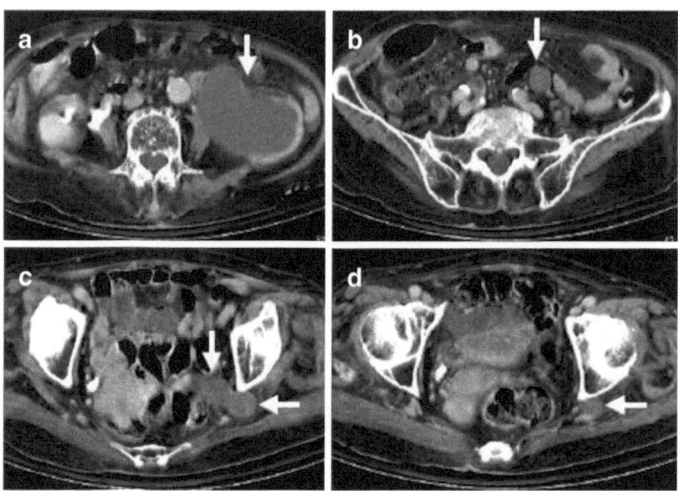

FIGURE 10.2 (**a–d**) A Computer tomography showing marked hydronephrosis of the left kidney and hydroureter to the level of the sciatic notch. The left ureter (*arrow*) is herniating through the greater sciatic foramen and is seen posteriorly and lateral to the ischial spine. From Tsai PJ et al. [8], with permission from Elsevier

exhibiting this syndrome often wander from hospital to hospital in an attempt to renew attention to their condition. They may also present false calculi picked up on the ground in an attempt to make their drama credible [11].

Some characteristic features differentiate Munchausen syndrome from malingering or hysteria [11]:

- Imposture: bizzare stories with fantastic past experiences and unusual life-styles
- Patients wandering from place to place
- Intelligent patients: For example, they will claim to have history of radiolucent stone and to be allergic to IV-contrast in order to avoid being

proven wrong by investigations.[1] They anticipate the questions and answers of young inexperienced doctors.

- Masochistic and self-destructive behavior. The patients accept painful and potentially dangerous diagnostic and operative procedures in order to preserve their "cover".[1] This extremist or die-hard attitude is not seen in malingering and hysteric patients.

2. Dysuria: Lower urinary tract infection and obstruction.
3. Haematuria: Renal arteriovenous malformation, renal vein thrombosis, renal cell carcinoma, upper tract urothelial carcinoma, urinary tuberculosis, haematological disorders (Henoch-Shönlein purpura), nutcracker syndrome, etc. Haematuria arising from the upper tract can also give colicky pain due to blood clots passage. In Munchausen Syndrome, patients may bite their lips or prick their gums or fingers with a needle to provoke bleeding that is then used to stain their urine [11].
4. Hydroureteronephrosis: PUJ obstruction (usually unilateral), retroperitoneal fibrosis (bilateral), urinary tuberculosis, advanced pelvic malignancy, any cause of ureteral stricture, ureteral herniation, etc. There is a dull continuous pain accompanying these pathologies.
5. Entities that can be mistaken for stones on imaging studies include:

   (a) Phleboliths: These are mostly encountered in the pelvic region and can mimic a lower ureteric stone on a KUB

---

[1]Nowadays, with the widespread use of Unenhanced CT-scans, it is extremely rare to undertake surgical procedures for urinary stone without confirmation of the diagnosis. The comedy of patients with Munchausen syndrome has become easy to discover obliging them to frequently change hospitals, cities or even states in order to regain attention from a new audience elsewhere.

X-ray. An old study of 1000 subjects aged 16–79 years showed a prevalence of pelvic phleboliths in 44.2% of the subjects (37.3% of the males and 50.1% of the females) [12]. Phleboliths number increase with age and their distribution in the pelvic region is not symmetrical, being more frequent on the left side than on the right (Fig. 10.3). They are also found in association with venous malformations (Maffucci and Klippel-Trenaunay syndromes etc.) [13, 14].

Phleboliths can also be seen in the suprapelvic or abdominal area where their frequency was shown to reach 2% of plain radiographs, raising confusion with upper ureteric stones. Herein the affected patients were all multiparous females, and the underlying

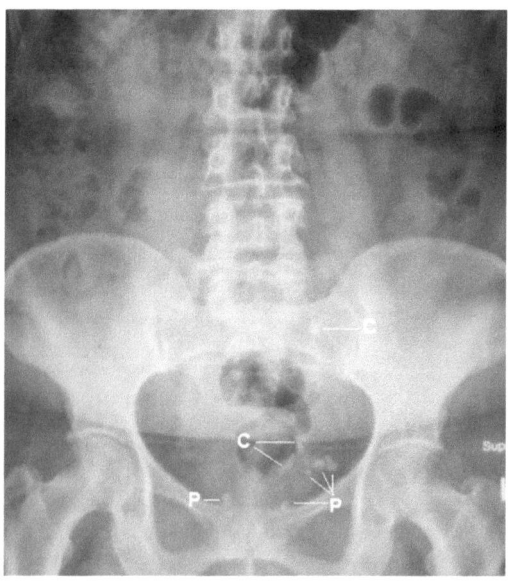

FIGURE 10.3 X-ray KUB showing multiple left mid and lower ureteral calculi (C) and phleboliths (P). Note the characteristic roundish shape and radiolucent center of phleboliths as well as their predominance on the left side (Courtesy Salim Al-Busaidy, Urology, the Royal Hospital, Muscat, Oman)

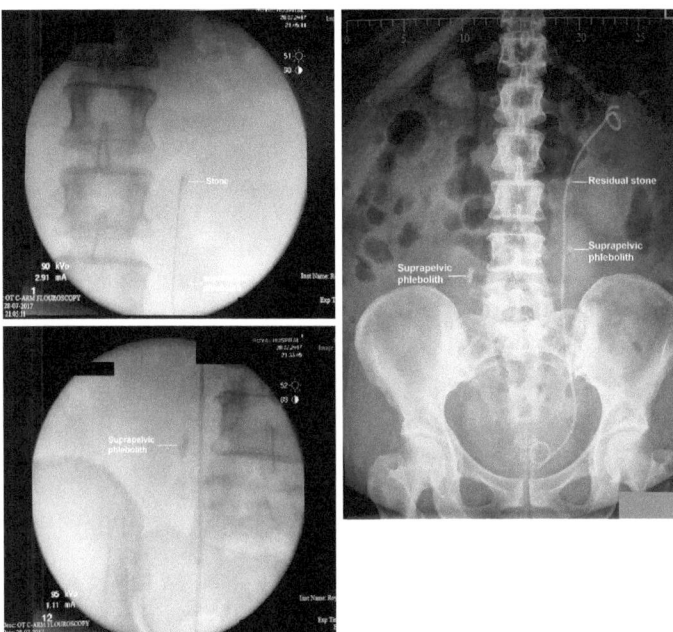

FIGURE 10.4 1 and 2. Intra-operative fluoroscopies showing an open-ended ureteral catheter abuting on a left upper ureteric calculus while suprapelvic phleboliths (of ovarian veins) are well seen lateral to its path on both sides. 3. X ray KUB of the same patient showing a DJ stent in situ with a small residual left upper ureteric stone (partially fragmented during ureteroscopy) and the suprapelvic phleboliths seen laterally. The patient was a 54-year old multiparous and diabetic woman who presented with an obstructed left kidney. Courtesy Salim Al-Busaidy, Urology department, The Royal Hospital, Muscat, Oman

pathologies were pelvic masses, hepatic disease, portal hypertension, or varices [15] (Fig. 10.4).

Some radiological features help to differentiate between ureteral calculi and phleboliths:

- The roundish shape and the characteristic radiolucent center of phleboliths are generally easily noticeable on plain X-ray KUB (Fig. 10.3).

However it is important to remember that the low attenuation-center of phleboliths is not present on routine clinical CT examinations [16].

• The rim and comet-tail signs: A soft tissue rim sign around a calcific focus helps identifying ureteral stones while phleboliths have a comet-tail shape. However there are interobserver discordances even among Radiologists raising questions about the reliability of these signs [17].

To reduce the interobserver bias, a recent study has demonstrated a good correlation between phleboliths and cut-off values of less than 171 mm^3 volume and 643 HU density (Table 10.1) [18].

Phleboliths can also be encountered in remote anatomical regions, such as the calves, but these will not be discussed as a differential diagnosis with urolithiasis.

(b) Renal vein thrombosis with calcification [19] (Fig. 10.5a–d).

TABLE 10.1 Differentiation of distal ureteral stones and pelvic phleboliths using cut-offs of 171 mm^3 size and 643 HU density

Density and size of pelvic radio-opacities	Phlebolith [n (%)]	Distal ureteral stone [n (%)]	Total [n (%)]	p Value
<643 HU and <171 mm^3	48 (92.3 %)	6(11.5 %)	54 (51.9 %)	0.0001
<643 HU and >171 mm^3	0 (0 %)	7 (13.5 %)	7 (6.7 %)	0.0126
>643 HU and <171 mm^3	4 (7.7 %)	7 (13.5 %)	11 (10.6%)	0.5256
>643 HU and >171 mm^3	0 (0 %)	32 (61.5 %)	32 (30.8 %)	0.0001
Total	52 (100%)	52 (100%)	104	

From Tanidir Y et al. [18] with permission from Springer

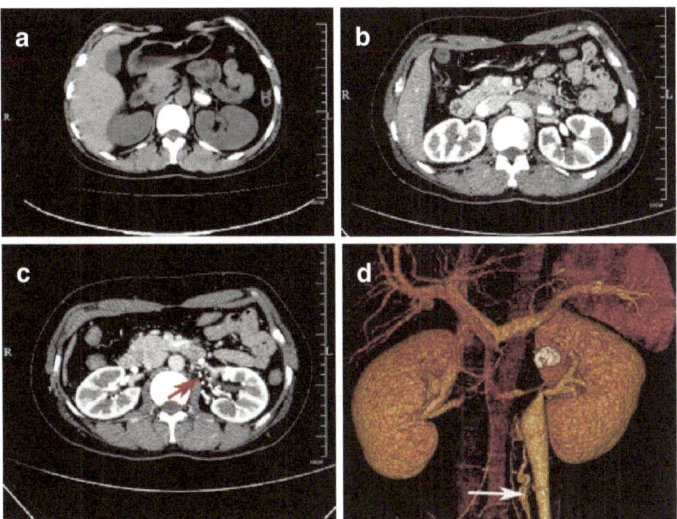

FIGURE 10.5 (**a–d**) Computed tomography (CT) of left renal vein calcified thrombus. (**a**) The NCCT suggests a left upper ureter calculus (but no hydronephrosis!). (**b**) The contrast enhanced CT indicates a hyperdense mass in the left renal vein. (**c**) The contrast-enhanced CT reveals peripheral veins (*red arrow*) around the left renal hilum. (**d**) The three-dimensional CT clearly displays the calcified left renal vein thrombus with varicose ovary vein (*white arrow*). Note: This 38-year-old woman presented with sudden onset of left flank pain and nausea, and was found to have microscopic hematuria. Initial diagnosis of a "left kidney stone" was made after Ultrasonography in a regional hospital and the patient underwent ESWL which failed. She was then referred to a tertiary care hospital for PCNL. A NCCT-scan showed the "stone" to be in the upper ureter but surprisingly no hydronephrosis was noted. Only CECT and CT-angiography allowed the treating team to reach the correct diagnosis!. Further management consisted of active monitoring with periodic ultrasonography and symptomatic treatment, and the patient had a good clinical course. From Wang Y et al. [19]. Creative Commons Attribution License

(c) Calcified renal artery aneurysm. This can mimic a renal pelvis stone on 2-D dimension representations, such as X ray KUB, U/S and IVP. A CT-scan is of paramount importance to rule out this rare pathology before embarking in a dangerous extracorporeal shockwave lithotripsy (ESWL) for what is believed to be a stone [20, 21] (Fig. 10.6a–c).

(d) Renal milk-of-calcium (MOC) cysts: This entity was first described in the literature by Lüdin and Howald in 1940 [22]. Formerly reported rare findings, MOC cysts

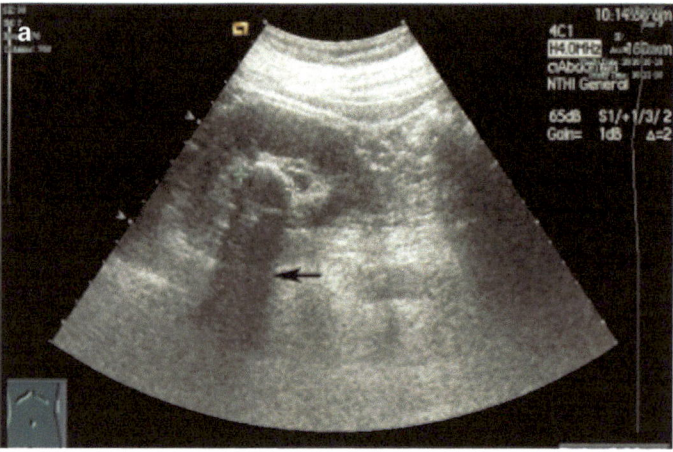

FIGURE 10.6 (**a**) Duplex ultrasonographic examination shows a hyperechoic focus in the left renal pelvis with acoustic shadow (*arrow*). (**b**) Images from intravenous pyelography. (*A*) A plain abdominal radiograph showed a left-sided renal calcification (*arrow*). (*B*) After injecting contrast medium, intravenous pyelography showed left hydronephrosis due to compression of the pyelo-ureteral junction by a 25-mm calcification (*arrow*). (**c**) Images from computed tomography. (*A*) The noncontrast scan shows a mass with a calcified rim. (*B*) The contrast-enhanced scan shows partial filling of the mass. (*C, D*) The coronal image and 3-dimensional reconstruction clearly show the aneurysm, which was located at the first bifurcation of the left renal artery and involved the posterior segmental artery. From Chen S et al. [21] with permission from Elsevier

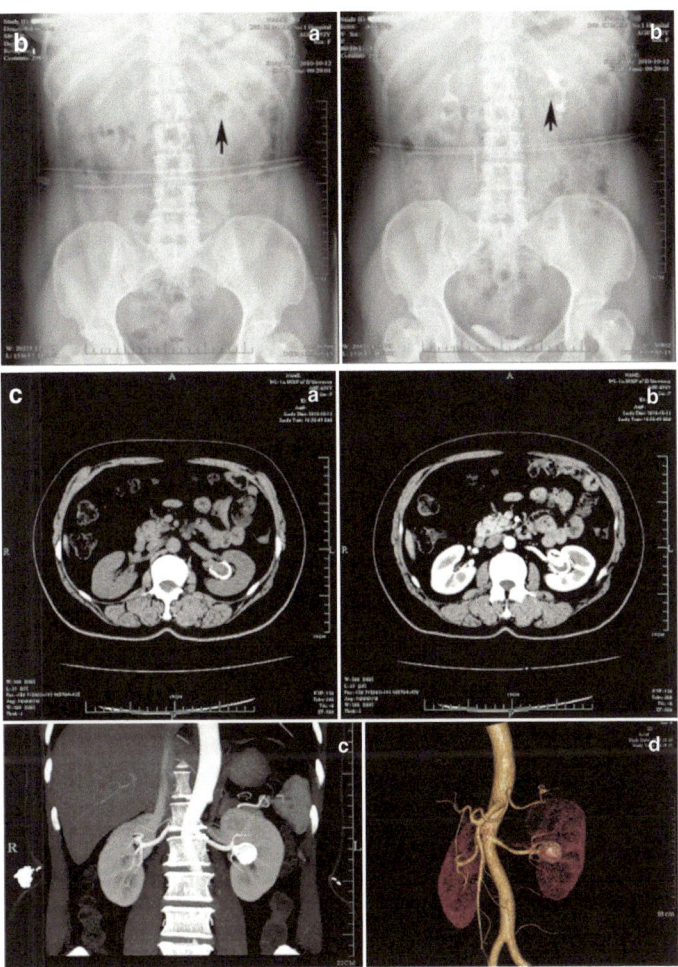

FIGURE 10.6 (continued)

are observed quite often nowadays with the increase awareness of Radiologists and Urologists. They consist of colloidal suspensions of calcium salts to which the predisposing factors are stasis, obstruction (by a true stone for example), and infection. They typically appear as spherical radiopaque structures on supine

X-ray KUB and are "half-moon-shaped" on standing beam radiography. These gravity-dependent structures appear on U/S as echogenic shadowy material in calyceal cysts or diverticula, and exhibit on CT-scan either a fluid level or a semi-lunar pattern with characteristically low density values, ranging from 100 to 600 HU [23–26] (Figs. 10.7a, b, 10.8a–c, and 10.9a, b). It is important to recognize this entity in order to avoid unnecessary and potentially hazardous procedures like ESWL. The terminology of milk-of-calcium stone has also been used by some authors [26]. MOC cysts generally don't require any treatment or further follow-up. However they can be associated with a UTI, and may also become symptomatic. In these scenarios, they may justify a PCNL with suction and retrieval of their contents; however the open approach appears to be an overtreatment for these colloidal microliths-containing materials [26].

(e) Gallbladder stones: these are rarely radiopaque and can then be mistaken for right renal stones on a KUB X-ray (Fig. 10.10a–c).

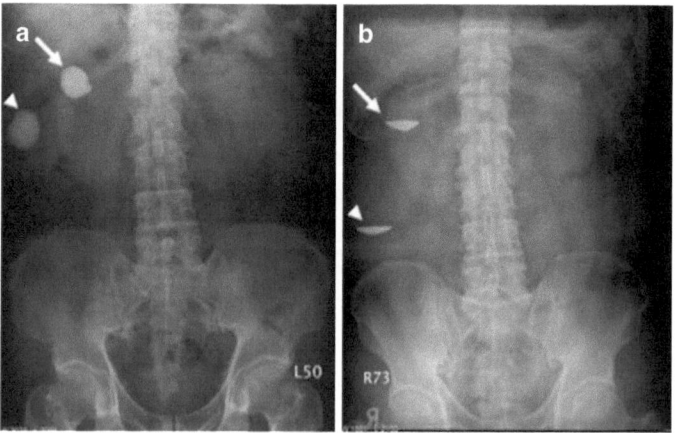

FIGURE 10.7 (**a**) Milk of calcium in supine abdominal radiograph. (**b**) Milk of calcium in standing abdominal radiograph. From Liu KL et al. [25]. With permission from Elsevier

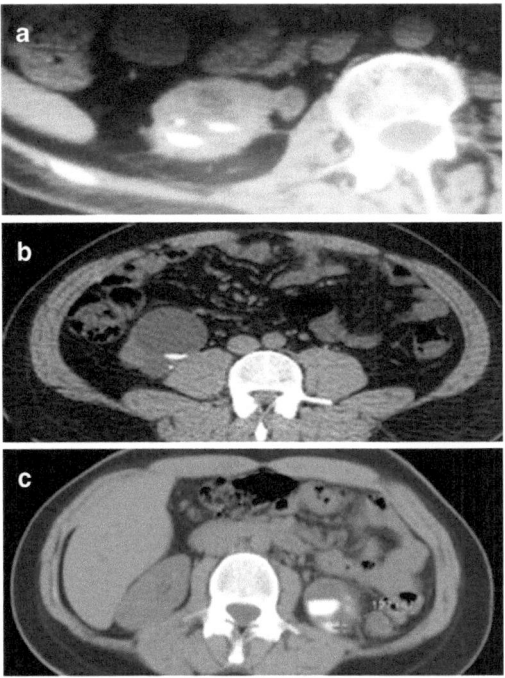

FIGURE 10.8 (**a–c**) CT-scan from three different patients showing MOC with typical fluid level. From El-Shazli [26], with permission from Springer-Verlag

(f) Others: Gastro-intestinal foreign body, fecalith or fecolith or coprolith, -especially appendicolith[2] [27, 28], paragonimus calcified ova [29].

---

[2]Appendicoliths are generally seen well lateral to the sacroiliac joint on abdomen radiographs and have roundish shapes avoiding confusion with a ureteric stone but not with an ectopic kidney stone. However they may sometimes be more medial when located at the tip of a long and mobile appendix. Moreover in case of appendicular perforation, an appendicolith can extrude outside the appendix lumen and become free in the peritoneal cavity. If inadvertently forgotten during surgery, this "retained appendicolith" may migrate to ectopic sites (even in the chest cavity!) where it has the potential to cause localized infection and abscess formation [30]. An abdominal X ray may show this "wandering radio-opaque structure" lying over the ureteric path, adding to confusion with a urinary stone. CT-scan is indicated to clarify this diagnosis.

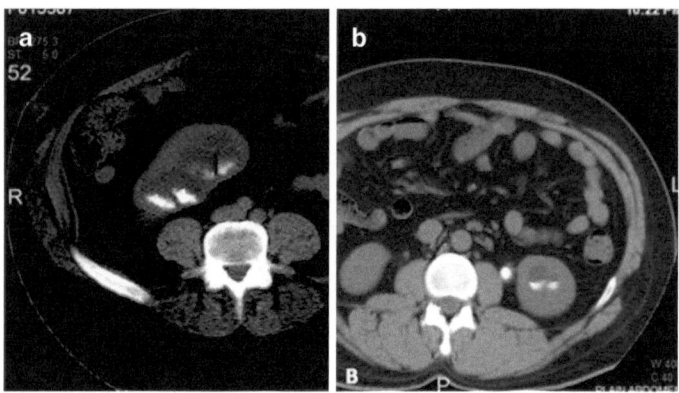

FIGURE 10.9 (**a** and **b**) CT-scan showing MOC with semilunar pattern in two different patients. An associated left upper ureteral stone is seen on the figure (**b**). From El-Shazly M. [26] with permission from Springer-Verlag

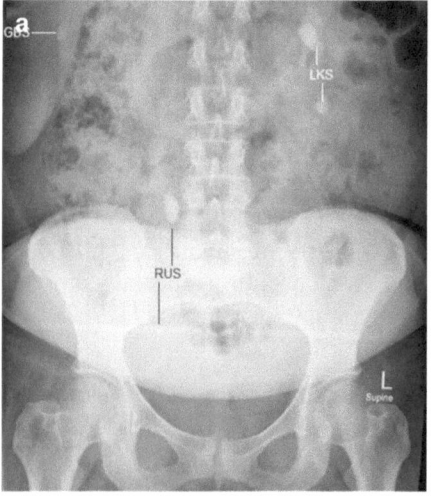

FIGURE 10.10 The KUB Radiograph (**a**) of a 53-year old woman shows multiple left kidney (LKS) and right ureteral stones (RUS). The patient was also thought to have a right renal calculus until plain NCCT scan showed that it was in reality a gall-bladder stone (GBS) (**b** and **c**) (Courtesy Salim Al-Busaidy, Urology, The Royal Hospital, Muscat, Oman)

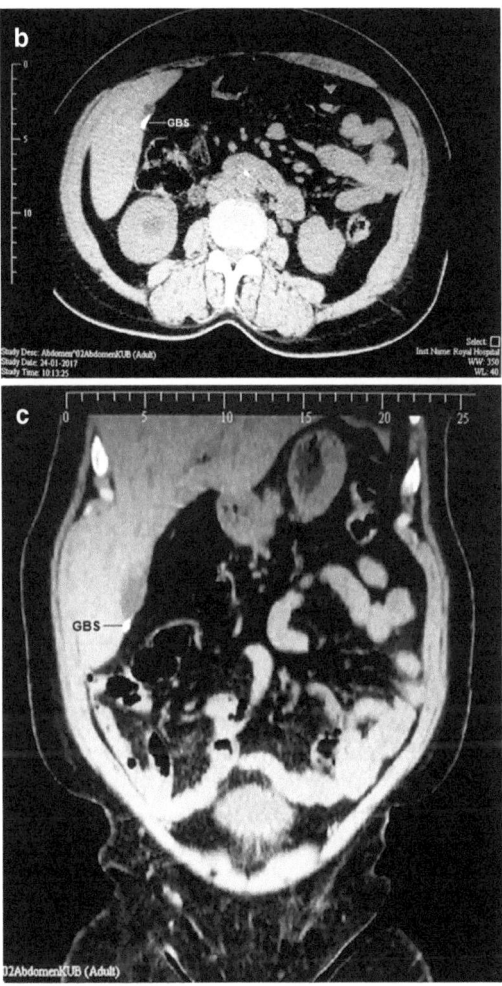

FIGURE 10.10 (continued)

References

1. Smith AE, Bhatti IN, Hester T, Ritchie JF. Loin to groin pain: the importance of a differential diagnosis. Int J Surg Case Rep. 2015;16:122–6.
2. Nash EF, Ohri CM, Stephenson AL, Durie PR. Abdominal pain in adults with cystic fibrosis. Eur J Gastroenterol Hepatol. 2014;26(2):129–36.

3. Robson WL, Leung AK, Mathers MS. Renal colic due to Henoch-Schönlein purpura. J S C Med Assoc. 1994;90(12):592–5.
4. Salih SB, Al Durihim H, Al Jizeeri A, Al Maziad G. Acute renal infarction secondary to atrial fibrillation—mimicking renal stone picture. Saudi J Kidney Dis Transpl. 2006;17(2):208–12.
5. Kurklinsky AK, Rooke TW. Nutcracker phenomenon and nutcracker syndrome. Mayo Clin Proc. 2010;85(6):552–9.
6. Skeik N, Gloviczki P, Macedo TA. Posterior nutcracker syndrome. Vasc Endovasc Surg. 2011;45(8):749–55.
7. Weintraub JL, Pappas GM, Romano WJ, Kirsch MJ, Spencer W. Percutaneous reduction of ureterosciatic hernia. AJR Am J Roentgenol. 2000;175:181–2.
8. Tsai PJ, Lin JT, Wu TT, Tsai CC. Ureterosciatic hernia causes obstructive uropathy. J Chin Med Assoc. 2008;71(9):491–3.
9. Anjamrooz SH, Azari H, Abedinzadeh M. Abnormal patterns of the renal veins. Anat Cell Biol. 2012;45(1):57–61.
10. Raspe RE, et al. Singular travels, campaigns, and adventures of Baron Munchausen. New York: Dover Publications Inc; 1960.
11. Jones WA, Cooper TP, Kiviat MD. Munchausen syndrome presenting as urolithiasis. West J Med. 1978;128(2):185–8.
12. Mattsson T. Frequency and location of pelvic phleboliths. Clin Radiol. 1980;31(1):115–8.
13. Enjolras O, Wassef M, Merland JJ. Maffucci syndrome: a false venous malformation? A case with hemangioendothelioma with fusiform cells. Ann Dermatol Venereol. 1998;125(8):512–5.
14. Casanova D, Boon LM, Vikkula M. Venous malformations: clinical characteristics and differential diagnosis. Ann Chir Plast Esthet. 2006;51(4–5):373–87.
15. Curry NS, Ham FC, Schabel SI. Suprapelvic phleboliths: prevalence, distribution and clinical associations. Clin Radiol. 1983;34(6):701–5.
16. Traubici J, Neitlich JD, Smith RC. Distinguishing pelvic phleboliths from distal ureteral stones on routine unenhanced helical CT: is there a radiolucent center? AJR Am J Roentgenol. 1999;172(1):13–7.
17. Guest AR, Cohan RH, Korobkin M, et al. Assessment of the clinical utility of the rim and comet-tail signs in differentiating ureteral stones from phleboliths. AJR Am J Roentgenol. 2001;177(6):1285–91.
18. Tanidir Y, Sahan A, Asutay MK, et al. Differentiation of ureteral stones and phleboliths using Hounsfield units on computerized

tomography: a new method without observer bias. Urolithiasis. 2016;45(3):323–8. doi:10.1007/s00240-016-0918-1.

19. Wang Y, Chen S, Wang W, et al. Renal vein thrombosis mimicking urinary calculus: a dilemma of diagnosis. BMC Urol. 2015;15:61.

20. Sallami S, Mizouni H, Mnif E. An unusual case of a calcified renal artery aneurysm mimicking a renal calculus. Tunis Med. 2014;92(4):287–8.

21. Chen S, Meng H, Cao M, Shen B. Renal artery aneurysm mimicking renal calculus with hydronephrosis. Am J Kidney Dis. 2013;61(6):1036–40.

22. Lüdin M, Howald R. Eine eigenartige intrarenale Zyste. Schwiezerisches medizinisches Wochenschrift. 1940;70:230–2.

23. Heidenreich A, Vorreuther R, Krug B, et al. Renal milk of calcium: contraindication to extracorporeal shockwave lithotripsy. Tech Urol. 1996;2(2):102–7.

24. Khan SA, Khan FR, Fletcher MS, Richenberg JL. Milk of calcium (MOC) cysts masquerading as renal calculi—a trap for the unwary. Cent European J Urol. 2012;65(3):170–3.

25. Liu KL, Chueh SC, Lee WJ, et al. Full moon and new moon. Milk of calcium in renal cysts. Kidney Int. 2008;73(4):515–6.

26. El-Shazly M. Milk of calcium stones: radiological signs and management outcome. Urolithiasis. 2015;43(3):221–5.

27. Kaya B, Eris C. Different clinical presentation of appendicolithiasis. The report of three cases and review of the literature. Clin Med Insights Pathol. 2011;4:1–4.

28. Teke Z, Kabay B, Erbiş H, Tuncay OL. Appendicolithiasis causing diagnostic dilemma: a rare cause of acute appendicitis (report of a case). Ulus Travma Acil Cerrahi Derg. 2008;14(4):323–5.

29. Lin CM, Chen SK. Paragonimus calcified ova mimicking left renal staghorn stone. J Urol. 1993;149(4):819–20.

30. Betancourt SL, Palacio D, Bisset GS III. The 'wandering appendicolith'. Pediatr Radiol. 2015;45(7):1091–4.

Chapter 11
Treatment of Urolithiasis

"Challenges in medicine are moving from 'Treat the symptoms after the house is on fire' to 'Can we preserve the house intact?'"

Elizabeth Blackburn (1948–) (Nobel Prize in Physiology/ Medicine in 2009)

This section will be approached systematically starting with the management of incidentally discovered urinary stones, then the treatment of a painful episode of urinary stones presenting in the emergency department as well as the management of obstructed kidneys with sepsis. Thereafter we will discuss the various active modalities performed when symptoms persist, or when at first glance the stone appears not to be prone for spontaneous passage. Active stone removal is also recommended when there is stone growth, de novo obstruction, or associated infection [1]. We will also develop the topic of dietary and medical preventive measures and will give a brief account on phytotherapy.

11.1 Management of Incidentally Discovered Urinary Stones (Non-obstructive and Asymptomatic)

1. Renal or ureteral stone ≤5 mm: **Active surveillance (AS)** is the best and the most cost-effective way to manage these stones as long as they remain asymptomatic, due to their likelihood to pass spontaneously.

© Springer International Publishing AG 2017   177
S.A. Al-Mamari, *Urolithiasis in Clinical Practice*,
In Clinical Practice, DOI 10.1007/978-3-319-62437-2_11

2. Renal stones 5–10 mm: **Extracorporeal ShockWave Lithotripsy** (ESWL) is the first-line treatment [1, 3]. **AS** still applies but the patient must be warned about the possibility of these stones persisting in their position and, more worrisomely, the potential to get stuck during their descent through the ureter and cause obstruction. A study of the natural history of 160 nonobstructing asymptomatic renal stones measuring around 3–11 mm (average 7 mm) was conducted over an average period of 3 and a half years; symptoms developed in 28% of cases during follow-up and obstruction occurred in 3% only. Less than 20% of the cases underwent surgery and 7% of stones passed spontaneously, while the rest of the stones remained unchanged [2]. In this study, besides the stone size, the only significant predictor of spontaneous passage or symptom was shown to be the stone location; upper and mid polar renal stones being more likely to become symptomatic and to pass spontaneously than lower pole stones.

3. Uncomplicated ureteral stones ≤10 mm: Observation, and in distally located stones, medical expulsive therapy with α-blockers is advised [3].

4. Renal stones 10–20 mm: **ESWL, except for lower calyceal position**, where flexible URS and PNCL are more effective options [1, 3]. Again AS can apply in special cases: patient reluctance or lack of medical fitness.

5. Ureteral stones >10 mm: Rigid ureteroscopy and in-situ lithotripsy. ESWL is an option if the patient is unwilling or unfit for endourology (very advanced age) [3].

6. Renal stones 20–30 mm: No place for ESWL here [3]. **RIRS or PCNL are the best solutions** [2, 3]. Again AS can apply in special cases: Patient unwillingness or unfitness (very advance age etc.).

7. Stones >30 mm: PCNL or open pyelolithotomy/nephrolithotomy. Rarely multi-sessions RIRS can be proposed (high volume center), but not for stone >40 mm.

When renal stones are kept under active surveillance, it is recommended to re-evaluate the disease after 6 months, then perform an annual follow-up of symptoms and stone status using U/S, X-ray KUB or CT [1].

11.2 Treatment of a Painful Episode of the Stone Disease

11.2.1 Symptomatic Treatment

A Cochrane meta-analysis including 87 studies for a total of 10,217 participants has shown that **Nonsteroidal anti-inflammatory drugs (NSAIDs) significantly reduced pain compared to antispasmodics (Hyoscine)**; and among NSAIDs, Indomethacin and Lysine acetyl salicylate (Aspegic®, a soluble salt of Aspirin) were found to be the least effective. Conflictual results were obtained when comparing combination therapy of NSAIDs plus antispasmodics with NSAIDs alone, however the majority showed that **the addition of antispasmodics to NSAIDS does not result in a better pain control**. No significant difference in pain recurrence at 72 h was observed when comparing IM Piroxicam (Feldene®) alone with the combination of IM Piroxicam with Phloroglucinol (Spasfon-Lyoc®), and none between IM Piroxicam and IV paracetamol. No major adverse effects were reported in the literature during the use of NSAIDs for treatment of renal colic [4].

We can conclude from this study that NSAIDs such as IM Diclofenac (Olfen®, Voltaren®), or IM Piroxicam (Feldene®), as well as IV Paracetamol can be considered as the **first-line drugs** for pain control in renal colic. However when the pain is severe and doesn't respond to these drugs, narcotics should be used as a **second line**, namely Tramadol, or Pethidine, or even Morphine as recommended by the EAU panel [1]. There should be a constant reminder that NSAIDs are to be avoided in the presence of renal failure and their repetitive or continuous use should be avoided in all patients.

11.2.2 Medical Expulsive Therapy

Medical expulsive therapy (MET) is indicated for distal ureteral stones. The drugs act by relaxing the smooth muscle of the ureter, causing an increase in the physical force proximal to the calculus and a decrease of resistance distally, enhancing the antegrade stone progression.

The two most important factors in predicting stone passage are the size and the site of the stone:

(a) Passage rates of **68 and 47%** have been reported for stones measuring **<5 mm and 5–10 mm** respectively [1, 5].
(b) Stone passage is more likely for **vesicoureteric stones** than for more proximal stones with reported passage rates **of 89.7%** and 75.2% respectively [6].

The most used drugs are α-1 adrenergic receptor blockers which have the biggest effect on anatomical sites known to harbor the highest α-adrenoreceptors density, i.e. the distal ureter and the bladder neck. **Nowadays Tamsulosin (Omnic®) is the most widely prescribed drug of this family at an adult dose of 400 μg HS daily**. Other drugs of this family which demonstrated effectiveness are 5-methylurapidil [7] and Alfuzosin [8].

However the effects of Tamsulosin are hindered by its **slow action**: **It does not increase the stone passage rate within a week** [9]. Moreover the effect of 0.4 mg of Tamsulosin daily was not proved to be superior over placebo for distal ureteric stone less than or equal to 5-mm in terms of spontaneous passage and **its effectiveness was shown only for larger stones (5–10 mm)** [6].

Further controversy was raised by the SUSPEND trial conducted in 24 British NHS hospitals in 2015 which showed that the use of Tamsulosin does not increase the rate of ureteric stone passage even over a 4-week period [10]. However a recent meta-analysis including 55 randomized controlled trials has supported the current guidelines on the use of alphablockers for ureteric stones measuring ≥5 mm, and also showed effectiveness of these drugs regardless of the stone location (including upper, middle or lower ureter) [11].

Silodosin (Rapaflo®) is a novel highly selective α1A-adrenoceptor blocker with promising effectiveness in MET for ureteral stone as shown in another meta-analysis [12].

This study suggested superiority of Silodosin at the dose of 8 mg/day for 3–8 weeks over other selective α1-adrenergic receptor antagonists such as Tamsulosin 0.4 mg/day or Naftopidil (Flivas®) 50 mg/day, and compared to inactive placebo, in terms of stone expulsion rate, time to stone expulsion, and analgesic requirements. However the number of studies included in this meta-analysis was small and the authors themselves do recognize the need for more high-quality trials with larger sample sizes to fully establish the role of Silodosin in the treatment of distal ureteral stones.

A common side effect of alpha-blockers is the retrograde ejaculation; however patients should be reassured that this is a reversible side effect and normal ejaculation is restored after cessation of the medication.

Another family of drugs used in MET consists of calcium–channel blockers which aim at "softening" the ureteral smooth muscles, resulting in the dilatation of this hollow tubular organ. The most frequently mentioned drug in this family in Nifedipine (Adalat®) [7].

Cortico-steroids form the third group of drugs proposed for stone expulsion because of their anti-edematous effect; however NSAIDs were shown ineffective for this purpose [13].

11.2.3 Management of an Obstructed Kidney with Sepsis

An acute kidney obstruction should be suspected whenever the patient presents with severe pain and U/S or CT-scan shows a dilated pelvicalyceal system (PCS) and ureter proximal to the stone. When in addition to the above signs, the patient develops fever or chills often associated with a high leucocyte count and/or raised C-reactive protein, this indicates sepsis. Pain control is no longer the sole goal, and direct treatment of the stone is not a priority, and the focus of attention must be to decompress and drain the obstructed kidney urgently. In this scenario, blood should be rapidly taken for urea and electolytes, full blood count, aerobic and anaerobic cultures and coagulation profile. Empirical Intravenous (IV) broad spectrum antibiotics are initiated such as third Generation Cefalosporin or Tazocin, and vitals sign monitored.

The urgent need for kidney drainage cannot be over emphasized in order to prevent serious complications associated with pyonephrosis such as septic shock and multiorgan failure especially in elderly or debilitated patients.

Two options exist to decompress the obstructed kidney: **percutaneous nephrostomy (PCN) and retrograde placement of a ureteral stent.** It is commonplace to prefer the insertion of a PCN tube in a septic scenario as it appears to be a rapid procedure not requiring general anesthesia, availability of an Operating Theater (OT) room, or pre-assessment by an Anesthetist. It is also more adequate for a vitally unstable patient or one with uncorrected significant electrolytes imbalance as there would be a high risk for general anesthesia. However a PCN tube insertion can be technically challenging if the pelvi-calyceal system (PCS) is not well dilated and in a morbidly obese patient, and is contra-indicated when there is a coagulation disturbance. Moreover randomized controlled trials failed to show the superiority of PCN over Double-J (DJ) stent insertion in terms of complications (septicemia) [14]. Retrograde DJ stenting doesn't require dilatation of the PCS and can be performed even with an impaired coagulation. It can be safely performed in OT under general anesthesia (GA) and after initiation of an empirical IV antibiotic; **however no attempt should be made to remove the stone at this stage**. Not surprisingly, experts panels have decided to treat equally these techniques of kidney decompression [15, 16]. The first urine drained by either method should be sent for culture and antibiogram, as a guide for further antibiotic adjustment.

11.3   Direct Treatment of the Urinary Stone

The indications for an active stone removal can be divided into two categories [15]:

- Stone characteristics:
    - a stone which at first glance appears not prone to pass spontaneously due to its size (>15 mm)
    - a stone which fails to pass after a reasonable observation time,
    - an obstructing stone de-novo,
    - a stone associated with persistent sepsis,
    - a stone associated with persistent symptoms,
    - a growing stone,

- Patients characteristics:

    - high-risk for recurrent stone formation (cystinuria, primary oxaluria etc.),
    - renal function impairment,
    - single kidney,
    - special professional constraints (pilots, businessmen with frequent travels, etc.).

Depending on the above characteristics, a urinary stone can be directly treated either with a non-invasive modality, namely the Extracorporeal ShockWave Lithotripsy (ESWL), or through invasive means. The latter may be minimally invasive such as endourological surgery, PCNL, laparoscopic, or robotic-assisted surgeries, or may consist of open procedures. The antegrade stone chemolysis was a minimally invasive procedure reported up to two decades ago and is now obsolete.

As shown by a French survey the number of surgical procedures performed for urolithiasis has doubled or trebled during the last three decades. ESWL was the main treatment until 10 years back, but has been supplanted by Ureteroscopy which represents now the leading procedure for urolithiasis in many French institutions, while PCNL remained stable. Nowadays open surgery for stone has become extremely rare there, representing only 0.1% in this study [17]. The same trends were observed by British researchers who found a near 50% increase in the number of ureteroscopies, especially ureterorenoscopy (i.e. flexible ureteroscopy) from the year 2009 to 2015. Although ESWL is still the most frequent treatment in the United Kingdom, its use has remained stable during the 5-year study interval and the gap with ureteroscopy continues to shrink, while the decline of the open stone surgery continues to deepen with only 30 reported cases in the period 2014–2015 for all the United Kingdom health systems [18].

11.3.1   Extracorporeal ShockWave Lithotripsy (ESWL)

The term "Lithotripsy" derives from Greek words "lithos" (stone) and "tribein" or "tripsis" (to rub, to pulverize, to dissolve).

11.3.1.1   History

The first ESWL machines were manufactured by the German aircraft manufacturing company Dornier. Its human clinical application was first reported by **Chaussy et al**. in 1982 [19] after a successful trial on dogs in 1980 [20]. The safety and efficacy of ESWL were also confirmed in children [21] as well as in solitary kidneys [22].

Dornier lithotripters were originally designed to test supersonic aircraft parts. Then human models (HM) were developed, starting with HM1 [23] (Fig. 11.1). The first clinical experiences were performed with HM3, based on an **electrohydraulic shockwaves generator**. The shocks were triggered underwater by spark plug (F1) discharges. The discharges which lasted one micro-second each caused an explosive evaporation of water triggering the shockwaves [24]. The shockwaves then bounced on an ellipsoidal reflector and were focused on the stone (F2) through a water-filled metal tub in which both the patient and the generator were

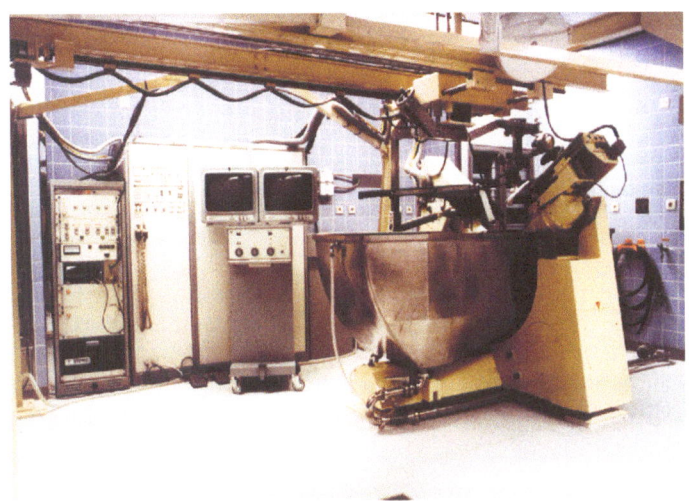

FIGURE 11.1 HM1 at the Munich University Hospital Grosshadern. From Tailly et al. [23] Copyright Dornier MedTech Systems

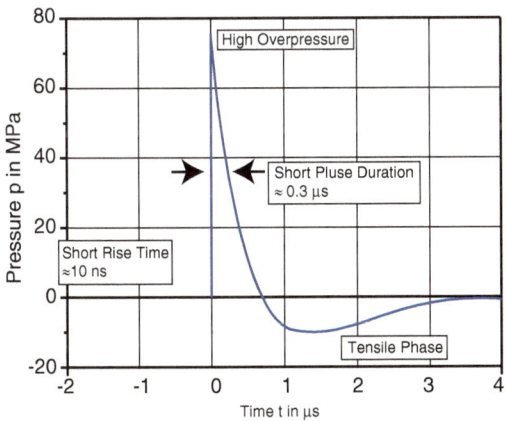

FIGURE 11.2 Shock wave pressure pulse as function of time measured in the shock wave focal zone F2. From Tailly et al. [23] Copyright Dornier MedTech Systems

immersed. A single shock can generate a peak positive pressure of 30–100 megapascals (1 megapascal equal to 9.87 Atm or 10 Bars) [23, 25] (Fig. 11.2).

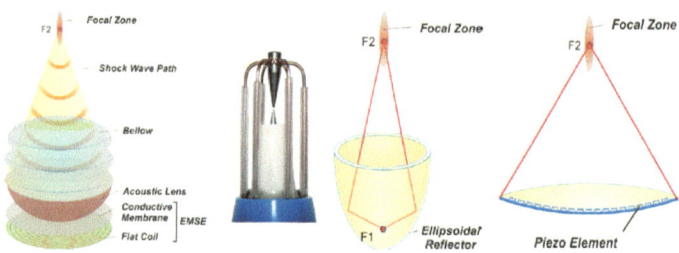

FIGURE 11.3 Principles of shock wave generators used in lithotripters. *Left*: Electro-Magnetic Shock wave Emitter (EMSE). *Centre:* Electrohydraulic Shock wave emitter. *Right*: Piezoelectric Shock wave emitter. HM1 at the Munich University Hospital Grosshadern. From Tailly et al. [23] Copyright Dornier MedTech Systems

With Dornier HM3, the treatment was very painful and had to be performed under either general or regional (epidural/spinal) anaesthesia. In the last three decades, the manufacturer presented further generations, where the used energy source is provided by **piezoelectric,**[1] **electrohydraulic, or electromagnetic generators** (Fig. 11.3), and the water-filled tub is replaced by a more comfortable silicone-encased water cushion that coapts to the patient anatomical region of interest. The stone can be localized either by Fluoroscopy or Ultrasound means (Fig. 11.4). There is a trend for the new generation lithotripters to have larger focal zones and lower shock wave pressure. Another sophistication being introduced is the automated localization or the use of optical and acoustic stone-tracking systems aiming at reducing the

---

[1]Piezoelectricity is an adjective coming from Greek words "piezein" (to press or to squeeze) and "electron" (amber: a shining fossilized tree resin). The principle of Piezoelectricity can be summarized as "production of electricity by pressure application". Indeed when submitted to high pressure, various solid materials such as quartz, ceramics, crystals, etc. accumulate a potential energy that is instantly delivered as an alternating electric current. Piezoelectricity was reportedly discovered by the French Physicists Jacques and Pierre Curie in 1880 and its simplest example nowadays is a gas lighter. "Reverse or inverse piezoelectricity" is the faculty of the same solid materials to become mechanically stressed, i.e. deformed in shape when submitted to electricity.

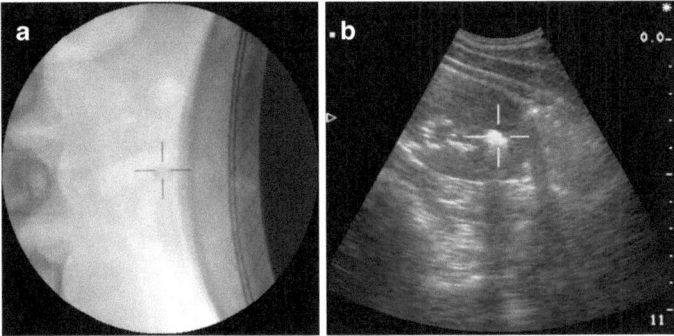

FIGURE 11.4 (**a**, **b**) Images of stone localization using X-ray (fluoroscopy) (**a**) and ultrasound (**b**) means. On both pictures, the stone is optimally localized within the crosshairs. The coupling cushion of the therapy head is seen at the right of the image (**a**) and the bright reflection of the stone is well seen on the image (**b**) accompanied by an acoustic shadow. HM1 at the Munich University Hospital Grosshadern. From Tailly et al. [23] Copyright Dornier MedTech Systems

fluoroscopy time [25]. Many adult patients can tolerate the pain related to new ESWL machines and just need be given IM Narcotic drugs as premedication. However children are still to be treated under general anesthesia.

Nowadays not less than ten other companies have been licensed to produce their own models (Siemens, Karl STORZ, Richard WOLF, EMD, Cellsonic, HYDE-medical, Elite, ELMED, GEMSS, US healthcare solutions).

11.3.1.2   Mechanisms of Action

Various different mechanisms have been proposed for stone comminution:

- Mechanical stress: When the shockwaves reach the patient's skin, they pass evenly through the anatomical soft tissues which have acoustic impedance not significantly different from that of the water. However when they reach the stone surface, part of the shockwave is absorbed and the remaining is reflected. The sudden change in acoustic impedance creates pressure gradients which trigger shear and tear forces resulting progressively in stone disintegration [20, 24].

- Cavitational microbubbles: This mechanism can be summarized by the following sequence [26]: Shockwaves hitting the stone → fissures in the stone material → liquid penetration through small cracks → formation of cavitation microbubbles within these small split lines → imploding of the microbubbles → fragmentation or disintegration of the stone.
- Other mechanisms are quazi-static squeezing and dynamic squeezing [25].

The critical role of the cavitation has been confirmed in a recent in-vitro study which also introduced the principle of controlled cavitation at strategic time points in order to enhance stone fragmentation during ESWL [27]. Furthermore when slow shockwaves frequency is applied (60 shocks per minute), there is a significantly greater likelihood of a successful treatment outcome that when high frequency (120 shocks per minute) is used [28].

11.3.1.3   Indications and Limitations of ESWL

It was written in 1995 that "ESWL remains the treatment of choice for moderately sized, uncomplicated renal calculi" [29]. It was also mentioned ibidem that this treatment should not be indicated for large calculi, those within obstructed or dependent portions of the collecting system, and those composed of calcium oxalate monohydrate. Both statements are still valid today [15]. Obstructed portions of the collecting system include a calyx or a calyceal diverticulum with a steep infundibular-pelvic angle, and/or with a narrow infundibulum or neck <5 mm. On the other hand a dependent portion is well exemplified by a long lower pole calyx (>10 mm) [15].

ESWL is currently the procedure of choice for treating most renal stones in the pediatric population, for whom it is the best option for the following situations [30]:

- all stones <1 cm or <150 mm^2,
- all soft renal stones (<900 HU on CT scan) >1 and <2 cm, provided the renal function is normal, there is no infection, and the stones are in a favorable anatomical location.

It is also indicated in small ureteral stones >10 mm and even for bladder calculi in patients unwilling or unfit for ureteroscopy and/or general anesthesia [31].

11.3.1.4   Contraindications

The contra-indications for the use of ESWL have not changed since long and can be described as absolute or relative [32, 33].

- Absolute contraindications:
  - Pregnancy,
  - Uncontrolled coagulation disorders,
  - untreated urinary infection, overt tuberculosis,
  - anatomical obstruction distal to the stone.

- Relative contraindications:

  - major deformities, such as severe skeletal malformations (difficult or impossible coupling with the water balloon),
  - morbid obesity (impossibility to localize the stone and weight in excess of the maximum withstandable by the machine table),
  - proximate calcified aortic aneurysm: this is a recommendation by precaution although experience did not actually show significant pathological damage to aneurysmal tissue submitted to shock waves [34].
  - implanted cardiac pacemaker or defibrillators: Here ESWL can be safely performed using ECG-triggered

shocks that are synchronized with R/S waves, i.e. the terminal portion of the QRS complex which represents the absolute refractory period of ventricles [35]. ECG-triggered ESWL has been shown to significantly lower the occurrence of ventricular arrhythmias compared to respiratory-triggered ESWL [36].

11.3.1.5   Complications

Despite being a non-invasive procedure, ESWL often causes some self-limited complications reported to reach a total of about 15%, a figure inferior to that seen with percutaneous pyelolithotomy (PCNL) and ureteroscopy [37].

The most commonly encountered complications are [15]:
– asymptomatic cardiac dysrhythmia (11–59%),
– bacteriuria (7.7–23%),
– asymptomatic renal hematoma (4–19%),
– steinstrasse[2] (3.6–7%),

---

[2]The word "Steinstrasse" is a German term which means "stone street", and its plural is "steinstrassen". It was coined by Chaussy C et al. [19] to refer to a post-ESWL adverse event where multiple stone fragments get jammed in the ureter eventually causing an obstruction. In a large Egyptian series of patients treated with ESWL (n = 2954), steinstrassen were observed in 4.9% of cases [38]. They mostly form in the pelvic or lower ureter (74%), then in the lumbar or upper ureter (18.5–21.7%), and rarely in the iliac or mid ureter (4.3–7.4%). Suggested risk factors for their formation are: renal stone size >2 cm, renal pelvis or upper calyceal location, a dilated system, and use of high power (>22 Kv) for disintegration [39, 40]. In the pediatric population, it is also associated with age <4 years. Some authors have proposed to classify steinstrassen into three types: type I is made up of tiny particles (≤2 mm), type II has a large leading fragment of 4–5 mm with a tail made of tiny particles, and type III is composed of large fragments [41]. Asymptomatic steinstrassen are managed conservatively, and Tamsulosin has been suggested [42]. Complicated steinstrassen (i.e associated with pain, hydronephrosis, fever) may require percutaneous nephrostomy, or ureteroscopy, or both [41, 43].

Steinstrassen can rarely form spontaneously in patient with nephrocalcinosis associated with distal RTA [44, 45] and have also been reported even in the urethra after ESWL for a renal stone, after cystolitholapaxy in a post-renal transplant patient, in association with stricture, or de-novo in children [46–49] (Fig. 11.5).

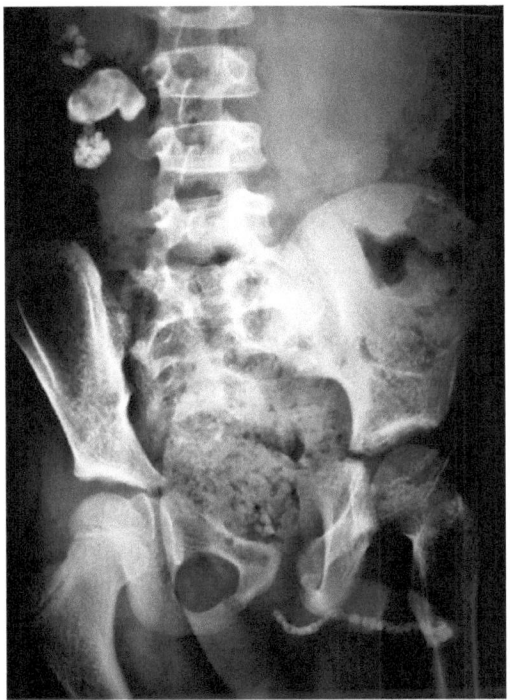

Figure 11.5 X-ray KUB showing multiple right renal calculi and a urethral steinstrasse in a child. From Vaddi SP et al. [49] with permission from Elsevier

- renal colic (2–4%), and
- urosepsis (1–2.7%)
- limited transient skin bruising in almost all the patients

Other complications of ESWL have been reported sporadically including bowel perforations, liver or spleen haematomas, and severe retroperitoneal haemorrhage.

Beside the above mentioned complications, the deleterious effect of the X-rays widely used in ESWL should not be overlooked. The mean total effective radiation exposure received by the patient per year varies according to the stone number, size and localization. It was calculated to be around 15.9, 13.3 and 27 milliSieverts (mSV) for renal stones, ureteric stones, and multiple stone locations respectively [50]. The International Commission on Radiological Protection (ICRP) guidelines recommends the occupational radiation dose not to exceed the safe threshold of 50 millisieverts (mSv) through a single year, or 20 mSv per year for a 5-year period for long-term treatment [51]. Therefore, considering that the average effective radiation exposure dose of 20 mSv per year should not be surpassed when the treatment has to be further treated for recurrent stones, one can easily deduct that localization of multiple stones should safely be performed using non-radiating means, namely ultrasonography for renal stones group, or the patient be offered alternative treatment, i.e. ureteroscopy for ureteral stones group.

11.3.1.6   Success Rate of ESWL

After excluding anatomical abnormalities of the kidney and urinary tract, the overall success rate for well-selected patients has been reported to reach 90% in many series and depends on the stone site, size, and composition (see below) [33, 52–54]. However many of these studies have ignored small residual renal fragments of less than 4 mm, and a study assessing the absolute stone clearance reported a "corrected" stone fragment-free rate of 57.5% [55].

11.3.1.7   Factors Influencing the Outcome of ESWL Treatment

- Higher BMI: Obesity increases the skin-to-stone distance (SSD). However the cut-off of the SSD above which a stone is unlikely to be fragmented is not clearly defined, **varying from 9 to 14 cm** [56, 57]. **SSD was shown to be the only independent predictor of success on multivariate analyses** [56, 58]**, and a better correlation was found**

between stone clearance and a BMI of around 27, while a **BMI of around 31 was related to residual stones** [58].

- Stone attenuation values detected by NCCT: This is in relation with the stone composition and is a good predictor of ESWL resistence. However it is worth noting that this relation is not absolutely linear since the chemical composition and the crystal structure of stones are not strictly correlated to their attenuation to X rays. This would explain why Cystine stones are more resistant to ESWL than calcium oxalate dihydrate stones despite having less density on NCCT and also why Whewellite stones are more resistant to ESWL than Wheddelite despite having almost the same density (see Table 9.2).

  The cut-off of density above which a stone is unlikely to be fragmented is also not yet clearly defined. An old study has shown that stone clearance was observed for attenuation of around 580 HU, while higher attenuation of around 910 HU exposed to failure [59]. However a more recent prospective study proposed to consider a density of 970 HU as the threshold below which the stones are likely to be fragmented after one ESWL session [60].

- Other factors: smooth contour, lower calyceal location and stone >15 mm have less satisfactory result [61]. But no statistical difference was detected between upper and distal ureteral localization [58].

11.3.1.8   Patient's Satisfaction

A prospective evaluation of nearly 3000 patients revealed a higher than 90% satisfaction rate following ESWL treatment [62].

11.3.1.9   Place of a DJ Stent in the ESWL

Before the era of retrograde intra-renal surgery (RIRS), it was commonplace to insert a DJ stent for renal stones greater than 20 mm considered for ESWL, as a safety measure to prevent secondary stone fragments impaction and obstruction. This is still in practice in institutions where the technique of flexible ureteroscopy is not yet well developed. **For ureteric stones however, many studies have consistently shown that the presence of ureteral stents adversely affects the ESWL outcome**, either by unnecessarily increasing the number of sessions [63], or affecting the stone-free rate [64], or causing significant side effects (dysuria, urgency, frequency, and suprapubic pain) [53]. Even if the DJ stents are removed prior to the procedure, it has been shown that they would still impact negatively on the ESWL outcomes, because of the induced paralysis of the ureteral smooth muscle. Some authors advise therefore to consider patients with a recent ureteral stent history for intracorporeal lithotripsy rather than for ESWL [65]. Logically expert panels do not recommend routine stenting for patients considered for ESWL [15, 16]. Another complication resulting from the DJ stent is the liability of this foreign body to become incrusted with calcifications, and difficult to remove when left for several months. It can also be forgotten or neglected by a non-compliant patient for years, resulting in recurrent UTI, and even in spontaneous fragmentation and passage with urine, namely stenturia [66] (Fig. 11.6a, b).

11.3.2   Antegrade Stone Chemolysis (Percutaneous Irrigation Chemolysis)

This historical treatment has been abandoned since the advent of RIRS. It was indicated for persistent residual calculi after various standard therapies such as ESWL, PCNL, and pyelolithotomy or nephrolithotomy. It was credited with some positive results as an appropriate management for stones in inadequately drained sites, and for patients with high anesthetic risks [67]. It was mostly used for infective stones (struvite) in an attempt to render the patient completely stone-free,

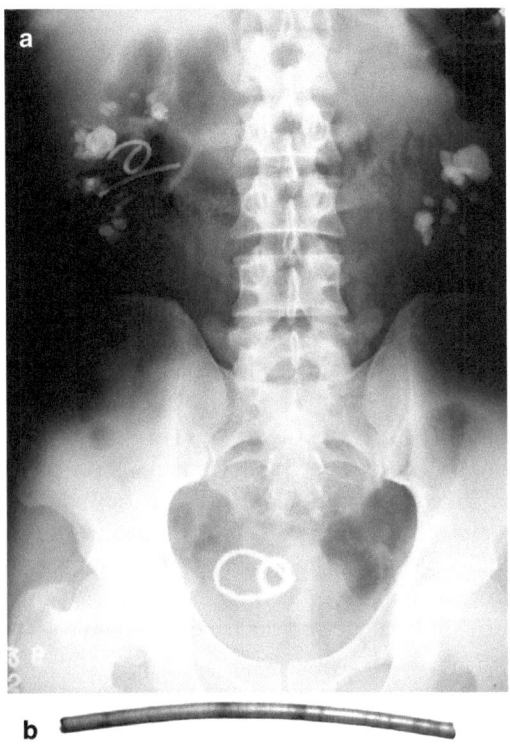

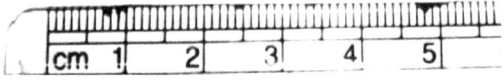

FIGURE 11.6 (**a**) Plain abdominal radiography showing fragmented pieces of a DJ stent in the bladder and the right kidney. From Singh and Gupta [66]. Creative Commons Attribution License. (**b**) An approximately 5-cm long piece of stent that has been passed through the urethra. From Singh and Gupta [66]. Creative Commons Attribution License

using Suby's G solution or 10% hemiacidrin, which is also effective in dissolving apatite and carbonate stones. Different solutions were used for other types of stones: Tromethamine-E or acetylcysteine for cystine calculi, sodium bicarbonate or potassium citrate solution for uric acid stones in combination with oral alkalinisation [68]. Renacidin® irrigation was used for struvite and apatite renal stones, but was also intravesically infused in an attempt to dissolve struvite or apatite bladder calculi, or as a preventive means against urethral and cystostomy catheters incrustations.

With the advent of RIRS, antegrade stone chemolysis approach has been neglected in the daily practice for the last two decades because it requires long hospital stay (2–4 weeks) and is not cost-effective. One of the last clinical studies attempting to revive this treatment approach was published in 2013 on 29 patients with infectious staghorn calculi [69]. It showed interesting results of the use of antegrade stone chemolysis as an adjuvant treatment after PCNL in patients deemed unfit for further interventions. More recently an in-vitro study suggested that several organic acids, namely hydroxyacetic acid, lactic acid, and α-ketoglutaric acid are superior to citric acid in dissolving urinary phosphate calculi, and could be regarded as promising solutions for chemolysis treatment [70]. The clinical echoes of these efforts are awaited.

11.3.3   Ureteroscopy

11.3.3.1   History

The first ureteroscopy was performed by **Young and McKay** in 1912, but was only reported by the year 1929 [71, 72]. The first ureteroscopic procedures were reported by **Goodman** in 1977 and **Lyon et al.** in 1978 [73, 74]. These early procedures were performed using pediatric cystoscopes and were merely limited to the lower ureteric end. Nonetheless they launched the concept of rigid ureteroscopy that was further developed later on with the advent of longer and thinner scopes.

Marshall reported on the first experience of the use of fiber optics in Urology in 1964 [75]. Flexible cystoscope was further developed with the introduction of actively deflectable ureteroscopes and irrigation channel, and the first series were published by **Bagley et al.** in 1987 [76] and **Kavoussi et al.** in 1989 [77]. This opened the era of Retrograde Intra-Renal Surgery (RIRS) which is defined as the use of a flexible ureteroscope to treat an intrarenal pathology such as a stone or a tumour. During the last decade, digital flexible ureteroscope with chip-on-the-tip technology was introduced and significantly improved the pictures and video quality compared to the fiber-optic flexible ureteroscopes [78].

11.3.3.2   Indications

In this paragraph, we will consider both the rigid and flexible ureteroscopies.

- Ureteral and renal stones resistant to ESWL.
- Obstructing ureteral stone: Here ureteroscopy is indicated ab initio.
- Large renal stone >20 mm: In our common practice a flexible Ureteroscopy is indicated in this scenario and we only consider PCNL for larger stones of >3–4 cm. However because of the increased need for multiple RIRS sessions and placement of a ureteral stent, expert panels recommend PCNL be considered as the first-line therapy for any stone >20 mm [3, 12].
- Solitary kidneys [79].
- Obesity and morbid obesity [80].
- Bilateral renal and/or ureteral stones: Safe treatment in one session [81].
- Lower calyceal stone.
- Horseshoe kidney [82].

11.3.3.3   Technique of Ureteroscope Insertion

As mentioned in the preface, the description of the operative steps provided here is not intended to replace more comprehensive and specialized manuals that should be used as references when one wants to start endourology practices or to improve his skills. However efforts were made here to provide to the reader the essential information and/or a practical reminder when he is preparing to enter the Operating Theatre for ureteroscopic procedures. Articles on "Tips and tricks" are produced every year by expert authors because surgery in general, and endourology in particular, is an ever-changing field where there is always something to improve. Herein let's share with some of those authors the following anonymous quoting sometimes attributed to Einstein: "the definition of insanity is doing the same thing over and over again and expecting different results" [83].

- Generally a first generation cephalosporin antibiotic (Cefazolin) is given on induction for prophylaxis. When anticipating a lengthy RIRS procedure, a mechanical thromboprophylactic measure should be started consisting of lower limbs intermittent pneumatic compression (IPC).
- As for almost all endourological procedures, the patient in placed in lithotomy position. After the introduction of a 30° cystoscope, the ureteral orifice corresponding to the stone side is identified and a standard PTFE (polytetra-fluoroethylene) guidewire is passed through the working channel into the ureteral orifice and advanced up to the renal pelvis, then eventually the superior calyx. At this point an open-ended 5-Fr ureteral catheter can be optionally inserted through the guidewire (which is removed immediately) for the injection of a diluted contrast material if one wishes to document the uretero-renal anatomy and locate any eventual obstruction or filling-defect on fluoroscopy. The guidewire is then replaced and the open-ended catheter is removed after this study. Before insertion of the ureteroscope, it is commonplace to introduce a 2-cm balloon to dilate the ureteric orifice for 1–2 min, but this practice is not encouraged by all authors and indeed is not always necessary, especially when a DJ-stent has been present, as the ureter will generally be well dilated in this circumstance. After its use, the balloon is deflated and removed along with the cystoscope taking care to leave the guidewire as a safety measure.

- Before the ureteroscope insertion, the bladder should be emptied to prevent compression of the intramural part of the ureter, which may preclude ureteroscope passage. Intermittent or continuous bladder emptying should also be ensured during a lengthy flexible ureteroscopy.
- For practical reason, the rigid or semi-rigid ureteroscope is preferred for ureteral stones and the flexible one is used for renal stones. This is simply because the ureteral stones are reachable by the rigid or semi-rigid ureteroscope which is easier to manipulate and quicker to insert. The semi-rigid ureteroscope also allows the use of various semi-rigid stone fragmentation tools (EKL, EHL, pneumatic, or ultrasound probe) resulting in a rapid stone disimpaction and fragmentation. The flexible ureteroscope will be necessary to reach the pelvi-calyceal system, being suitable to cross an angulated pelvi-ureteric junction, and being deflectable to reach all the calyceal groups (superior, mid-polar and inferior) allowing a full ureterorenoscopy. Nonetheless the use of flexible ureteroscopes requires more skill and only a limited number of tools can be used through this approach to treat a renal stone, including the laser fiber and the miniaturized electrohydraulic probe. Flexible ureteroscopy is a longer procedure than the rigid ureteroscopy and is generally not preferred for stone location attainable by the latter.
- When a rigid or semi-rigid ureteroscope is to be used, it is inserted beside the guidewire up to the level of the stone. If there is some initial difficulty to enter the ureteric orifice, turning the semi-rigid ureteroscope 90°–180° is a recommended maneuver to safely and successfully negotiate this critical point. This maneuver is called by French Urologists "technique du chausse-pied" (the shoehorn technique) and is also useful when inserting a flexible ureteroscope through a hydrophilic guidewire [84]. In some cases, the semi-rigid ureteroscope cannot be pushed upward due to ureteral edema generally encountered just below the level of the stone at the pelvic brim. It is then recommended to insert a second standard PTFE wire as a navigating guidewire through the working channel of the

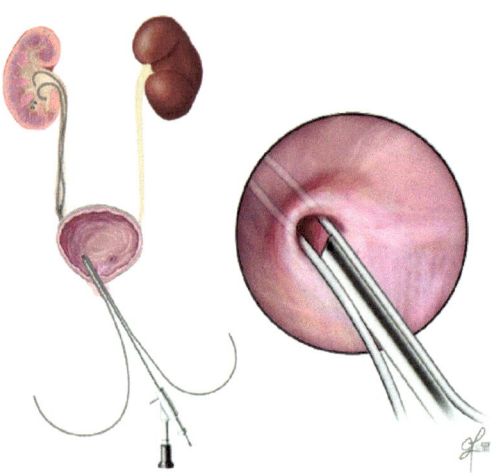

FIGURE 11.7 The semirigid ureteroscope is advanced between two wires into the ureteral orifice ("Ladder Technique"). Reproduced from Noble MJ and Esac WE [85], with permission from Springer

ureteroscope which is then progressively pushed up. Sometimes it may be necessary to retrieve the semi-rigid ureteroscope while leaving the second guidewire in-situ, then reinserting the instrument back between the two guidewires in a so-called "railroading or ladder technique" [85] (Fig. 11.7). If all the above maneuvers are ineffective, the lower ureter should be dilated with a balloon catheter (Boston® or Cook®). This can produce an effective dilatation upto 15-Fr from the ureteral orifice to the iliac level. It should always be kept in mind that when difficulty persists in the ureteroscope insertion despite the abovementioned maneuvers, calling for help from a more expert colleague, or terminating the procedure by inserting a DJ stent and coming back after 2–4 weeks is the safest decision [83]. Never forget the principle of "Primum non nocere" (first do no harm); so don't try to realize heroic exploits at the expense of the patient's safety; you will not impress anybody and, on the contrary, you will be the target of acrimonious criticisms, often beyond the harm you actually caused.

- When a flexible ureteroscope is used, the first ordinary guidewire should be changed to a hydrophylic (Nitinol) guidewire through an intermediate open-ended ureteral catheter, as the fragile flexible ureteroscope is to be inserted only through this slippery and atraumatic guidewire. As mentioned above, rotating the flexible ureteroscope may be necessary to allow its intramural passage. However this depends on the ureteroscope tip design: rotation is required if the working channel is eccentric in order to position the working guidewire ventrally; but this maneuver is not required for some newer ureteroscopes with smaller tips and centrally located working channel [86] (Fig. 11.8a, b). If there is narrowing or edema of the ureter, the use of a ureteral access sheath (UAS) is recommended to allow progression of the flexible ureteroscope up to the kidney.

- Gravity irrigation system with saline may sometimes be sufficient when one uses the rigid ureteroscope, but a manual or pump pressure is often necessary. However, due its narrow irrigating channel, a flexible ureteroscope almost always requires a direct irrigation under manual pressure using a 60-mL syringe. Intrarenal navigation with a flexible ureteroscope requires the Surgeon to be well oriented with regard to the 12 O'Clock position (the so-called "North" pole of the endourologist). This is particularly important when a fixed camera (such as with the digital ureteroscope) is used as opposed to a pendulous one, since it will turn during manipulation and produce an upside down image on the monitor. A proposed trick to detect the 12 O'Clock position is the injection of few air bubbles in the upper urinary tract [87].

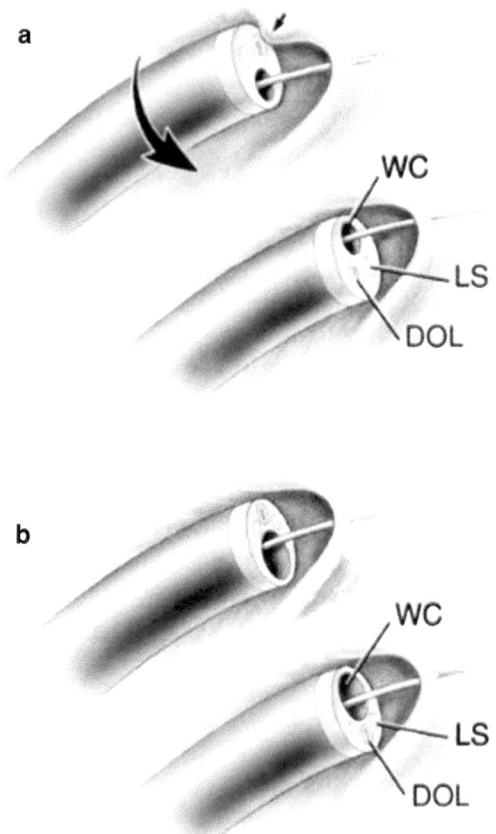

FIGURE 11.8 (**a**, **b**) The intramural passage of the flexible uretero-scope varies with ureteroscope tip design. If the working channel is eccentrically placed (**a**), the ureteroscope must be rotated to position the working guidewire ventrally. The newer scopes with smaller tips and centrally located working channel (**b**) do not require rotation to be passed in the intramural ureter. *WC* working channel, *LS* light source, *DOC* distal optical lens. From Rabah DM and Fabrizio MD [86], with permission from John Wiley and Sons

11.3.3.4   Energy Sources

The energy sources used for stone ablation and their mechanisms of action can be summarized as follows [88–90]:

- Ballistic lithotripsy: The term "ballistic" comes from the Latin word "Ballista" (a military machine used for throwing heavy stones) which derived from the Greec verb "ballein" (to throw). In Military language, this term refers to projectiles propelled by air drag, gravity, or rocket power. In our context, it represents a stone destruction method in which the pulsatile compression produced by air (pneumatic lithotripsy) or electromechanical forces (EKL: Electrokinetic lithotripsy) is transmitted through a semi-rigid metallic rod whose tip is in contact with the stone (Fig. 11.9). Pneumatic lithotripter is well exemplified by

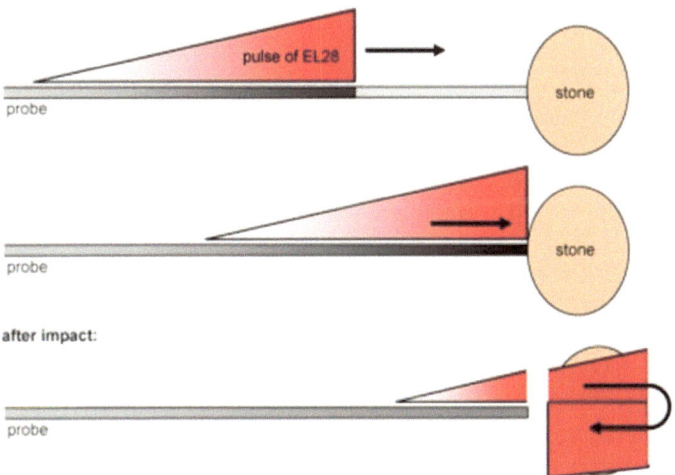

FIGURE 11.9 Mechanism of action of Electrokinetic Lithotripsy: fast kinetic pulses are generated in an electromagnetic field and transmitted to a rigid rod. In the rod steep longitudinal shock pulses are forwarded to the tip. The stone which is in close contact to the tip is effectively fragmented. Can be used in the ureter (tight ureter stones), urinary bladder and for percutaneous kidney stone fragmentation (From and with permission of Walz Elektronik, Germany)

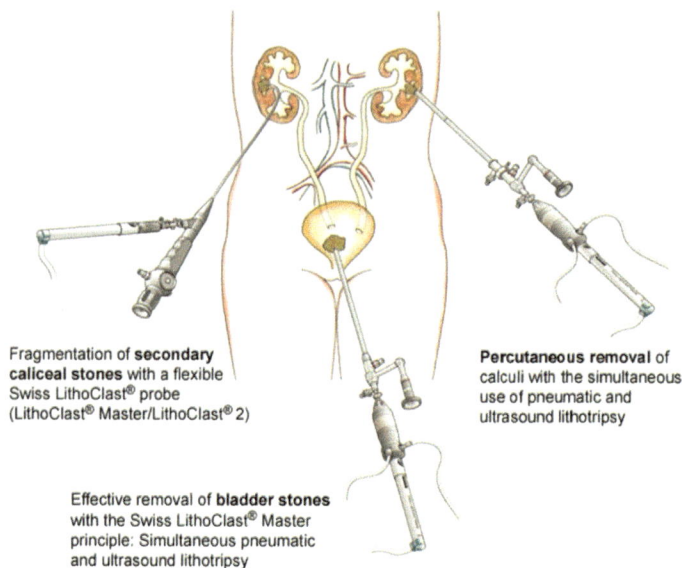

Fragmentation of **secondary caliceal stones** with a flexible Swiss LithoClast® probe (LithoClast® Master/LithoClast® 2)

Percutaneous removal of calculi with the simultaneous use of pneumatic and ultrasound lithotripsy

Effective removal of **bladder stones** with the Swiss LithoClast® Master principle: Simultaneous pneumatic and ultrasound lithotripsy

FIGURE 11.10 The Swiss Lithoclast®Master. Credit E.M.S. Electro Medical Systems S.A

the Swiss Lithoclast®. Flexible pneumatic lithotripsy probes have also been developed, but their use is still limited.

- Ultrasonic Lithotripsy: The principle of ultrasonic lithotripsy consists of transforming electrical energy into ultrasound energy through the excitation of a piezoelectric crystal. Acoustic waves with frequency of 23–25 kHz are produced and transmitted through the rigid sonotrode to the stone which vibrates and fragments. The Swiss Lithoclast ®Master combines both ultrasonic and pneumatic energies and has also an incorporated Suction System, namely the Swiss LithoVac® technology (Fig. 11.10).

- Electrohydraulic lithotripsy (EHL): The mechanism of this energy can be summarised as follows: electrical discharge released in a liquid medium → spark at the tip of the probe which is in direct contact with the stone → thermal energy

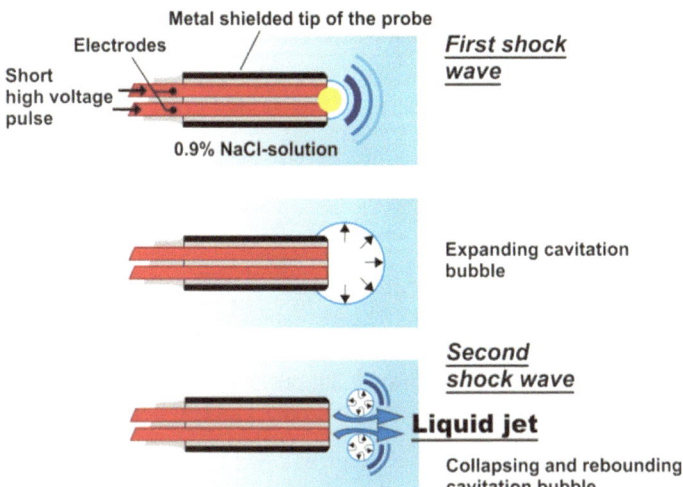

FIGURE 11.11 Disintegration of urinary or common bile duct calculi by a shock wave that results from an intracorporeal electric discharge. The probe is advanced to the stone through the working channel of an endoscope. The position is monitored via direct endoscopic view and via x-ray. A controlled, very fast electric discharge centered at the tip of the probe generates a spark plasma. This expanding plasma and later the collapse of a cavitation bubble create sharp rising shock waves which disintegrate the stone in seconds (From and with permission of Walz Elektronik, Germany)

→ large amount of caloric energy in a small space → vaporization of a small quantity of the irrigation fluid → gas bubble formation at the tip of the probe → rapid bubble expansion (4–11 mm in 400–500 µs) pushing the liquid with force → hydraulic shockwaves → stone fragmentation (Fig. 11.11). This energy can be used for ureteric as well for renal stones because of the availability of miniaturized 2–3 Fr flexible electrode usable for RIRS as well as antegrade percutaneous access [89] (Fig. 11.12).

- Lasers: The term "Laser" is an acronym for "**l**ight **a**mplification by **s**timulated **e**mission of **r**adiation". The first working Laser was invented by the American Engineer and Physicist Theodore Harold Maiman (1927–2007) in

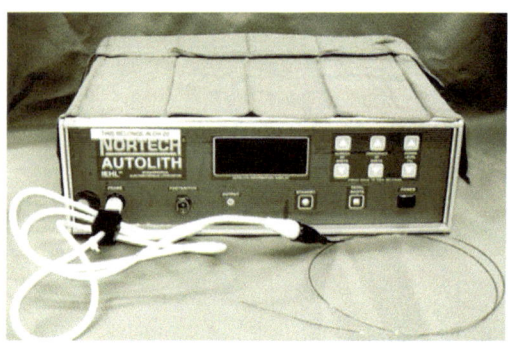

Figure 11.12 Electrohydraulic lithotrite (note the miniaturized flexible probe). Reproduced from Miller J and Stoller ML [89] with permission from Springer

1960. The first clinically successful laser lithotrite was the coumarin pulse dye laser reported in 1987 [91]. However this Laser could not fragment cystine stones. Successful early clinical experiences of the holmium:YAG laser for intracorporeal lithotripsy of urinary calculi were reported in the middle of the 1990s.

Lasers with pulsatile-type emission are particularly used for stone ablation due to their potential to deliver short bursts of energy, creating therefore a high power with less or no heating of the surrounding tissue. These include:

- "Pulsed-dye" laser: has 1 µs pulse duration and 504 nm wavelength.
- FREDDY Nd:YAG laser: This is the so-called Frequency-doubled double-pulse Nd:YAG with 532–1064 ng wavelength. FREDDY Nd:YAG laser causes stone fragmentation through the generation of plasma bubbles which collapse and generate a mechanical shock [92].
- Holmium-yttrium aluminum garnet (Ho:YAG) laser: With its 2150 nm wavelength, Ho:YAG laser is now considered the most efficient and cost-effective energy source for intracorporeal lithotripsy, being effective

even for cystine, calcium oxalate monohydrate and Brushite stones. It causes stone destruction by vaporisation [92].

- Erbium:YAG laser: This is a newer laser type having 2940 nm wavelength. Initial reports showed that the Er:YAG could be more efficient than the Ho:YAG laser [93, 94] but is still not yet widely used probably because of the larger wavelength which precludes its transmission through the standard available silica fibres and requires special mid-infrared fibres which are typically less flexible, more expensive and less biocompatible than silica fibres [95].

- Thulium laser: This is another new fiber still under evaluation. It has the advantages of having a tunable wavelength and a diameter of only 18 µm which allows an easy coupling of the laser radiation into small-core optical fibers [95].

- As opposed to the above Lasers featured with a pulsatile-type energy emission, Nd:YAG is a continuous emission laser. This 1064 nm — wavelength laser exposes therefore to a high risk of tissue damage and is not suitable for stone ablation. Nonetheless its high coagulative necrosis potential and excellent hemostasis capacity have opened other surgical applications to this Laser source: it is used to perform tissue incisions or tumour resection and destruction.

Advantages and Disadvantages of Various Energy Sources

- Ultrasonic and ballistic lithotripters such as Electrokinetic Lithotripsy (EKL) and pneumatic Swiss Lithoclast are used with the rigid ureteroscope for ureteral stones. They have the advantages of a quick fragmentation of impacted stones, but these energies expose to an increased risk of stone retropulsion. EKL was shown to have a very high efficacy in fragmenting the stones (99.3%), including some stones that have resisted to Electrohydraulic (EHL) lithotripter, but the stone-free rate was only 80% after a single procedure because of stone retropulsion (12%) and retained ureteric fragments (8%) [96]. Because of the risk of retropulsion, it is advised to have a flexible uretero-scope available when treating a proximal ureteral stone with ballistic lithotripsy means. Authors have advocated the injection of K-Y or Lidocaine jelly 2% above the stone or the insertion of a Stone Cone™ device as means to minimize stone retrograde migration [97, 98]. Other proposed means are the Ntrap®, the Accordion®, BackStop® [99], etc.

- EHL and pneumatic lithotripsy were shown to have comparable efficacy when performed for ureteral stones with success rate of 85.3% and 89.5% respectively, but the former exposed to a significantly higher rate of ureteral injury than the latter with 17.6% and 2.6%, respectively [100]. **Consequently AUA experts recommend the avoidance of EHL as first-line modality for in-situ lithotripsy of a ureteral stone** [16].

- Urological Surgeons may opt for a Holmium:YAG Laser fragmentation when aiming to minimize ureteral mucosal injury and stone retropulsion. The use of a Holmium-YAG Laser fiber is a time-consuming procedure compared to ballistic lithotripsy [101], but this drawback is compensated by its 100% stone fragmentation rate and a better safety profile as shown in an ex-vivo pig ureter model [102]. The Holmium:YAG Laser is the most frequently energy means used in association with the flexible ureteroscope due to its diameter and better flexibility. Laser fibers exist in two different groups: Small (200–275 μm) and large diameters (365–500 μm). The two groups perform equally in term of stone ablation, but the advantage of the formers is the better irrigation and deflection potentials and less stone retropulsion, and their drawback is the more rapid "burn-back" effect with a subsequent rapid tip degradation requiring more frequent trimming [87]. A safe strategy is to start with low pulse energy and frequency settings, such as 0.6 J at 6 Hz. The energy settings can then progressively be increased upto 1–1.2 J if the stone is very hard [90].

11.3.3.5 Technique for Stone Ablation Using a Holmium Laser and Stone Fragments Retrieval

Several techniques can be applied for stone ablation with Holmium laser: initially it is recommended to perform "painting" of the stone, and at the end to proceed to "popcorning" of the multiple small residual fragments. Other techniques such as "dancing", "chipping", or "fragmenting" need to be adapted to the stone characteristics. The stone "drilling" or "perforation" should be avoided to prevent formation of large multiple fragments, as these will increase the work load and the duration of the procedure [103]. After an in-situ lithotripsy the resulting fragments of a ureteral stone can be removed using a forceps or a Nitinol basket (Dormia). Renal stone fragments can only be removed using a long Nitinol basket, but as for the ureteral stone, they can also be left in place if they appear small enough to pass spontaneously.

11.3.3.6 Safety Measures When a Mucosal Injury Occurs

When a ureteral or pelvi-calyceal mucosa injury occurs, a diluted contrast material should be injected to exclude the possibility of extravasation which calls for immediate termination of the procedure and insertion of a DJ stent. Retrograde pyelography is also advisable at the end of every procedure for documentation purpose.

11.3.3.7 Controversies About the Use of Ureteral Access Sheaths (UAS) in RIRS

UAS may be helpful to ensure an absolute stone-free status (required for infective stones) by allowing multiple and rapid flexible ureteroscope removals and reintroductions into the ureter along with the Nitinol Dormia basket. They lower the intra-renal pressure and eliminate the need to drain the bladder during prolonged procedures. It has been calculated that the average baseline pressure within the collecting system was 13.6 mmHg, and when the ureteroscope reaches the renal pelvis, the pressure rises to 40.6 mmHg and 94.4 mmHg respectively when a UAS is used or not [104]. This fact should not be overlooked when considering that by minimizing the rise of intrapelvic pressure, the UAS is potentially protective against pyelovenous and pyelolymphatic backflow, lowering thereby the risk of an infection spreading into the bloodstream in struvite stones or undiagnosed UTI. Additionally UAS offers a mechanical protection against the burst of an atrophied thin renal parenchyma frequently seen in long-standing stones with recurrent pyelonephritis. Outside the urolithiasis field, working in a low intrapelvic pressure also provides a safer management of upper-tract urothelial carcinoma minimizing the risk of hematogenic or lymphatic spread of malignant cells [104]. A UAS remains very useful in facilitating the insertion of a flexible ureteroscope through a narrow ureteral lumen and they are more cost-effective than balloon dilatation. Indeed some high-volume centers have reported the use of UAS in the great majority of their cases (around 90%), especially when dealing with large stone burdens [87].

However studies did not show any advantage from the UAS use with regard to the outcome, i.e. the stone-free rate, complication rate or average number of procedures per patients [105]. Moreover it should be remembered that UAS are not required when one is not planning to basket retrieve the stone fragments, and their use have been sometimes associated with ureteral trauma and perforation in inexperienced hands. They are suspected to have potentials to induce segmental ischemia of the ureter and secondary stenosis [72]. Ureteral wall injury associated with UAS was reported in as much as 46.5% of cases, including severe injury up to the smooth muscle layers in 13.3%; associated risk factors were male gender and older age, while a pre-operative Double-J stenting was shown to significantly decrease the occurrence of severe injury [106]. It should be remembered however that expert panels plead against the routine use of a D-J stent prior to ureteroscopy, reserving it only for specific indications (ureteral stenosis, impacted stone with sepsis, etc.) [1, 3].

Some tricks have been proposed to decrease the risks associated with the use of UAS [87, 107]:

- performing an initial semi-rigid ureteroscopy which will enable the ureteric orifice to be dilated, will detect any ureteric stone and will assess whether the ureter has enough capacity to accommodate the UAS without damage or not.
- advancing the sheath slowly through a guidewire under pulsed fluoroscopy monitoring and watching for any eventual buckling in the bladder or any early resistance or failure to progress.
- positioning the upper end of the UAS just below the PUJ, to allow full deflexion of the flexible scope.
- retrieving the scope and the UAS simultaneously at the end of the procedure, while keeping the scope's tip a few centimeters out of the sheath. This strategy allows one to detect any eventual ureteral mucosal injury.

11.3.3.8   Results

- Stone-free rates
  - Rigid ureteroscope: A large retrospective study conducted in 2007 and including 2129 patients with ureteral stones showed an initial stone-free rate of 73.3%, then further 5% of patients passed the residual stones spontaneously, while 21% needed ESWL, and ureterolithotomy or PCNL were required only in 14 patients (0.7%) [108]. Nowadays the results have been significantly improved and most recent studies frequently report success rate of over 85% after a single intervention [109, 110].
  - Flexible ureteroscope (RIRS): This largely depends on the size of the stone and the experience of the surgeon.

High-volume centers reported a stone-free rate of 77–79% after one session in the immediate post-operative period, which increased up to 82% and 95% 3 months after the procedure, respectively for stones larger and smaller than 2-cm diameter [87, 111, 112]. Encouraging results were achieved even with larger stones of 3–4 cm, where the primary stone-free rate was only 55%, but could improve to 80% after repeat sessions [87].

- Complications
  The overall intra-operative complications rate is 4.4–5.9% and the post-operative rate may reach 7.3% [110, 113]

  - Frequent: transient hematuria, fever, flank pain, urinary tract infection, and need for rehospitalisation. It is strongly recommended to exclude or treat UTI before any endourological stone removal, and also to give prophylactic antibiotics to all patients [15, 16]
  - Rare: Ureteral mucosal tear (2.4–2.7%), persistent haematuria for few days (0.7%), ureteral perforation (0.6–1%), ureteral stricture, mucosal eversion (0.08–0.4%), complete ureteral avulsion requiring nephrectomy (0.1–0.2%), urethral injury (0.08%), rupture of the Dormia basket catheter (0.16%).

- Predictive factors for intraoperative complications [110, 113, 114]:

  - Larger stones,
  - proximally located stones (for ureteral stones),
  - previous history of in situ lithotripsy,
  - longer operation duration,
  - lack of experience of the operator,
  - multiplicity of stones,
  - congenital renal abnormalities

Note: A further important factor significantly associated with complications is the non-compliance to the break'n'leave policy. When the surgeon aggressively endeavors to remove all the stone fragments after their breaking, including those who can easily pass spontaneously (<3 mm), he unnecessary lengthens the operation duration and increases the risk of iatrogenic injury [110].

11.3.3.9   The Need for DJ Stenting After Ureteroscopy (URS)

Uncomplicated ureteroscopy for distal ureteral calculi can safely be performed without placement of a ureteral stent, especially if an intraoperative ureteral dilation was not performed [115].

According to the AUA experts, a DJ stent insertion can safely be omitted when all of the following criteria are met: no suspicion of ureteric injury during URS, no evidence of ureteral stricture or other anatomical obstacles to stone fragment clearance, no impaired renal function, presence of a normal contralateral kidney, and no plan for a secondary URS procedure [16]. It is commonplace in this favorable scenario to insert a simple open-ended 5-Fr ureteral catheter that is fixed outside to the urethral catheter, and to remove both catheters at the same time after an inpatient 24-h observation.

However the insertion of a DJ stent is recommended after the treatment of large renal stones with incomplete clearance, or when a ureteral of calyceal mucosal injury has occurred, and is also advisable when a UAS has been used, based on the hypothesis that a mucosal edema secondary to the UAS visceral dilatation could cause temporary obstruction and pain [87].

11.3.3.10   RIRS vs PCNL

RIRS has shown comparable surgical results with single-session PCNL for patients harbouring a main stone size of 15–30 mm and located in the lower-pole calyx. However, RIRS can be performed more safely than PCNL with less bleeding. Stones in the lower-anterior minor calyx should be carefully removed during these procedures [116].

RIRS is a safer alternative to PCNL in patients with coagulopathy because the bleeding risk in these patients persists even after an apparent pre-operative normalization of the clotting disorder [117].

A recent study performed in our institution also demonstrated the feasibility and safety of a multistage RIRS for stones measuring 2–4 cm. Seventy-one patients were included and an 81% stone-free rate was achieved after a mean procedure number of 2.1 per patient [118].

Further advantages of the flexible ureteroscopy with holmium laser are the possibility to successfully treat stones in calyceal diverticula with stenotic infundibulum [119], the feasibility of a bilateral same-session procedure [81], the relative safety to deal with solitary and/or ectopic kidneys, and the possibility of an effective treatment in morbidly obese and severely kyphoscoliotic patients [120].

11.3.3.11   RIRS Combined with PCNL

A combined PCNL-RIRS approach has been introduced for over a decade ago aiming at reducing the number of access tracts, the retrograde treatment being used for stones not accessible percutaneously [121]. This combination has traditionally been performed with the patient in supine position. However it was also proved to be possible with the patient in prone split-leg position [122, 123].

Recently the prone flexible ureteroscopy was proposed in the University of Vermont to treat large renal stones with the advantage of a rapid conversion to prone PCNL when required without the need to change the patient's position. Seventy-five percent of patients were treated with ureteroscopy alone and 80% of those were rendered stone-free after one session only [124]. Experiences from another center confirmed the feasibility of this approach in the reverse way: PCNL was first performed in prone position and stone clearance was achieved in combination with RIRS without changing position [125].

11.3.3.12   The Future of Ureteroscopy

After the successful introduction of digital flexible uretero-scopes, two further steps are being tried: single-use uretero-scopes and robotic manipulation of the endoscope. These two technologies have proven advantages, but are still evaluated for cost-effectiveness and are not yet widely distributed. Furthermore, the developement of nanotechnology and robotics may open many other perspectives in the future which are well beyond our imagination [126].

11.3.4   PCNL

11.3.4.1   History

The technique of percutaneous nephrolithotomy (PCNL) was first described in 1976 by Fernstrom and Johannson [127], and became rapidly developed and standardized in the following years [128].

11.3.4.2   Indications

Guy's grade III or IV,[3] i.e. complete or partial staghorn renal calculi. In the pediatric population, a stone burden of >2 cm

---

- [3]The Guy's classification helps to predict the outcome of PCNL. It comprises of four grades [129]:

  - grade I: solitary stone in mid/lower pole or solitary stone in the pelvis with simple anatomy
  - grade II: solitary stone in upper pole or multiple stones in a patient with simple anatomy or a solitary stone in a patient with abnormal anatomy
  - grade III: multiple stones in a patient with abnormal anatomy or stones in a caliceal diverticulum or partial staghorn calculus
  - grade IV: staghorn calculus or any stone in a patient with spina bifida or spinal injury.

- Other stone scoring systems include the Clinical Research Office of the Endourological Society (CROES) nomogram, the S.T.O.N.E. (stone size, tract length, obstruction, number of involved calices, and essence/stone density) nephrolithometry, and the Seoul National University Renal Stone Complexity (S-ReSC) score [130].

is a sufficient indication for PCNL. For hard stones (>900 HU on CT scan), even stones within 1–2 cm size can be considered for PCNL, when the anatomy of the kidney or the stone location are unfavorable for an endourological approach. Other indications are significant renal obstruction and infected stones [30].

It is strongly recommended to obtain a non-contrast CT scan before any stone-targeting procedure in general. For PCNL in particular and especially for patients with complex stones or anatomy, a contrast-enhanced CT scan is also required to better define the collecting system and the ureteral anatomy [16]. A functional isotope study, preferably performed with MAG-3 radiotracer, is also indicated when there is a clinical suspicion of a significant loss of renal function of the kidney to be treated. This is important not only to justify the treatment when a satisfactory function of the renal unit is proven, but also as a medico-legal caution to prove that some deterioration of the renal function pre-existed before the intervention.

11.3.4.3   Contraindications

- Coagulopathy
- Infection/fever
- Pregnancy
- Abdominal wall tumour at or near the puncture site
- Ipsilateral renal or upper tract urothelial tumour
- Solitary kidney: The recommendation to avoid PCNL in solitary kidneys still stands valid despite some investigators have published successful series of this procedure where the stone-free and complication rates (mainly bleeding) were 67% and 30% respectively [131]. In this study, factors associated with increased bleeding were operative time and increased number of tracts.
  Although some damage does occur to the nephrons, as shown by renal scintigraphy studies [132], this remains negligible and the strongest reason for the contra-indication of PCNL in solitary kidney remains the risk of vascular injury.

11.3.4.4   Surgical Technique

After antibioprophylaxis (third generation cephalosporin) and mechanical thrombophylaxis measures (intermittent pneumatic compression), retrograde insertion of a ureteric tube (5-Fr open-ended catheter) into the kidney of interest is generally performed to allow for contrast material or methylene blue dye injection during surgery.

Then the PCNL proper will start by a needle puncture of the calyceal system under U/S and/or fluoroscopy guidance. The fully anesthetized patient is either in prone (classical) [133] or in supine position technique. The latter approach is also called "Valdivia technique", named after the Spanish Urologist Valdivia-Urìa, who introduced it in 1987 using a 3-L serum bag below the ipsilateral flank and advocated it for its anesthesiological benefit among other advantages. However the first series was reported only 11 years later [134]. The popularity of this approach was enhanced several years later when a so-called Galdakao-modified Valdivia position was introduced, featured by a modified lithotomy position allowing combination of a retrograde flexible ureteroscopic access with the percutaneous approach [135–137] (Fig. 11.13a, b). To date not less than five different supine positions have been described, including the "complete supine", the Valdivia proper, the Galdakao-modified Valdivia, the Barts modified Valdivia and the Barts flank-free modified supine position [138].

The prone position implies changing the patient posture after insertion of the ureteral catheter from the lithotomy position, i.e. from the supine to prone position using a side trolley parallel to the operating table in a co-ordinated manner.

In the majority of cases, the puncture aims at the lower posterior calyceal group. Puncturing a posterior calyx is likely to cross the Brödel's bloodless line of the kidney, therefore causing less bleeding risk, but also provides a direct path to the renal pelvis [133]. With the patient in prone position, a good starting point for this puncture is situated 1 cm inferior and 1 cm medial to the tip of the 12th rib [139] (Fig. 11.14a).

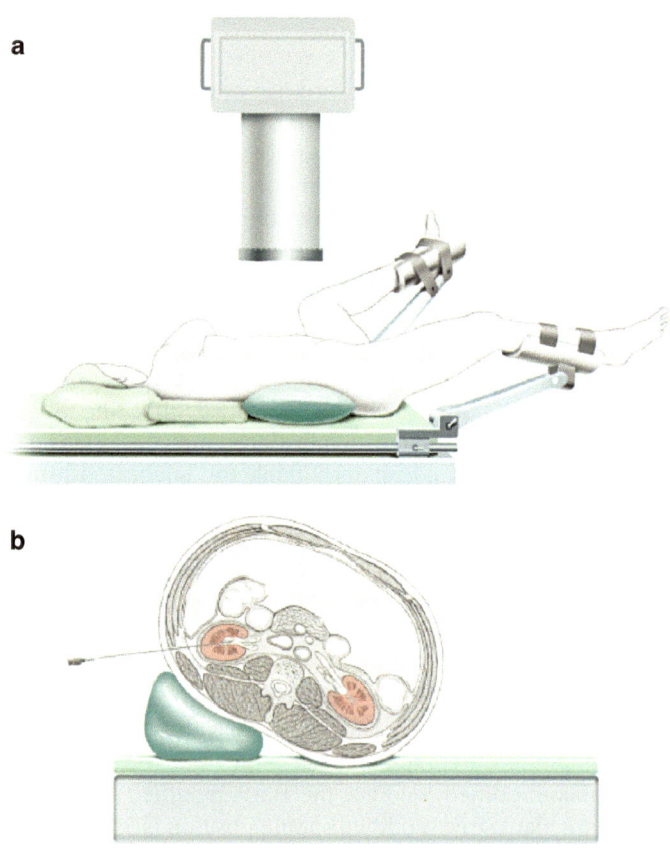

FIGURE 11.13 (**a**) The Galdakao-modified Valdivia position. (**b**) Direction of the needle in the Galdakao-modified Valdivia position. From Ibarluzea G [135]. With permission from John Wiley and Sons

In some circumstances, it is advisable to aim at the upper pole as this is favourable for a complete staghorn removal and also allows a direct access to the PUJ if desired [140]. Obviously the risk associated with an upper pole puncture is the possibility of a pleural injury. A trick to minimize this risk is to avoid any puncture above the 11th rib and to stay in the lateral half of the 12th rib, flush to the lateral border of the paraspinal muscles, in order to ensure an extrapleural needle

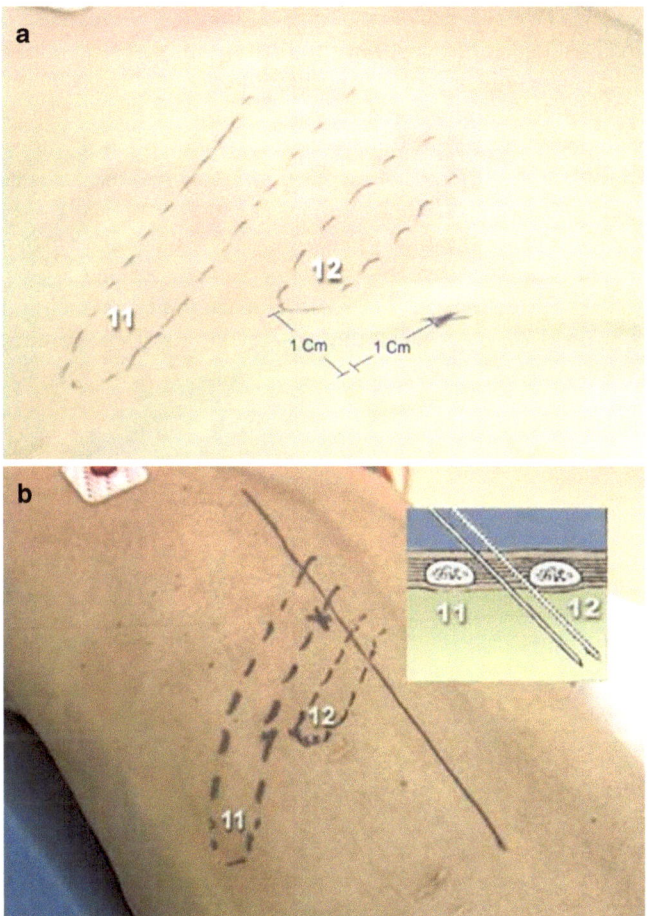

FIGURE 11.14 (**a**) For a lower pole puncture, a good starting point is 1 cm inferior and 1 cm medial to the tip of the 12th rib. The starting point is marked with an X. From Kim SC and Lingeman JE [139], with permission from Springer. (**b**) For a supracostal upper pole puncture, the point of entry at the skin is at the inferior border of the 11th rib and just lateral to the paraspinal muscles. This point of entry will allow the needle to enter the middle of interspace (solid needle of inset). If the entry point at the skin is at the midpoint between the 11th and 12th rib, the needle will come too close to the 12th rib (dashed needle of inset), and the rigid sheath will be difficult to place. From Kim SC and Lingeman JE [139], with permission from Springer

passage [139–142]. The puncture should also be carried out flush to the lower border of the 11th rib in order to avoid the rigid sheath hitting the 12th rib [139] (Fig. 11.14b). When the upper pole is approached from below the 12th rib through a so-called infra-costal puncture, the risk of pleural injury is minimized but the puncture angle is less favorable for subsequent intra-renal stone treatment [139].

When using the fluoroscopy guidance, one can either use the Bull's eye appearance of the needle (also called the Eye of the Needle technique) (Fig. 11.15), the triangulation technique, or even the hybrid technique where the angle of the needle

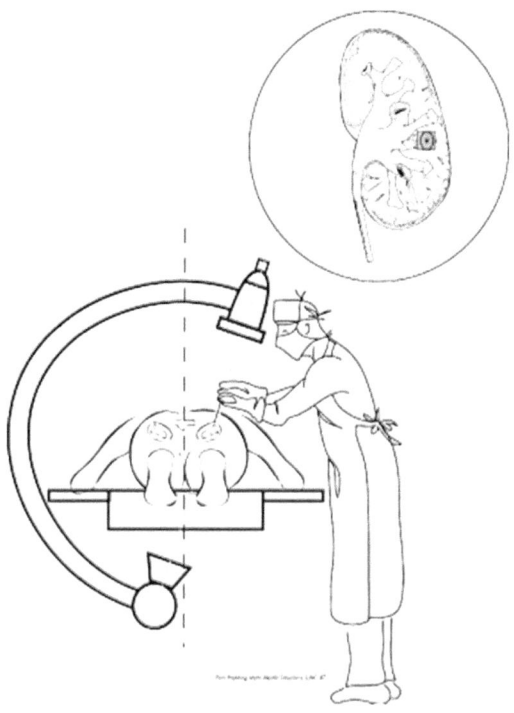

FIGURE 11.15 The C-arm rotation toward the surgeon to align the needle tip with the desired entry calyx. The inset shows the 'bull's eye' appearance of the needle on the fluoroscopy monitor. From Ko R et al. [140]. With permission from John Wiley and Sons

puncture on the skin surface is measured using a protractor [133, 140]. PCNL under a sole ultrasound-guidance is feasible and, with increased experience, carries a high stone-free rate (85.5%) with a very low complication profile as shown by a large Chinese study including over 8000 patients [143].

Dilatation of the tract is performed either using rigid dilators or balloon dilators. Rigid dilators include the sequential (Amplatz dilators) or telescopic coaxial dilators (Alken dilators).

The supine position has the following advantages:

- not necessitating to change the patient's positioning from the lithotripsy posture (hence less risk of central and peripheral nervous injury),
- being time-saving,
- avoiding the cardio-vascular restrictions caused by prone position, especially in obese patients,
- being an option for patients suffering from ankylosing spondilytis who cannot lie in prone position (risk of neck fracture), and
- reducing the X-ray exposure to the Surgeon.

However, as every medal has its reverse, the supine position has also some disadvantages:

- the rigid dilators and nephroscope can abut to the operating table as they will have an upward direction to the puncture site. The Galdakao-modified supine Valdivia position (see below) aims at avoiding this problem which can also be overcome by bringing the patient flush to the operating table edge, but the latter maneuver may create the second disadvantage below.
- X-ray blocking by the operating table edge inline with the treated kidney.

After a successful access to the calyceal system has been confirmed either by the observation of the retrogradely injected methylene blue exiting through the nephrostomy access, or by the contrast medium injected directly in the PCS, the tract is progressively dilated using a balloon, a metal telescopic, or Amplatz serial dilatation. Finally a sheath is inserted through which the nephroscope will be deployed to visualize and break the stone using either pneumatic, EKL, EHL, or a Holmium Laser fiber. Smaller stone fragments will be flushed out through the Amplatz by fluid pressure, and larger ones will be removed with a grasper.

The standard access sheaths are 24–30 Fr. However several centers have successfully performed mini-PCNL ('Miniperc') consisting of the use of smaller sheaths of 11–20 Fr with small rigid nephroscope and this technique has gained interest especially when dealing with pediatric population [144–146].

The miniaturization has been further developed up to the use of the so-called "Micropercutaneous nephrolithotomy" ('Microperc') using as small as a 4.85-F (1.6 mm outer diameter) 'all-seeing needle' with a 272-μm laser fibre and a 0.9 mm flexible fiberoptic [147–151] (Fig. 11.16a–c).

Tubeless PCNL has also been proposed for selected patients, where no post-op nephrostomy tube is left, nor a ureteral DJ stent, with the advantages of a shorter hospitalization and lower analgesic requirement while carrying similar outcomes to standard PCNL technique, i.e comparable stone-free and complications rates [151–154].

When considering the three main critical steps of PCNL, namely accurate puncture, passage and location of the guidewire into the pelvicalyceal system in such a way as to prevent its slipping out (the most ideal being passage of guidewire into the ureter), and tract dilatation, some authors have proposed a novel technique to help passage of the guidewire down the ureter in order to ensure a safe and accurate dilatation of the tract [155]. In this technique a semi-rigid ureteroscope is introduced percutaneously through the puncture and helps in maneuvering the guidewire into the upper ureter. However it should be remembered that having the guidewire secured in the PCS despite not progressing down the ureter is sufficient to proceed to a safe tract dilatation [156].

The concept of daycare PCNL was recently introduced by combining the micropercs and tubeless techniques with the use of a composite hemostatic tract seal [157].

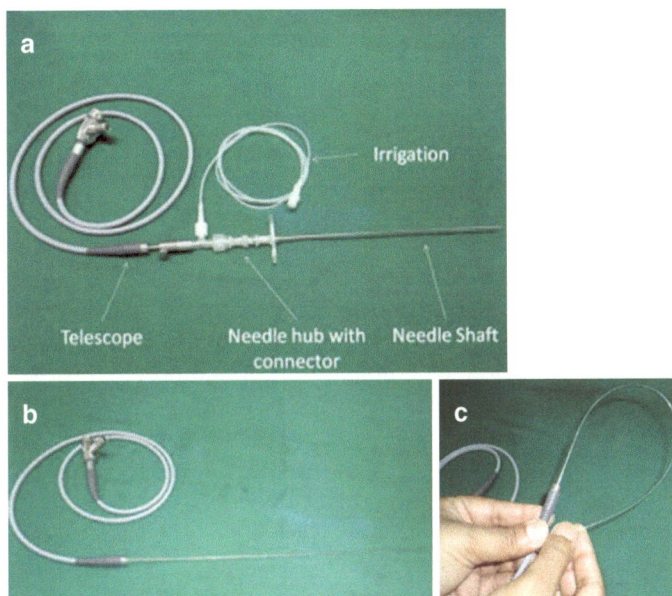

FIGURE 11.16 (**a**) 4.85 Fr "All seeing" needle in preparation for puncture. (**b**, **c**) Flexible fibreoptic telescope (0.9 mm). From Ganpule AP and Desai MR [147]. With permission from the Arab Association of Urology

Finally it is noteworthy remembering that the learning curve needed to master the PCNL technique is long and can only be completed in high volume institutions; it was observed that the mean operating time, the stone-free and the complication rates improved gradually to reach a plateau only after 60 cases [158].

11.3.4.5   Complications

In a review of 5750 PCNL procedures performed in English Institutions over a 5-year period, infections and hemorrhage were found to be the commonest complications of PCNL occurring in 5.5% and 1.4% respectively. The emergency readmission rate within 1 month post-operatively was 9% (almost one in ten patients), mainly due to UTI, sepsis, hemorrhage and acute urinary retention. The mortality rate within the first 30 post-operative days was 0.2% [159].

A Japanese study of nearly equal size (5537 cases) conducted over a 2-year period revealed that the median operating time using balloon dilation was significantly longer than with other techniques, and was also associated with more bleeding (9.4% vs 6.7%) and more transfusions (7.0% vs 4.9%) compared to other dilatation means, namely metal telescopic dilation, or Amplatz serial dilation [160]. In this study sheath size, operating time, stone load, and case load were shown to be independent factors associated with bleeding/transfusion.

Hereafter is a summary of complications that can occur after PCNL:

- Sepsis and fever
- Bleeding and need for transfusion and/or embolization. Herein a computed tomography angiography prior to the procedure was suggested in order to define the vascular anatomy and reduce the bleeding rate as well as the need of transfusions [161], but its use is not widely accepted.
- Urinary leak and urinoma
- Organ injury (colon, liver, spleen, pleura with pneumothorax)
- Major kidney injury with the need for conversion to open surgery
- Nephronic mass loss (it results in an apparently negligible loss of renal function, but may be of concern for initial borderline renal function).
- death

11.3.5   Cystolitholapaxy

Bladder stones account for 5% of urinary stones in the developed countries and the incidence is thought to be higher in developing countries.

Cystitholapaxy is traditionally indicated for bladder stone ≤4 cm and its safety has also been proven for children [162].

Conventional mechanical lithotripsy with serrated, jawed instruments is preferred for smaller stones (<2 cm) that can be trapped in the jaws and broken manually. For larger stones electrohydraulic lithotripsy in the preferred option with proven safety, effectiveness, and technical ease [163].

However even stones larger than 4-cm have been successfully and safely treated using Ho:YAG laser in an effort to spare patients the morbidity of open cystolithotomy [164] and the 550-μ side-firing fiber was shown to perform better for this purpose.

The AH-1 Stone Removal System (SRS) invented by Aihua Li in 2007 was recently presented as an effective tool to treat larger bladder stones [165] (Fig. 11.17a–c). It comprises of a jaw

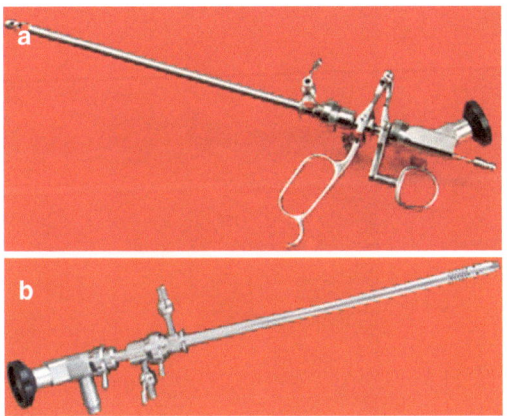

FIGURE 11.17 (**a**) AH-1 stone removal system (SRS). From Li A [165]. BMC Urology. Creative Commons Attribution License. (**b**) The outer sheath with inner sheath and endoscope. From Li A [165]. BMC Urology. Creative Commons Attribution License. (**c**) **Characteristics and functions of the jaw**. (**A**) The jaw in endoscope; (**B**) Stone stabilized with the jaw and lithotripsy performed with holmium laser; (**C**) Fragments retrieved using the jaw through outer sheath. From Li A [165]. BMC Urology. SRS was designed by Aihua Li, M.D., and manufactured by Hangzhou Tonglu Shikonghou Medical Instrument Co., Ltd

FIGURE 11.17
(continued)

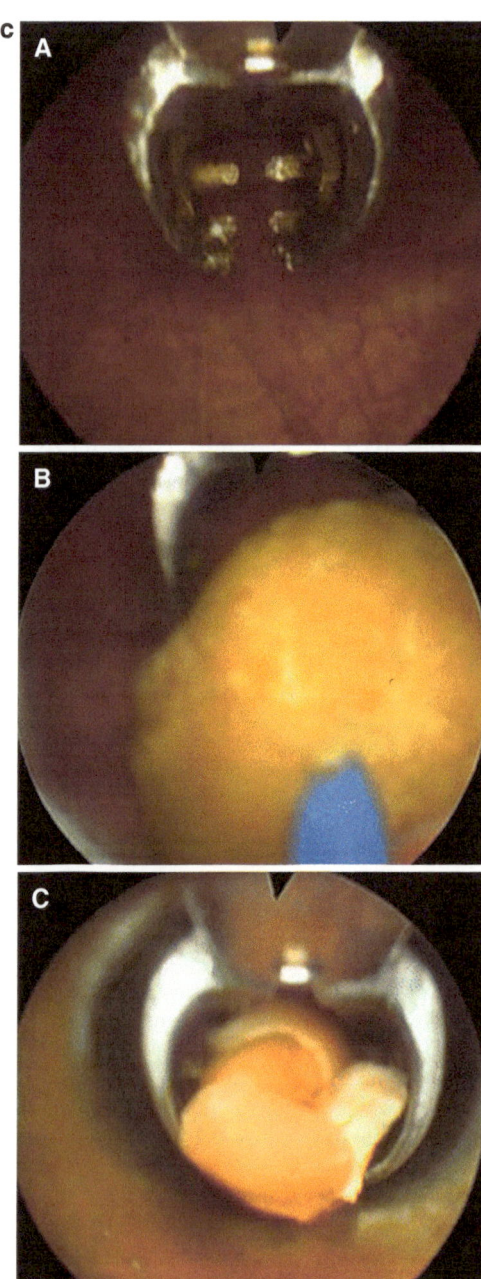

which can grasp and stabilize stones measuring even 60-mm in diameter, and their ablation is performed using Holmium Laser. The fragments are grasped with the jaw and rapidly evacuated through the outer sheath, avoiding multiple entries of the outer sheath and potential urethral injury. If there are more residual smaller fragments, an Ellik's evacuator can be connected to the outer sheath for suction. However this system is yet to be evaluated further by multiple independent centers.

Our readers should keep in mind that open cystolithotomy remains the safest and most effective method for the majority of cases with stone >4-cm diameter [166].

When the stone is secondary to a bladder outlet obstruction, commonly caused by a hypertrophied prostate, cystitholapaxy can safely be performed in one session along with the surgical treatment of the cause, namely transurethral resection of the prostate.

Cystolitholapaxy is also particularly useful in augmented bladder, and can be performed in an ileal conduit and in the bladder through a Mitrofanoff catheterizable stoma in expert hands [167, 168].

Caution must be taken in patients with spinal cord injury to avoid autonomic dysreflexia which is associated with larger or multiple stones, spinal injury level above T6, greater hydraulic irrigation height, longer operation time and the use of local anesthesia [169].

11.3.6   Percutaneous Cystolithotomy

Percutaneous cystolithotomy has been successfully performed in children and showed comparable results with open cystolithotomy and cystolitholapaxy [170].

When the calculus size in inferior to 1 cm in children, a novel technique consists of stone crushing with an artery forceps percutaneously inserted through a suprapubic puncture under cystoscopy guidance. As per the reports available, it is a rapid technique that carries a 100% stone-free rate [171]. In the adult population, single or multiple bladder stones with a burden larger than 3 cm can successfully be treated using a pneumatic lithotripter (Swiss Lithoclast) through a rigid nephroscope inserted percutaneously. The access is created according to the same technique used for PCNL: needle puncture → guidewire insertion → dilatation of the tract using Alken coaxial dilators → insertion of the Amplatz sheath [172]. At the end of the procedure, the fragments are removed with a peanut forceps, a bladder flushing or Ellik's evacuator. Bladder malignancy, history of radiotherapy or abdomino-pelvic surgery, and huge prostatomegaly (>80 cm^3) are considered contraindications to this treatment.

11.3.7 Laparoscopic Pyelolithotomy (LP)

11.3.7.1 Indications

The place of LP has shrunk nowadays with the advent of PCNL and RIRS. It is a more technically challenging and time-consuming procedure compared to PCNL which remains the gold standard for most large pelvic stones [173, 174].

However LP can still be a better alternative in the following situations:

• Very large or complex staghorn calculi de novo or after failure of other treatment modalities [175].
• Infective staghorn stones that are particularly known to have a high recurrence rate and are to be completely removed.
• Ectopic kidneys, horseshoe kidney, and concomitant PUJ obstruction where a dismembered pyeloplasty is to be performed at the same time [176–180].
• Patients at high risk for PCNL, i.e. those with severe comorbidities such as coronary artery disease (CAD) or chronic liver disease (CLD) [181].
• Patients in whom a maximal preservation of renal function is necessary [174].

LP was also shown to be safe and feasible in the pediatric population [182].

11.3.7.2   Surgical Technique

In this minimally invasive procedure, the renal pelvis dissection follows the same principle described by Gil-Vernet for the open counterpart (see below), i.e. performing a pyelotomy in a V-shaped manner, and creating a flap [181] (Fig. 11.18).

LP is most frequently carried out through an intraperitoneal approach. However the retroperitoneal route can also be performed and was even presented as a preferable option by authors who found it more rapid to complete, and associated with a shorter patient's hospital stay [183]. Nonetheless the anatomical unfamiliarity of the retroperitoneal approach remains a barrier for many laparoscopic surgeons.

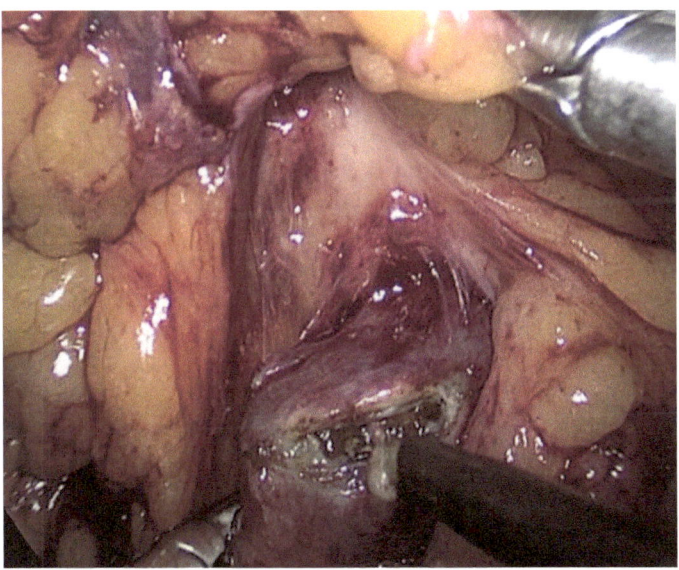

FIGURE 11.18 LP using the Gil-Vernet technique for dissecting the renal parenchyma and pyelotomy performed with a monopolar hook cautery. From Gandhi HR et al. [181], with permission from the Arab Association of Urology

LP is generally performed alone, but a recent study mentioned its successful combination with Ho:YAG laser lithotripsy, using a flexible cystoscope introduced through a 12-mm trocar. This allowed to clear calyceal stones that were not accessible to the rigid laparoscopic instruments [184].

Even the more complex laparoscopic anatrophic nephrolithotomy has been performed successfully in some centers but remains a major surgical challenge [185].

11.3.7.3   Results

LP is credited with an approximately 90% stone-free rate in large stones, but this rate decreases with the stone burden. The operation doesn't require blood transfusion, but exposes to a 4–12% urinary leak [173, 181].

11.3.8   Robot-Assisted Anatrophic Nephrolithotomy

This minimally-invasive technique avoids the need for multiple tracts or multiple sessions PCNL in complex staghorn calculi. It also avoids the high invasiveness of the open counterpart while producing comparable stone-free rates. Similar to the open surgery (see below), cold ischemia is performed with ice slush. However it is an extremely rare procedure and only scarce cases and small series have been published from centers of excellence [186–188].

11.3.9   Laparoscopic Ureterolithotomy (LU)

When ureteral stones are not amenable to ureteroscopy due to their large size, the laparoscopic approach is definitely the preferred technique and is more frequently performed than the open counterpart [189]. This is because laparoscopy in general is associated with significantly less postoperative pain, less analgesic requirement, a shorter hospital stay and a short convalescence in comparison to the open surgery. Moreover laparoscopy performed for a ureteral stone in particular is a less challenging and less stressful procedure than when performed for a renal stone.

(a) Indications: large impacted ureteral stones (>15 mm) or failed ESWL and ureteroscopy.
(b) Technique: Both intraperitoneal and retroperitoneal approaches are effective but the transperitoneal route was shown in one study to have significantly higher stone-free rate, shorter operative time and lower rate of conversion to open surgery, but with the drawback of exposing to a longer time to oral intake [190].
(c) Results: As shown by a meta-analysis of six randomized controlled trials, laparoscopic ureterolithotomy is credited with a high stone-free rate compared with uretero-scopic lithotripsy especially for larger proximal ureteral calculi, but has a longer operative time and hospital stay, with equal complication rates [191]. A 99% stone-free rate was reported in a monocentric study which included as much as 213 patients treated over a 9-year period, with the majority of patients being treated through a retroperitoneal approach [192]. Perhaps the largest series of LU to date has been published by a Chinese study comprising of 1171 cases with the following outcome [193]:

  – 1142 successful cases in one session (97.5%),
  – Conversion to open surgery in two cases (0.17%),
  – Calculi moving retrogradely to the pelvis in 27 cases (2.3%).
  – Ureteral stricture (the most worrisome complication) in 12 patients (1%), 5 (0.44%) of whom developed progressive renal atrophy, and 3 of those (0.26%) had nephrectomy due to recurrent loin pain and persistent urinary infection.

11.3.10   Surgery for Urethral Stones

Urethral stones are very rare comprising less than 0.3% of urolithiasis cases [194].

Impacted stones in the proximal urethra are treated endoscopically whereby they are pushed back in the bladder and crushed in the same way like bladder stones. The same technique applies for impacted distal urethral stones that are still far from the external meatus. When the stone is impacted at the external meatus, a ventral midline meatotomy can be performed under a local anesthesia in the emergency department and the stone be removed. For small stones in the anterior urethra with no documented urethral stricture, we frequently perform an instillation of 2% lidocaine jelly into the urethra under pressure using the dominant hand, while the non-dominant hand compresses the base of the penis proximal to the stone. Milking the urethra antegradely upon release of the lidocaine pressure is very effective to eject these stones. For impacted anterior urethral stone in children that cannot be safely flushed back or milked out, a urethrolithotomy should be performed under general anesthesia: the penile skin and urethra are incised over the stone. The stone is retrieved, then the periurethral tissues are closed over a urethral catheter (8-Fr) using 5/0 interrupted polyglycolic acid sutures (Vicryl®, PolySyn®, Surgicryl®, Polysorb®, Dexon®) and care taken not to penetrate urethral mucosa [195]. The urethral catheter is kept indwelling for 1 week. In-situ Holmium laser lithotripsy can also be performed for impacted urethral stones at any anatomic levels after failure to push back the calculus. In expert hands, this was proven to be a safe and effective procedure [196].

11.3.11   Open Procedures

We will describe them in an orderly manner, from proximal to distal: anatrophic nephrolithotomy, pyelolithotomy (combined or not to the former), ureterolithotomy and cystolithotomy.

11.3.11.1 Open Pyelolithotomy and Open Anatrophic Nephrolithotomy (OAN)

The intrasinusally *extended pyelolithotomy* was pioneered by JM Gil-Vernet in 1965.[4] However the anatrophic nephrolithotomy[5] for the treatment of staghorn stones was first performed by Smith and Boyce in 1968 [197]. Both operations are now seldom performed.

A simple pyelolithotomy may be all that is required if the stone to be removed has a relatively small size (around 2 cm) whether located in the pelvis or in an upper or middle calyx from where it can be retrieved using a straight or a curve forceps. It remains also sufficient for multiple small stones in these locations. Nevertheless such relatively small stone burden is now effectively dealt with by less invasive techniques and should not be addressed primarily by an open surgery. Practically the open approach is only justified by the complexity of the stone in the renal pelvis and its multiple coralliform extensions into the calyces (Fig. 11.19a, b). Consequently when performing pyelolithotomy, the dissection should be extended under the renal parenchyma to maximally expose the renal pelvis and the calyceal infundibula as described by Gil-Vernet. It should be noted that the incision to the renal parenchyma is better avoided. However when there are multiple coralliform extensions of the stone into the calyces, additional radial paravascular nephrotomies are necessary to ensure its complete removal. These paravascular nephrotomies can sometimes be performed without the need for vas-

---

[4]The Spanish Professor Josep María Gil-Vernet Vila is credited with many other original urological contributions, such as a technique for renal homotransplantations [198], hypospadias correction [199], vesicoureteral reflux correction [200], pelvic floor repair [201], complex vesico-vaginal fistula repair [202], orthotopic renal transplantation [203], etc. He is the son of the late Professor Salvador Gil-Vernet who proposed a model for the description of the prostate anatomy in 1953 [204].
[5]Anatrophic is an adjective related to what is used in order to prevent or correct atrophy of cells, tissues, or organs. However this adjective has become almost obsolete nowadays, being merely used in the context of nephrolithotomy.

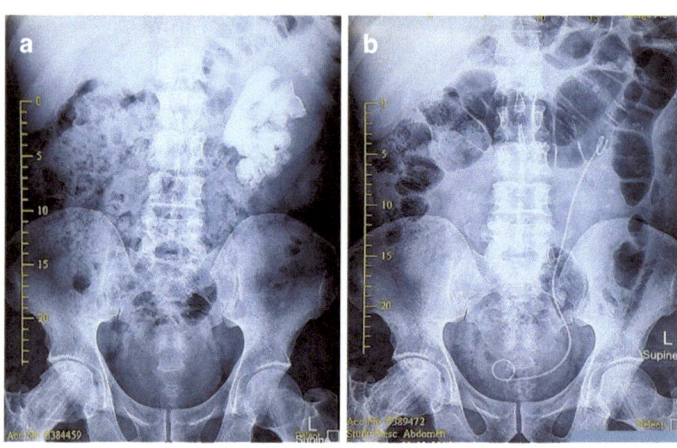

FIGURE II.I9 (**a**, **b**) A complexe left staghorn calculus. (**a**) Pre-operative view. (**b**) Post open pyelo-nephrolitotomy status with a DJ stent left in situ (Courtesy Salim Al-Busaidy, Urology, The Royal Hospital, Muscat, Oman)

cular clamping. Yet the main renal artery must be identified, dissected and controlled beforehand with a silastic loop. This safety measure allows immediate clamping of the renal artery should an uncontrollable bleeding occur during nephrotomies.

The bleeding can also be anticipated by performing the so-called "anatrophic nephrolithotomy" whereby the renal artery is occluded prior to the parenchymal incision and renal hypothermia is achieved by cooling the kidney with sterile ice slush. Here a single curvilinear incision will be made along the avascular Brödel's line[6] (or Brödel's bloodless line),

---

[6] The eponym Brödel's line is used in the USA and the UK, being given after the Germano-American medical Illustrator Max Brödel, *"the man who put art into medicine"* [205]. Brödel depicted this line in 1901 (Fig. 11.20a, b) [206]. However in Continental Europe and Latin America, preference is sometimes made for the eponym Hyrtl's line, given after the Austrian anatomist Josef Hyrtl who described this line in 1882, almost 20 years earlier than Brödel [207]. Hyrtl was the first to suggest the "natürliche Teilbarkeit der Niere" (natural divisibility of the kidney) through this avascular line and Brödel credited him for this fact [206].

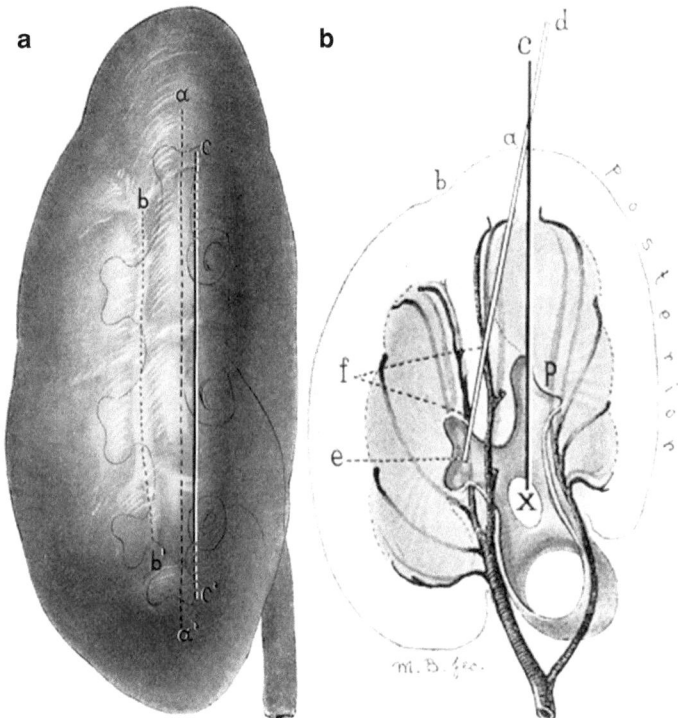

FIGURE 11.20 (**a**) Lateral view of left kidney, showing the location of the most advantageous incision through the parenchyma in kidneys which have a normal arterial arrangement. *aa´*: Lateral convex border of kidney. *bb´*: Position of lateral column of cortical substance containing the vessels. *cc´*: Best incision. (**b**) *de*: Incorrect direction of incision. *cx*: Correct direction of incision. From Max Brödel [206]. Original illustration 1901 Brödel Publication, reproduced with permission from the Collection of the Max Brödel Archives, in the Department of Art as Applied to Medicine, The Johns Hopkins University School of Medicine, Baltimore, Maryland, USA

located 5–10 mm posterior to the lateral convex border of the kidney (Fig. 11.20a, b).

Performed through a lumbar incision, this technique was "en vogue" in the past, but has progressively lost ground with the advent of endourological procedures and PCNL for the last two decades. However there are still some indications for the open anatrophic nephrolithotomy, including in developed countries, where it is sometimes the preferred choice for complex staghorn calculi due to its high stone-free rate after a single procedure and in presence of co-morbidities [208, 209].

OAN was shown to have the highest stone-free rate (92.85%) compared to laparoscopic approach (80%) and PCNL (43.75%), but carries the greatest deleterious effect on the function of the operated kidney (minus 8.66%) compared to the laparoscopic counterpart (minus 6.04%) and PCNL (minus 2.12%) [210]. However with increased experience in PCNL, the stone-free rate can be significantly improved. The long hospital stay and longer convalescence period are negative points inherent to the open surgery, but the reduced need for ancillary procedures pleads in favor of the open procedure for complex staghorn calculi, while PCNL may expose to readmissions for repeat sessions and the need for a combined RIRS and a DJ stent reinsertion.

11.3.11.2   Open Ureterolithotomy

This procedure is exceptionally performed nowadays as it has been supplanted by ureteroscopy for small ureteral stones while laparoscopic ureterolithotomy is the preferred option for larger and impacted ureteral stones not manageable endourologically.

11.3.11.3   Open Cystolithotomy[7]

Very few publications have compared cystolithotomy with cystolitholapaxy. It is known that in both routes the stones are removed successfully, but the hospital stay is significantly less after endourological approaches [211].

The indications of open cystolithotomy are:

• large stone size (>4 cm) [212] (Fig. 11.21a–c)
• stone in ileal conduit,

---

[7]The percutaneous cystolithomy has been mentioned above (see section number 11.3.6).

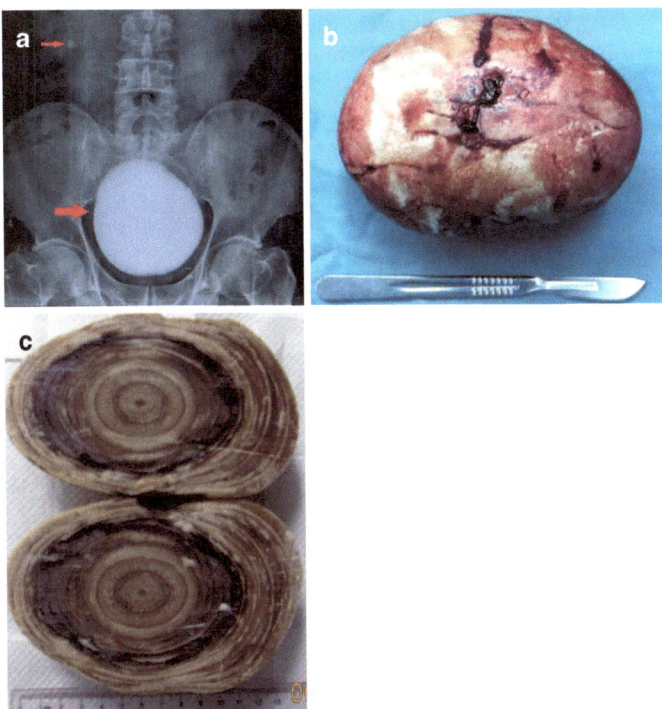

FIGURE 11.21 (a) An extremely large bladder stone and a small renal stone (*red arrow*) seen on a KUB X ray of a 54-year-old man with >9-year history of urinary frequency and urgency and who presented with recent occurence of gross hematuria. (b) The oval-shaped stone was extracted through open vesicolithotomy: It measured 13.3 × 8.0 × 9.7 cm and weighted 1048 g. (c) Stone transection showing many compartments of stratified lamellae, composed of magnesium ammonium phosphate. For Ma C et al. [212], with permission from Wolters Kluwer Health, Inc.

Note: The above specimen is still far from the largest stones reported in the literature. Alexander Randall presented in 1919 what he considered to be the largest bladder stone ever documented [213, 214]. The patient was a 61-year old male who presented with gross hematuria and constipation and died 36 h after cystolithotomy. The stone measured 48-cm circumference and weighed 64 oz (1814 g or 4 lb). More recently an even larger stone was removed from a neo-bladder in a 71-year-old man in 2010, 20 years after a radical cystectomy with continent orthotopic diversion. It weighed 160 oz (4.5 kg or 10 lb) and was essentially made of struvite [214]

• Any condition where there is impossibility to access the bladder through a retrograde endourological route (traumatised or severely strictured urethra etc.)

11.3.11.4   Urethrolithotomy

A succinct account on this technique has already been given above in the paragraph "Surgery for urethral stones".

11.4   Specific Dietary and Medical Treatment of Stones

11.4.1   Fluid Intake

To prevent stone recurrence, the minimal daily urine output target slightly varies according to expert panels, being 2.5 L for the AUA and the EAU and 2 L for the CLU[8] working group [1, 215, 216].

The fluid intake needed to promote this urine output varies from 2.5 to 3 L/day for sedentary adults in cold weather to as much as 1.5 L per work-hour for militaries, manual workers or sportsmen subjected to outdoor performance in extremely hot conditions. When exercising in summer, the daily sweat volume of professional sportsmen can exceed 2 L/h, and the sodium loss in the sweat can reach 4.8–6 g, equivalent to 10–15 g salt (NaCl), and must be replaced [217–219].

11.4.2   Medical and Dietary Measures

Despite the abundant research and publications on urolithiasis, no new drug with proven effectiveness has been produced for stone prevention since the introduction of potassium citrate in the 1980s [220, 221].

---

[8]CLU (Club della litiasi Urinaria) is the Italian expert committee for urinary lithiasis.

Modification of the pH is an essential part of the treatment. Herein readily available beverages have shown an effective action **mainly due to their bicarbonate and citrate content** and can replace alkalinization therapy with potassium citrate. However, although citrus[9] and non-citrus[10] juices have good concentrations of citrate, results of their long-term efficacy in the prevention of various types of stones are conflictual [216, 222].

Fruits and vegetables consumption are included in the general recommendation to prevent urolithiasis [215]. As stated by the CLU Working Group, the conjugate base of potassium salts present in **fruits and vegetables** represents the main **dietary source of alkali** while **dietary acid** is mainly provided by the **non-dairy animal proteins**, such as those present in meat, poultry, fish and eggs, which contain amino acids with sulfur moieties [216]. In a very large study of near 84,000 post-menopausal women, **higher intake of fruits, vegetables and fibers** was proven effective to decrease the risk of incident kidney stone formation, and was independent from other factors such as BMI, water, sodium, calcium, and animal protein intake [223]. Herein pears may be particularly useful due to their high content of malic acid, a precursor of citrate. A comprehensive review article has recently emphasized the favorable action of pears in preventing renal stone formation, in association with high fluid intake and low consumption of meat and salt, but more evidence is needed to establish their specific role [224].

After the above general measures about fluid intake and urinary pH modification, further approach must be individualized according to the stone composition.

---

[9]Citrus fruits: lemon, orange, mandarin, clementine, grapefruit, lime, sudachi, calamondin, etc.

[10]Non-citrus fruits: melon, grapes, apricots, pears, peaches, blackberries, raspberries, plums, etc.

11.4.2.1   Calcium Stone Associated with Idiopathic Hypercalciuria

The **thiazide diuretics** are the standard treatment here, especially for preventing idiopathic calcium-containing kidney stone recurrence [215, 225, 226]. **Hydrochlorothiazide (Esidrex®, Microzide®)** is the reference-drug of this group, and is given at the dose of 25 mg twice daily. Other agents are: chlorthalidone (Hygroton®) 25–50 mg/day, indapamide (Lozol®) 2.5 mg/day, bendroflumethazide (Naturetin®, Aprinox®) 2.5 mg thrice a day etc.

The daily dietary calcium intake for patients with calcium stones and hypercalciuria should be limited to 1000–1200 mg [215]. A Cochrane study on diet has recently found that **long-term (5 years) adherence to diets** consisting of normal levels of calcium, low protein and low salt may reduce the number of stone recurrences, decrease the relative supersaturation indexes of oxaluria and calcium oxalate in people with idiopathic hypercalciuria who experience recurrent kidney stones [227]. However it should be remembered that a previous Cochrane study showed that **Thiazides** produce a significant decrease in the number of new stone recurrences compared with increased water intake or specific dietary recommendations alone [228].

11.4.2.2   Calcium Oxalate Stone Associated with Hypocitraturia

Citrate is known to inhibit calcium oxalate crystallization by complexing calcium and also by directly affecting nucleation [229]. The efficacy of potassium citrate in the prevention of calcium stone formation in idiopathic hypocitraturia has been proven by a randomized trial [230]. The maximal recommended dose of **potassium citrate** is 60 mEq/day in divided doses, which is enough to induce a daily citraturia of >500 mg/day. However this treatment should be avoided when the urinary pH is above 6.5 because of the risk of increasing calcium phosphate supersaturation [231, 232].

11.4.2.3   Hyperoxaluria

It is of paramount importance to clinically differentiate between primary and secondary hyperoxaluria, and also between the various types of primary hyperoxaluria in order to initiate the most suitable treatment. Therefore one should proceed to an **early screening** in patients with recurrent calcium oxalate nephrolithiasis or in those developing this disease at young age, since delay in diagnosis in primary hyperoxaluria is common and carries a high risk for chronic kidney disease and systemic oxalosis.

a. Primary Hyperoxaluria (PH)

This is also referred to as the idiopathic form, and comprises of types I (the most severe and most frequent), II and III [232].

Pyridoxine (Vitamin B6) is a co-factor of alanine glyoxylate aminotransferase, a liver-specific enzyme which normally converts glyoxylate to glycine, but which is deficient in type I primary hyperoxaluria (PH I). **Therefore Pyridoxine is recommended in PH I where it can reduce hyperoxaluria in about 30% of patients** [232]. The initial recommended dose of Pyridoxine is 50 mg daily, to be titrated up to 200 mg or until a therapeutic response in urinary oxalate is observed [233].

Adjunctive treatment options aiming at reducing urinary CaOx supersaturation are alkaline citrate, orthophosphate, or magnesium which will also bind to the intestinal oxalate; however magnesium salts supplementation are contraindicated in the presence of renal insufficiency [234].

It is essential to initiate early conservative management of this disease such as high liquid intake, pyridoxine, and to aggressively treat any stone with acute presentation in order to prevent renal failure and oxalosis crisis [235, 236]. Unfortunately despite optimal medical management, many patients will develop recurrent nephrolithiasis and will need to undergo multiple urologic procedures to ensure a stone-free status.

When renal insufficiency is established, dialysis is ineffective in removing excess oxalate, and even after kidney transplantation, there is a rapid oxalate deposits in the graft leading to its failure [236]. Consequently pre-emptive liver transplantation in PH I, or combined liver and kidney transplantation in patients with irreversible renal damage, is the treatment of choice to treat this disease (Table 11.1).

TABLE 11.1 Transplantation methods in primary hyperoxaluria and possible indications

Isolated kidney transplant	Early: not appropriate due to the uncertainty of renal deterioration in slowly progressing cases. If there is rapid renal deterioration or the patient is on dialysis, the best option is dual transplantation. It may be considered in cases of slow renal deterioration, usually in older patients
Simultaneous liver-kidney transplant	The best option in patients with advanced renal failure or on dialysis. It should be carried out at the earliest possible stage (GFR 15–20 mL/min). The donor must obviously always be deceased
(Split) partial liver transplant	Not recommended, due to the liver's excess residual oxalate production. Transplantation would be from a living donor and would be carried out using one of three methods: partial liver (when GFR >15–20 mL/min), simultaneous liver-kidney or sequential liver-kidney. Consider in exceptional and critical situations
Isolated liver transplant	Ideal when there is not yet advanced renal failure (GFR >20 mL/min) in young adults or children
Sequential liver and kidney transplant	This option requires two donors, but it is less aggressive from the surgical perspective. If GFR >15–20 mL/min, the option is liver first and assessment of subsequent kidney progression. If GFR <15–20 mL/min, the option is kidney first. Consider in cases of advanced kidney damage but with very slow progression

GFR Glomerular filtration rate. From Lorenzo V et al. [236], with permission from the authors and Revista Nefrologia

b. Secondary Hyperoxaluria

This is also referred to as absorptive or enteric hyperoxaluria. Dietary calcium influences the bioavailability of ingested oxalate which accounts for a non-negligible part of urinary oxalate excretion; when the calcium load of an oxalate-containing diet is reduced, the urinary oxalate excretion increases [237]. **Therefore a normal dietary calcium intake should be recommended, as opposed to a poor calcium diet.**

The treatment (T) of absorptive hyperoxaluria can be summarized by the following equation:

$$T = \text{Low oxalate diet} + \text{normal calcium.}$$

A summary of dietary values for fluid and some foods in relation with CaOx stone prevention can be proposed as follows [216, 233, 234]:

- Daily fluid: Minimum urinary output per day is 2.5 L for an adult. To reach this output, the required intake should be about 3 L. In children, an oral fluid intake of >1.5 L/m² body surface area is advised. Obviously extra fluid will be necessary to compensate increased sweat loss in a hot environment and during intensive physical activity as already discussed above. Along with water, give preference to lemon juice 4 oz per day (113 g). Alternatively one can take melon juice or orange juice, but avoid tomato (sodium ++), grapefruit (oxalate ++), and cranberry juice (oxalate++). Carbohydrate-electrolyte sports beverages (Gatorade) do not affect the urinary stone risk profile.
- Avoid low-carbohydrate high-protein diets because they deliver a marked acid load to the kidney with the secondary risk of stone formation. These are specifically animal proteins contained in meats, fish, poultry, cheese, and eggs. A low-normal protein intake decreases calciuria and could be useful in stone prevention and preservation of bone mass. When facing high animal protein consumption as a "fait accompli", one should compensate with extra fruit/vegetables.

- Parsimonious consumption of spinach, potatoes, and nuts, as well as chocolate, because they are significant sources of dietary oxalate.
- Dietary calcium restriction is not recommended for stone formers with nephrolithiasis. A daily calcium intake of 1000–1200 mg should be reached (equal to a 225-g glass of milk taken four times per day). Preference should be given to non-diary calcium-fortified products beverage or food such as orange juice, coagulated soy milk (tofu), dark leafy greens, broccoli, bock choy (Chinese cabbage), okra, almonds, and fish canned with their bones.
  Diets with a calcium content ≥ 1 g/day (and low protein-low sodium) could be protective against the risk of stone formation in hypercalciuric stone forming adults
- As mentioned above, low sodium intake should be avoided because it increases the fraction of unbound oxalate in the intestinal tract → increased oxalate absorption and urinary oxalate excretion → increased risk of developing symptomatic kidney stones.
- Pyridoxine (Vit B6) intake is beneficial when one aims at reducing oxaluria. Pyridoxine-containing foods are sunflower seeds, pistachio nuts, cooked tuna or halibut, bananas, avocados, soybeans, mangoes, oatmeal, dried prunes, cooked spinach, fortified ready-to-eat cereal (corn flakes, Froot Loops™, etc.). The administration of pyridoxine in oral doses of 250–500 mg daily to both normo- or hyperoxaluric calcium renal stone formers decreases urinary oxalate excretion.
- Bran of different origins (rice, oat, wheat, etc.) decreases calciuria, but the impact on the urinary stone risk profile is uncertain.
- Fish oil contains eicosapentaenoic acid (EPA). This n-3 fatty acid is a competitor of arachidonic acid (an n-6 fatty acid present in vegetable oil and animal fats). Arachidonic acid breakdowns to produce prostaglandins including PGE_2 → increased intestinal calcium absorption + decreased reabsorption in the renal tubules + increased bone resorption → hypercalciuria. Sources of EPA are

cold-water fish (salmon, tuna, mackerel, menhaden, herring and sardines), fish oil and cod liver. EPA is also contained in walnuts, flax seeds, and canola oil. Omega-3 fatty acids decrease calciuria, but the impact on the urinary stone risk profile is uncertain.

11.4.2.4   Calcium Oxalate (CaOx) Stone and Hyperuricosuria

The effectiveness of Allopurinol (Zyloric®) at the dose of 100 mg thrice a day has been demonstrated since long by a randomized control trial [238] and this drug is therefore recommended in patients with recurrent calcium oxalate stones who have hyperuricemia and normal urinary calcium [215]. However the major concerns in the use of Allopurinol is the large inventory of the side effects including skin rash, gastro-intestinal upsets, and hepatic toxicity. Febuxostat[11] (Uloric®, Adenuric®) is a promising new drug proposed for its better toxicity profile [239] at the dose of 40 mg/day per os initially, to be increased to a maintenance dose of 80–120 mg/day per os.

11.4.2.5   Calcium Phosphate (CaP) Stones

These stones are often found in association with distal renal tubular acidosis. Treatment is similar to that of CaOx stones and consists of reduced dietary sodium and protein, increased fluid intake, and use of thiazides [231, 232]. Citrate is also recommended in the treatment of distal renal tubular acidosis, where it is effective in alleviating both acidosis and hypocitraturia, thence preventing recurrent calcium nephrolithiasis [240]. However careful monitoring through 24-h urine collections should be undertaken to avoid an excessive rise in urinary pH and a potential worsening of CaP supersaturation [232].

---

[11]Febuxostat is FDA-approved since 2009.

11.4.2.6   Uric Acid (UA) Stones

Most patients with UA stones have a low urinary pH rather than hyperuricosuria as the predominant risk factor [241]. Therefore reduction of urinary UA excretion with the use of Allopurinol in patients with UA stones will not prevent stones in presence of unduly acidic urine, and **the AUA panel recommends not giving this drug as a first-line therapy in these patients** [215]. **The first-line therapy here is alkalinization of the urine with potassium citrate**. Allopurinol may only be considered as an adjunct when alkalinization is not successful (e.g., patients with inflammatory bowel disease, chronic diarrhoea and ileostomies) or for patients who continue to form UA stones despite adequate alkalinization of the urine.

Urine alkalinization is the corner stone of the treatment and urine pH should rise to 6.0–6.5 to increase the solubility of uric acid in urine. Increasing the fluid intake and lowering the protein diet to reduce concentration of UA are other important measures. To raise the urinary pH, potassium citrate is preferred over sodium citrate and its recommended dosage is 30–40 mEq/day.

Weight reduction is essential to successfully treat and prevent uric acid-containing stones as these have a significant association with obesity. A BMI between 18 and 25 in the adult category of age is the ideal target that the patient should be encouraged to strive for [234]. Remember that the metabolic syndrome (MS) is considered as the most common cause of uric acid stone formation and obesity is one of its main components.

As already mentioned, antegrade infusion of dissolving agents through percutaneous nephrostomy access is obsolete. The use of Allopurinol and Febuxostat has been discussed above [239].

11.4.2.7   Cystine Stones

Their treatment remains a major challenge. Despite extensive research and publications in this field with a better understanding of the molecular basis of cystinuria, no or little progress has been achieved in the last 30 years in the treatment of this entity. The preventive management still consists merely of urinary alkalinization and adequate fluid intake (generally >4 L/day), while available chelating agents should be cautiously proposed for selected patients due to their excessive side effects. **There is still no curative treatment for cystinuric patients who are at lifelong risk of urolithiasis, often requiring repeated surgeries and being highly exposed to impaired renal function in the long run.**

Not surprisingly the most effective cystine stone-prevention measure is still **hyperdiuresis** with the aim to decrease the urinary cystine concentration. It has been estimated that a homozygous cystinuric patient excretes between 600 and 1400 mg of cystine per day. Knowing that the solubility of cystine is 250–300 mg/L at a pH of 7.0, a simple calculation indicates that **a urine output of 4–5 L/day is to be promoted** if one wants to prevent urinary cystine precipitation for the majority of homozygous cystinurics. Indeed hydration alone can prevent stone recurrence in up to a third of patients [242] and a urine output of 3 L/day is considered as the minimal target. To achieve this goal, it is required to drink 4–4.5 L of water per day in order to cover the insensible loss. The following is a suggested practical regimen for daily water intake: 240 mL every hour during daytime and 480 mL before bed, and at least once during the night [242].

To increase the urinary pH, one can use potassium citrate at the dose of 10–20 mEq thrice daily. Cystine-binding thiols should be offered for patients who do not respond to dietary modifications and urinary alkalinization, or who have large recurrent stone burdens [243]. These chelating agents are: **D-Penicillamine**[12] (Cuprimine®, Cuprenyl®, Depen®) 1–2 g/day (known for more than 50 years) [244], **Tiopronin** (Thiola®) 800–1200 mg/day (this is the α-mercaptopropionylglycine; it has

---

[12]The chelating action of Penicillamine has been used for many other medical indications: Wilson's disease (where it binds with copper and allows its elimination with urine), arsenic poisoning etc. Penicillamine has also been used as a disease-modifying agent in scleroderma and rheumatoid arthritis. However in all these indications its use was progressively confined to exceptional cases or banned because of the potentially dangerous side effects.

a better tolerance than D-Penicillamine, especially with regard to allergy) [232], and **Captopril** (Capoten®) 75–100 mg/day. These drugs work by interrupting the disulfide bond of cystine and forming complexes with cysteine that are about 50-fold more soluble than cystine [245]. However cautions should be observed when prescribing these medicines because of the many side effects related to their use, especially D-Penicillamine: bone marrow suppression, dysgeusia, anorexia, vomiting, nausea, diarrhoea, itching, rash, mouth sores, poor wound healing, nephropathy, hemopathy, membranous glomerulonephritis, aplastic anemia, antibody-mediated drug-induced systemic lupus erythematous and myasthenia gravis, etc.

Captopril is an angiotensin-converting enzyme inhibitor, also containing a thiol group and with proven in-vitro efficacy in increasing cystine solubility, but with poor urinary excretion at usual dose to cause meaningful changes in cystine solubility [246, 247].

11.4.2.8   Struvite Stones

Struvite stones occur as a consequence of urinary infection with urease-producing (or urea-splitting) organisms which include a wide range of genera such as Proteus spp, Brucella spp, corynebacterium spp, Staphylococcus, Mycoplasma, Cryptococcus, etc.

Patients treated for struvite stones may still be at risk for recurrent urinary tract infections after stone removal, and in some patients surgical stone removal is not feasible. These patients are also at increased risk for stone recurrence or progression, and an aggressive medical approach is required to mitigate this risk [243]. The use of a urease inhibitor, Acetohydroxamic acid (AHA, Lithostat®), may be beneficial in these patients, but the striking side effect profile limits its use [248]. In particular, patients taking this medication should be closely monitored for phlebitis and hypercoagulability phenomena [249]. In view of its side-effects, AHA should be prescribed only for residual or recurrent struvite stones that cannot be managed surgically, and close monitoring of persistent or recurrent urinary tract infections is recommended in these patients [215]. Acidifying the urine to a pH between 5.8 and 6.2 with L-Methionine (200–500 mg three times a day) combined with an increased fluid intake are important adjuncts to stone removal procedures [234].

11.4.2.9 Summary of the Dietary and Medical Therapies

There are no specific dietary measures for cystine and struvite stones. The formers are addressed merely by urinary alkalinization and increased water intake to promote a diuresis of ≥ 3 L/day, and the latters by their complete surgical removal whenever possible and aggressive treatment of UTI with antibiotics and urinary acidification. As take-home messages, we reproduce the following two tables summarizing the diet and medication advices in relation to specific metabolic abnormalities associated with urolithiasis (Table 11.2) [233] and reminding the indications of the various drugs used to treat urinary stones (Table 11.3) [234].

TABLE 11.2 Summary of dietary and medical therapies for kidney stone prevention

Abnormality	Diet	Medications
General guidelines	Fluids, limit sodium, citrates	None
Hypercalciuria	Sodium restriction	Thiazide, fish oil
Hypocitraturia	Lemon, lime, melon, oranges	Potassium citrate
Hyperuricosuria	Protein moderation	Allopurinol
Hypernatriuria	Sodium limit 1500 mg/day	None
Hyperoxaluria	Limit spinach, nuts, berries	Pyridoxine (vitamin B-6)
Low pH	Increase fruits and vegetable	Potassium citrate

From Gul Z and Monga M. [233]. With permission from the Korean Urological Association

TABLE 11.3 When to use which medication

Medication/dose	Indication
Potassium citrate/9–12 g/day Sodium bicarbonate 1.5 g 3×/day	When adjustment of the acid/base towards the alkaline region is needed and dietary measures are not sufficient. This can be the case for patients with high uric acid production, low dietary acid tolerance (overweight, renal acidification disorders), high intrinsic oxalate production. Stone types: uric acid, calcium-oxalates, ammonium urate
Hydrochlorothiazide 25–50 mg/day	To correct hypercalciuria when that cannot be corrected by dietary advice (or by surgery in the case of primary hyperparathyroidism) Stone types: calcium-salts
Magnesium salts 200–400 mg/day	For patients with oxalate overproduction (hyperoxaluria that cannot be corrected by dietary advice) Magnesium salts should not be given to patients with renal insufficiency Stone types: calcium oxalates
Pyridoxine 5–20 mg/kg/day	Patients in whom hyperoxaluria remains present despite dietary restriction of oxalate and normalisation of calcium intake (primary hyperoxaluria) Goal: normo-oxaluria
L-Methionine 200–500 mg 3× daily	When acidification of the urine is needed. This can be to remove fragments of infection stones (struvite/calcium apatites) or patients with uric acid/ammonium urate stones Goal: urinary pH 5.8–6.2, where urine pH remains >6.2 despite advice to neutralise the dietary acid/base intake

TABLE 11.3 (continued)

Medication/dose	Indication
Allopurinol 100–300 mg/day	For patients with hyperuricosuria that is not corrected by dietary advice. These are patients who produce extra uric acid as a result of severe overweight or due to an enzymatic disorder. The high dose should be reserved for patients who have both hyperuricosuria and hyperuricosaemia

From Kok DJ. [234] with permission from the Arab Journal of Urology

11.5   Herbal Medicines

Phytotherapy (from Greek "Phytos", plant, and "Therapeia", treatment or cure) is as old as the mankind itself and has been intensively used for urolithiasis since ancient human civilizations (Greco-roman, Egyptian, Indian, Chinese, Persian, etc.). In the middle age the Persian Islamic polymath Ibn-Sina (known as Avicenna in Western countries) has listed in his "Canon of Medicine" (القانون في الطب) a total of 64 herbal, 8 animal, and 4 mineral medicines that were used to dissolve, expel, or prevent kidney calculi [250].

Pakistani researchers have endeavored to propose a rich taxonomy of herbs reportedly having a therapeutic or preventive effect against renal stones; they outlined not less than 35 medicinal plants whose active ingredients included flavonoids, terpenoids, and tannins [251]. More recently an Iranian group has inventoried 18 species of plants used by Shirazian herbalists to treat urolithiasis, among which Alhagi maurorum (Camelthorn, Persian mannaplant, etc.), Tribulus terrestris (goat's-head, bindii, etc.), and Nigella sativa (black-caraway or Kalonji) were the most frequently mentioned (Table 11.4 and Fig. 11.22a–c) [252].

Through the above mentioned studies alone, one can be impressed by the great number of plants proposed for urinary stone compared to the striking paucity of scientifically

TABLE 11.4 Medicinal plants recommended by the Shirazian herbalists for the treatment of kidney stone

Scientific name	Family	Persian names	Usable part of plant	How to use	Traditional therapeutic effect in Shiraz
Alhagi maurorum	Fabaceae	Kharshotor	Aerial parts	Decoction	Kidney stone
Tribulus terrestris	Zygophyllaceae	Kharkhasak	Aerial parts	Decoction	Kidney stone
Nigella Sativa	Caryophyllaceae	Siahdaneh	Seed	Decoction	Kidney stone
Althea aucheri Boiss.	Malvaceae	Khatmi-armanestani	Aerial parts	Decoction	Kidney stone
Lactuca sativa L	Compositae	Kahoo	Leave	Fresh	Kidney stone
Prunus cerasus	Rosaceae	Albaloo	Fruit	Fresh	Kidney stone
Alhagi camelorum	Papilionaceae	Taranjebin	Aerial parts	Decoction	Kidney stone
Mangifera indica	Anacardiaceae	Anbeh	Fruit	Fresh	Kidney stone
Prangos acaulis (DC.) Bornm	Apiaceae	Jashi-kotoleh	Aerial parts	Decoction	Kidney stone

Urtica dioica L	Urticaceae	Gazaneh	Aerial parts	Decoction	Kidney stone
Fumaria officinalis	Fumariaceae	Shah-tareh	Leave	Decoction and fresh	Kidney stone
Plantago psyllium	Plantaginaceae	Esfarzeh	Leave	Decoction	Kidney stone
Medicago sativa	Leguminosae	Yonjeh	Decoction	Decoction	Kidney stone
Apium graveolens	Umbelliferae	Karafs	Decoction	Decoction	Kidney stone
Rheum ribes	Polygonaceae	Rivas	Fruit	Fresh	Kidney stone
Arctium lappa	Compositae	Baba-adam	Aerial parts	Decoction	Kidney stone
Pimpinella anisum	Apiaceae	Anison	Aerial parts	Decoction	Kidney stone
Gundelia tournefortii	Asteraceae	Kangar	Leave	Fresh	Kidney stone

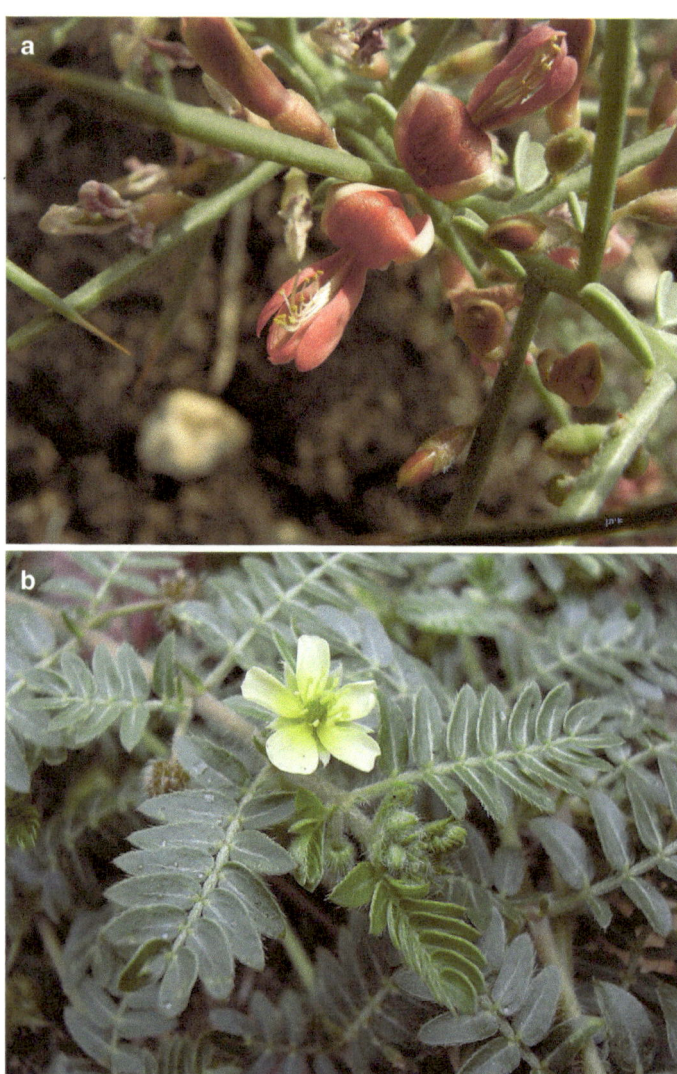

FIGURE 11.22 (**a**) Alhagi maurorum flowers. CC BY-SA 3.0. By Eitan f. (**b**) Tribulus terrestris flower and leaves. CC BY-SA 3.0. By Forest & Kim Starr. (**c**) Nigella sativa photographed in the Vienna Botanical Garden (Austria). By Andre Holz. CC BY-SA 3.0

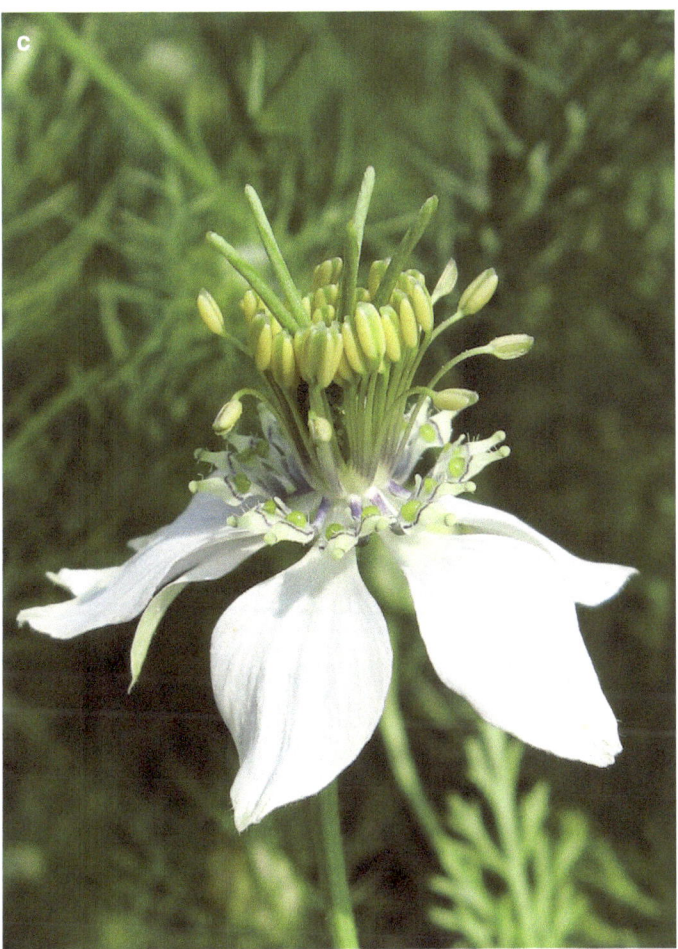

FIGURE 11.22 (continued)

proven drugs discussed in previous paragraphs and chapters of this book.

Not even included in the above publications is Phyllanthus niruri, one of the most studied botanic species used to treat the urinary stone disease. This ubiquitous tropical plant is commonly known in Brazil as 'Quebra-pedra', in Peru as 'Chanca

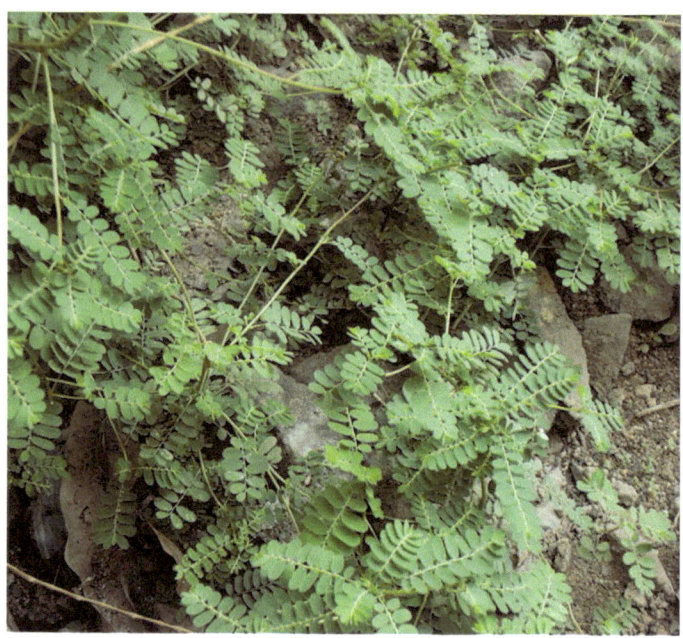

FIGURE 11.23 Phyllanthus niruri ('quebra-pedra') (Public Domain). File: Keezhanelli. JPG

Piedra' ('the stone breaker'), in India as 'Bhue Amala' or 'Keezhar Nelli', in Malaysia as "Dukung Anak" and in many other countries under different names (Fig. 11.23). It is known in the English language as "gale of the wind". Interestingly this plant is also mentioned as "bhumyamalaki" in ancient Ayurvedic texts in India where it is credited with many other medical indications including liver function strengthening and gastrointestinal tract cleansing.

Phyllanthus niruri has been proposed by several authors as a treatment for urolithiasis alone [253, 254], or in combination with ESWL [255], but further evidence is needed to confirm its therapeutic properties.

Another ayurvedic medicine reported to have activity against urinary lithiasis is Cystone®, a complex product comprising of herbs and minerals. Nevertheless two short-term studies (1-year duration each) failed to show any benefit in

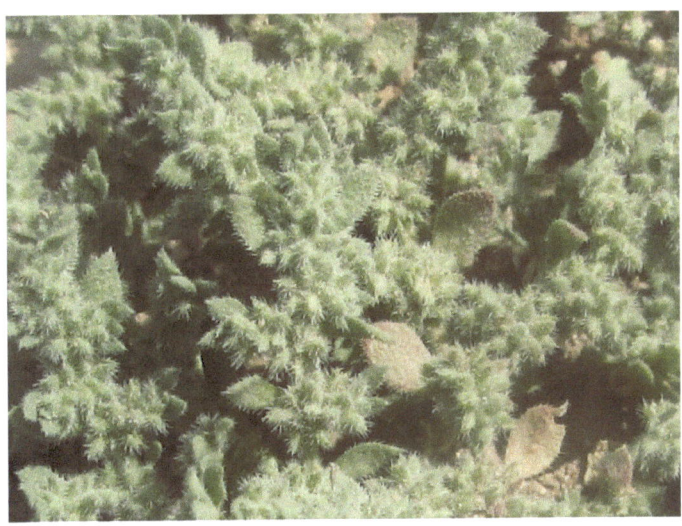

Figure 11.24 Herniaria hirsuta (hairy rupturewort). Courtesy of Pr. Atmani F, Laboratory of Biochemistry and Biotechnology, Department of Biology, University Mohammed the First, Oujda, Morocco

preventing kidney stone formation and growth in recurrent cystine and CaOx stone formers [256, 257].

A Moroccan herb, Herniaria hirsuta (hairy rupturewort) (Fig. 11.24) has also been reported to have beneficial effect in preventing calcium oxalate stones in rats; however human studies are still awaited [258].

A recent in-vitro study attempted to explore the effects of five herbal extracts on the crystallization of calcium oxalate in synthetic urine [259]. The selection included Folium pyrrosiae (a Chinese plant), Desmodium styracifolium, Phyllanthus niruri, Orthosiphon stamineus ("Java tea") (Fig. 11.25), and Cystone®. All these products showed a potential in the inhibition of calcium oxalate stone formation, the greatest effect being observed with Cystone®. Nonetheless a large meta-analysis showed that citrate is more effective than phytotherapy in decreasing the size of existing calculi in the urinary tract and in decreasing the urinary excretion rate of uric acid [260].

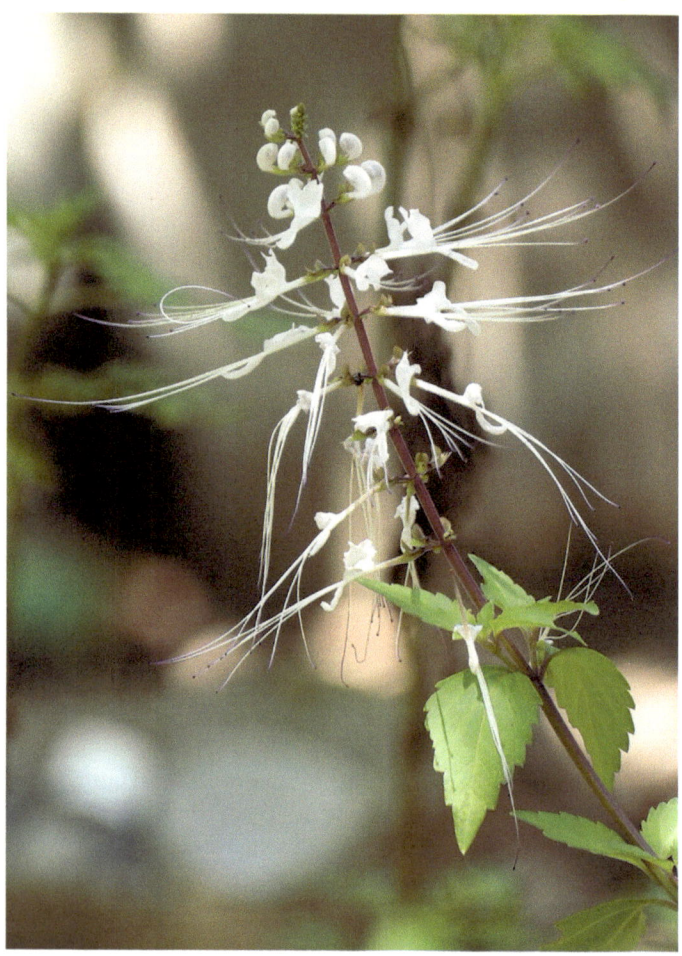

FIGURE 11.25 Orthosiphon stamineus ("Java tea"). <u>CC BY 3.0,</u> By Tu7uh

Therefore it should always be borne in mind that despite their popularity, herbal solutions suffer the lack of randomized scientific data on their exact pharmacodynamics, efficacy and safety to support their clinical use.

11.6   An Eye on the Future

- It is generally accepted that struvite (infectious) stones are not to be managed conservatively and there is no place for any dietary measure. It is essential to render the patient stone-free, and surgery is the mainstay here (either RIRS or PCNL, or sometimes open procedures) aiming at a complete stone removal, in combination with a urine culture-guided antibiotic therapy. However this attitude has recently been tempered by some investigators who found metabolic abnormalities even in pure struvite stone and reported on the positive effect of a directed medical therapy in these patients [261]. Additionally the advent of Proteus mirabilis vaccine would be a positive step for struvite stones prevention. Preliminary studies have shown effectiveness of hemolysin (HpmA) in a mouse model [262] and further trials are expected.
- A randomized, double-blind, placebo-controlled multicenter trial has evaluated the efficacy of Oxalobacter formigenes, an anaerobic oxalate-degrading bacterium, which naturally colonizes the colon of most humans. This study showed that orally administered Oxalobacter formigenes (Oxabact®) (not less than 10^7 CFU twice daily) with meals was safe and well tolerated [263]. Disappointingly however this study showed no significant change in urinary oxalate compared with placebo. Nonetheless a further study has reemphasized the interest of this probiotic therapy [264].
- Imposters that structurally mimic the L-Cystine, namely L-cystine dimethylester (L-CDME) and L-cystine methylester (L-CME), were identified through the use of atomic force microscopy, and were proven effective to inhibit L-cystine crystal growth in vitro and in a murine model [265–268]. Further trials in humans are warranted to confirm the effectiveness and evaluate the adverse effects of this novel therapy.
- A model of genetic manipulation has been developed using the antisense technology to reproduce cystinuria type 1 in vitro [269]. This research is based on the genes

encoding the two transporters, rBAT and b(0,+)AT, whose defects cause non-transport of cystine in proximal tubular cells resulting in cystinuria. The authors succeeded to artificially silence the rBAT gene using antisense oligonucleotides complimentary to human rBAT mRNA achieving a cystinuria type I phenotype in cultured human kidney cells. This model could open the door to gene therapy of cystinuria.

References

1. Türk C, Petřík A, Sarica K, et al. EAU guidelines on diagnosis and conservative management of urolithiasis. Eur Urol. 2016;69(3):468–74.
2. Dropkin BM, Moses RA, Sharma D, Pais VM Jr. The natural history of nonobstructing asymptomatic renal stones managed with active surveillance. J Urol. 2015;193(4):1265–9.
3. Assimos D, Krambeck A, Miller NL, et al. Surgical management of stones: American Urological Association/Endourological Society Guideline, PART I. J Urol. 2016;196(4):1153–60.
4. Afshar K, Jafari S, Marks AJ, et al. Nonsteroidal anti-inflammatory drugs (NSAIDs) and non-opioids for acute renal colic. Cochrane Database Syst Rev. 2015;(6). Art. No.: CD006027. doi:10.1002/14651858.CD006027.pub2.
5. Preminger GM, Tiselius HG, Assimos DG, et al. 2007 Guideline for the management of ureteral calculi. Eur Urol. 2007;52:1610–31. [PMID: 18074433].
6. Furyk JS, Chu K, Banks C, et al. Distal ureteric stones and tamsulosin: a double-blind, placebo-controlled, randomized, multicenter trial. Ann Emerg Med. 2016;67(1):86–95.e2.
7. Davenport K, Timoney AG, Keeley FX. A comparative in vitro study to determine the beneficial effect of calcium-channel and alpha(1)-adrenoceptor antagonism on human ureteric activity. BJU Int. 2006;98:651–5.
8. Liu C, Zeng G, Kang R, et al. Efficacy and safety of alfuzosin as medical expulsive therapy for ureteral stones: a systematic review and meta-analysis. PLoS One. 2015;10(8):e0134589.
9. Berger DA, Ross MA, Hollander JB, Ziadeh J, Chen C, Jackson RE, Swor RA. Tamsulosin does not increase 1-week passage rate of ureteral stones in ED patients. Am J Emerg Med. 2015;33(12):1721–4.

10. Pickard R, Starr K, MacLennan G, et al. Use of drug therapy in the management of symptomatic ureteric stones in hospitalised adults: a multicentre, placebo-controlled, randomised controlled trial and cost-effectiveness analysis of a calcium channel blocker (nifedipine) and an alpha-blocker (tamsulosin) (the SUSPEND trial). Health Technol Assess. 2015;19(63):vii–viii, 1–171.

11. Hollingsworth JM, Canales BK, Rogers MA, et al. Alpha blockers for treatment of ureteric stones: systematic review and meta-analysis. BMJ. 2016;355:i6112. doi:10.1136/bmj.i6112.

12. Yang D, Wu J, Yuan H, Cui Y. The efficacy and safety of silodosin for the treatment of ureteral stones: a systematic review and meta-analysis. BMC Urol. 2016;16(1):23.

13. Yuvanc E, Yilmaz E, Tuglu D, Batislam E. Medical and alternative therapies in urinary tract stone disease. World J Nephrol. 2015;4(5):492–9.

14. Ramsey S, Robertson A, Ablett MJ, et al. Evidence-based drainage of infected hydronephrosis secondary to ureteric calculi. J Endourol. 2010;24(2):185–9.

15. Türk C, Petřík A, Sarica K, et al. EAU guidelines on interventional treatment for urolithiasis. Eur Urol. 2016;69(3):475–82. doi:10.1016/j.eururo.2015.07.041. Epub 2015 Sep 4.

16. Assimos D, Krambeck A, Miller NL, et al. Surgical management of stones: American Urological Association/Endourological Society Guideline, PART II. J Urol. 2016;196(4):1161–9.

17. Doizi S, Raynal G, Traxer O. Evolution of urolithiasis treatment over 30 years in a French academic institution. Prog Urol. 2015;25(9):543–8.

18. Heers H, Turney BW. Trends in urological stone disease: a 5-year update of Hospital Episode statistics. BJU Int. 2016;118(5):785–9. doi:10.1111/bju.13520.

19. Chaussy C, Schmiedt E, Jocham D, et al. First clinical experience with extracorporeally induced destruction of kidney stones by shock waves. J Urol. 1982;127:417–20.

20. Chaussy C, Brendel W, Schmiedt E. Extracorporeally induced destruction of kidney stones by shock waves. Lancet. 1980;2:1265–8.

21. Gschwend JE, Paiss T, Gottfried HW, Hautmann RE. Extracorporeal shockwave lithotripsy in children. Complications and long-term results. Urologe A. 1995;34(4):324–8.

22. Zogović J. Extracorporeal shock wave lithotripsy in the urinary tract in patients with one kidney. Srp Arh Celok Lek. 2002;130(9–10):312–5.

23. Tailly G, Chaussy CG, Bohris C, et al. ESWL in a nutshell. 4th ed. Munich: Dornier MedTech Europe GmbH; 2014.

24. Pemberton J. Extra-corporeal shock wave lithotripsy. Postgrad Med J. 1987;63:1025–31.

25. Rassweiler JJ, Knoll T, Köhrmann KU, et al. Shock wave technology and application: an update. Eur Urol. 2011;59(5):784–96.

26. Sass W, Braunlich M, Dreyer H, Matura E. The mechanisms of stone disintegration by shock waves. Ultrasound Med Biol. 1991;17(3):239–43.

27. Duryea AP, Roberts WW, Cain CA, Hall TL. Controlled cavitation to augment SWL stone comminution: mechanistic insights in vitro. IEEE Trans Ultrason Ferroelectr Freq Control. 2013;60(2):301–9.

28. Semins MJ, Trock BJ, Matlaga BR. The effect of shock wave rate on the outcome of shock wave lithotripsy: a meta-analysis. J Urol. 2008;179:194–7.

29. Grasso M, Loisides P, Beaghler M, Bagley D. The case for primary endoscopic management of upper urinary tract calculi: I. A critical review of 121 extracorporeal shock-wave lithotripsy failures. Urology. 1995;45(3):363–71.

30. Mishra SK, Ganpule A, Manohar T, Desai MR. Surgical management of pediatric urolithiasis. Indian J Urol. 2007;23(4):428–34.

31. Telha KA, Alkohlany K, Alnono I. Extracorporeal shockwave lithotripsy monotherapy for treating patients with bladder stones. Arab J Urol. 2016;14(3):207–10.

32. Streem SB. Contemporary clinical practice of shock wave lithotripsy: a reevaluation of contraindications. J Urol. 1997;157(4):1197–203.

33. Lechevallier E, Traxer O, Saussine C. Extracorporeal shockwave lithotripsy for upper urinary tract stone. Prog Urol. 2008;18(12):878–85.

34. Vasavada SP, Streem SB, Kottke-Marchant K, Novick AC. Pathological effects of extracorporeally generated shock waves on calcified aortic aneurysm tissue. J Urol. 1994;152(1):45–8.

35. Atlee JL, Bernstein AD. Cardiac rhythm management devices (part II): perioperative management. Anesthesiology. 2001;95(6):1492–506.

36. Ector H, Janssens L, Baert L, De Geest H. Extracorporeal shock wave lithotripsy and cardiac arrhythmias. Pacing Clin Electrophysiol. 1989;12(12):1910–7.

37. Tonolini M, Villa F, Ippolito S, et al. Cross-sectional imaging of iatrogenic complications after extracorporeal and endourological treatment of urolithiasis. Insights Imaging. 2014;5(6):677–89.

38. Abdel-Khalek M, Sheir KZ, Mokhtar AA, et al. Prediction of success rate after extracorporeal shock-wave lithotripsy of renal stones--a multivariate analysis model. Scand J Urol Nephrol. 2004;38(2):161–7.

39. Madbouly K, Sheir KZ, Elsobky E, et al. Risk factors for the formation of a steinstrasse after extracorporeal shock wave lithotripsy: a statistical model. J Urol. 2002;167(3):1239–42.

40. El-Assmy A, El-Nahas AR, Elsaadany MM, et al. Risk factors for formation of steinstrasse after extracorporeal shock wave lithotripsy for pediatric renal calculi: a multivariate analysis model. Int Urol Nephrol. 2015;47(4):573–7.

41. Coptcoat MJ, Webb DR, Kellet MJ, et al. The steinstrasse: a legacy of extracorporeal lithotripsy? Eur Urol. 1988;14(2): 93–5.

42. Resim S, Ekerbicer HC, Ciftci A. Role of tamsulosin in treatment of patients with steinstrasse developing after extracorporeal shock wave lithotripsy. Urology. 2005;66(5):945–8.

43. Puppo P. Steinstrasse 20 years later: still a problem after ESWL? Eur Urol. 2006;50(4):643–7.

44. Van Savage JG, Fried FA. Bilateral spontaneous steinstrasse and nephrocalcinosis associated with distal renal tubular acidosis. J Urol. 1993;150(2 Pt 1):467–8.

45. Kok HK, Donnellan JP, Torreggiani WC. Spontaneous steinstrasse from multiple ureteric calculi. Br J Hosp Med (Lond). 2012;73(8):474.

46. Biyani CS, Bhatia V, Baliga D. Urethral steinstrasse—clinical experience and radiographic findings. Clin Radiol. 1993;48(4):273–4.

47. Brahmbhatt YG, Schulsinger DA, Wadhwa NK. Urethral steinstrasse in renal transplantation. Kidney Int. 2009;75(3):344.

48. Kumar S, Sharma S, Ganesamoni R, Singh SK. Urethral steinstrasse with urethrocutaneous fistula. Urology. 2012;79(2):e1–2.

49. Vaddi SP, Devraj R, Reddy V, et al. Urethral steinstrasse causing acute urinary retention. Urology. 2011;77(3):594–5.

50. Kaynar M, Tekinarslan E, Keskin S, et al. Effective radiation exposure evaluation during a one year follow-up of urolithiasis patients after extracorporeal shock wave lithotripsy. Cent European J Urol. 2015;68(3):348–52.

51. Wrixon AD. New ICRP recommendations. J Radiol Prot. 2008;28(2):161–8.

52. Ackermann D, Merz V, Marth D, Zehntner C. Clinical experiences with extracorporeal shockwave lithotripsy. Schweiz Med Wochenschr. 1989;119(26):935–40.

53. Ghoneim IA, El-Ghoneimy MN, El-Naggar AE, et al. Extracorporeal shock wave lithotripsy in impacted upper ureteral stones: a prospective randomized comparison between stented and non-stented techniques. Urology. 2010;75(1):45–50.

54. Matsuoka Y, Ishizaka K, Machida T, et al. Treatment of 2019 cases with upper urinary tract calculi using a piezoelectric lithotriptor ESL-500A. Nihon Hinyokika Gakkai Zasshi. 2002;93(3):476–82.

55. Bon D, Doré B, Irani J, et al. Results of extracorporeal lithotripsy with ultrasonography-guided hydroelectric lithotriptor: study on 546 patients, prognosis factors. Prog Urol. 1995;5(5):671–8.

56. Park BH, Choi H, Kim JB, Chang YS. Analyzing the effect of distance from skin to stone by computed tomography scan on the extracorporeal shock wave lithotripsy stone-free rate of renal stones. Korean J Urol. 2012;53:40–3.

57. Müllhaupt G, Engeler DS, Schmid HP, Abt D. How do stone attenuation and skin-to-stone distance in computed tomography influence the performance of shock wave lithotripsy in ureteral stone disease? BMC Urol. 2015;15:72.

58. Yazici O, Tuncer M, Sahin C, et al. Shock wave lithotripsy in ureteral stones: evaluation of patient and stone related predictive factors. Int Braz J Urol. 2015;41(4):676–82.

59. Pareek G, Armenakas NA, Panagopoulos G, et al. Extracorporeal shock wave lithotripsy success based on body mass index and Hounsfield units. Urology. 2005;65(1):33–6.

60. Ouzaid I, Al-qahtani S, Dominique S, et al. A 970 Hounsfield units (HU) threshold of kidney stone density on non-contrast computed tomography (NCCT) improves patients' selection for extracorporeal shockwave lithotripsy (ESWL): evidence from a prospective study. BJU Int. 2012;110:E438–42.

61. Bon D, Doré B, Irani J, et al. Radiographic prognostic criteria for extracorporeal shock-wave lithotripsy: a study of 485 patients. Urology. 1996;48:556–60. Discussion 560–1.

62. Bastian PJ, Bastian HP. Outpatient extracorporeal shock wave lithotripsy. Prospective evaluation of 2937 cases. Urologe A. 2004;43(7):829–35.

63. Kaczmarek K, Gołąb A, Słojewski M. Impact of ureteric stent on outcome of extracorporeal shockwave lithotripsy: a propensity score analysis. Cent European J Urol. 2016;69(2):184–9.

64. Argyropoulos AN, Tolley DA. Ureteric stents compromise stone clearance after shockwave lithotripsy for ureteric stones: results of a matched-pair analysis. BJU Int. 2009;103(1):76–80.

65. Sfoungaristos S, Gofrit ON, Pode D, et al. History of ureteral stenting negatively affects the outcomes of extracorporeal shockwave lithotripsy. Results of a matched-pair analysis. Prague Med Rep. 2015;116(3):225–32.

66. Singh V, Gupta A. Stenturia: a rare complication of indwelling ureteral stent. Urol J. 2009;6(3):226–7.

67. Heimbach D, Bäumler D, Schoeneich G, Hesse A. Percutaneous chemolysis: an important tool in the treatment of urolithiasis. Int Urol Nephrol. 1998;30(6):655–64.

68. Pfister RC, Dretler SP. Percutaneous chemolysis of renal calculi. Urol Radiol. 1984;6(2):138–43.

69. Kachrilas S, Papatsoris A, Bach C, et al. The current role of percutaneous chemolysis in the management of urolithiasis: review and results. Urolithiasis. 2013;41(4):323–6.

70. Zhang J, Wang S, Hong J, et al. New potential solutions for the chemolysis of urinary phosphate calculi determined by an in vitro study. Urolithiasis. 2015;43(2):147–53.

71. Young HH, McKay RW. Congenital valvular obstruction of the prostatic urethra. Surg Gynecol Obstet. 1929;48:509–12.

72. Rizkala ER, Monga M. Controversies in ureteroscopy: wire, basket, and sheath. Indian J Urol. 2013;29(3):244–8.

73. Goodman TM. Ureteroscopy with pediatric cystoscope in adults. Urology. 1977;9(4):394–7.

74. Lyon ES, Kyker JS, Schoenberg HW. Transurethral ureteroscopy in women: a ready addition to the urological armamentarium. J Urol. 1978;119(1):35–41.

75. Marshall VF. Fiber optics in urology. J Urol. 1964;91:110–4.

76. Bagley DH, Huffman JL, Lyon ES. Flexible ureteropyeloscopy: diagnosis and treatment in the upper urinary tract system. J Urol. 1987;138:280–5.

77. Kavoussi L, Clayman RV, Basler J. Flexible actively deflectable fiberoptic ureteronephroscopy. J Urol. 1989;142:949–54.

78. Gridley CM, Knudsen BE. Digital ureteroscopes: technology update. Res Rep Urol. 2017;9:19–25.

79. Jones P, Rai BP, Somani BK. Outcomes of ureteroscopy for patients with stones in a solitary kidney: evidence from a systematic review. Cent European J Urol. 2016;69(1):83–90.

80. Ishii H, Couzins M, Aboumarzouk O, et al. Outcomes of systematic review of ureteroscopy for stone disease in the obese and morbidly obese population. J Endourol. 2016;30(2):135–45.

81. Drake T, Ali A, Somani BK. Feasibility and safety of bilateral same-session flexible ureteroscopy (FURS) for renal and ureteral stone disease. Cent European J Urol. 2015;68(2):193–6.

82. Ishii H, Rai B, Traxer O, et al. Outcome of ureteroscopy for stone disease in patients with horseshoe kidney: Review of world literature. Urol Ann. 2015;7(4):470–4.

83. Rukin NJ, Somani BK, Patterson J, et al. Tips and tricks of ureteroscopy: consensus statement Part I. Basic ureteroscopy. Cent European J Urol. 2015;68(4):439–46.

84. Traxer O, Lechevallier E, Saussine C. Flexible ureteroscopy with Holmium laser: technical aspects. Progrès en urologie. 2008;18:929–37.

85. Noble MJ, Esac WE. Semirigid ureteroscopy: the Cleveland Clinic approach. In: Monga M, editor. Ureteroscopy: indications, instrumentation and technique. New York: Humana Press/Springer; 2013. p. 257–70.

86. Rabah DM, Fabrizio MD. Flexible fiberoptic ureteropyeloscopy. In: Smith AD, Badlani GH, Baglev DH, et al., editors. Smith's textbook of endourology. 2nd ed. Hamilton, London: BC Decker Inc; 2007. p. 237–42.

87. Giusti G, Proietti S, Villa L, et al. Current standard technique for modern flexible ureteroscopy: tips and tricks. Eur Urol. 2016;70(1):188–94.

88. Georgescu D, Multescu R, Mirciulescu V, et al. Instruments. In: Geavlete PA, editor. Retrograde ureteroscopy. Handbook of endourology: Elsevier; 2016. p. 29–35.

89. Miller J, Stoller ML. Intracorporeal lithotripsy: electrohydraulic, pneumatic, and ultrasonic. In: Monga M, editor. Ureteroscopy: indications, instrumentation and technique. New York: Humana Press/Springer; 2013. p. 149–60.

90. Knudsen BE. Flexible ureteroscopy: holmium:YAG laser and optical fibers. In: Monga M, editor. Ureteroscopy: indications, instrumentation and technique. New York: Humana Press/Springer; 2013. p. 161–8.

91. Dretler SP, Watson G, Parrish JA, Murray S. Pulsed dye laser fragmentation of ureteral calculi: initial clinical experience. J Urol. 1987;137(3):386–9.

92. Marguet CG, Sung JC, Springhart WP, et al. In vitro comparison of stone retropulsion and fragmentation of the frequency doubled, double pulse Nd:YAG laser and the holmium:YAG laser. J Urol. 2005;173:1797–800.

93. Teichman JM, Chan KF, Cecconi PP, et al. Erbium : YAG versus holmium : YAG lithotripsy. J Urol. 2001;165(3):876–9.

94. Lee H, Kang HW, Teichman JM, et al. Urinary calculus fragmentation during Ho: YAG and Er:YAG lithotripsy. Lasers Surg Med. 2006;38(1):39–51.

95. Matlaga BR, Lingeman JE. Surgical management of stones: new technology. Adv Chronic Kidney Dis. 2009;16:60–4.

96. Keeley FX Jr, Pillai M, Smith G, Chrisofos M, Tolley DA. Electrokinetic lithotripsy: safety, efficacy and limitations of a new form of ballistic lithotripsy. BJU Int. 1999;84(3):261–3.

97. Ali AA, Ali ZA, Halstead JC, et al. A novel method to prevent retrograde displacement of ureteric calculi during intracorporeal lithotripsy. BJU Int. 2004;94(3):441–2.

98. Bastawisy M, Gameel T, Radwan M, et al. A comparison of stone cone *versus* lidocaine jelly in the prevention of ureteral stone migration during ureteroscopic lithotripsy. Ther Adv Urol. 2011;3(5):203–10.

99. Kreydin E, Eisner B. Stone migration devices. In: Monga M, editor. Ureteroscopy: indications, instrumentation and technique. New York: Humana Press/Springer; 2013. p. 169–78.

100. Hofbauer J, Hobarth K, Marberger M. Electrohydraulic versus pneumatic disintegration in the treatment of ureteral stones: a randomized, prospective trial. J Urol. 1995;153:623.

101. Garg S, Mandal AK, Singh SK, et al. Ureteroscopic laser lithotripsy versus ballistic lithotripsy for treatment of ureteric stones: a prospective comparative study. Urol Int. 2009;82(3):341–5.

102. Santa-Cruz RW, Leveillee RJ, Krongrad A. Ex vivo comparison of four lithotripters commonly used in the ureter: what does it take to perforate? J Endourol. 1998;12:417.

103. Hecht SL, Wolf JS. Techniques for holmium laser lithotripsy of intrarenal calculi. Urology. 2013;81:442–5.

104. Auge BK, Pietrow PK, Lallas CD, et al. Ureteral access sheath provides protection against elevated renal pressures during routine flexible ureteroscopic stone manipulation. J Endourol. 2004;18(1):33–6.

105. Geraghty RM, Ishii H, Somani BK. Outcomes of flexible ureteroscopy and laser fragmentation for treatment of large renal stones with and without the use of ureteral access sheaths: results from a university hospital with a review of literature. Scand J Urol. 2016;50(3):216–9.

106. Traxer O, Thomas A. Prospective evaluation and classification of ureteral wall injuries resulting from insertion of UAS during RIRS. J Urol. 2013;189:580–4.
107. Rukin NJ, Somani BK, Patterson J, et al. Tips and tricks of ureteroscopy: consensus statement. Part II. Advanced ureteroscopy. Cent European J Urol. 2016;69(1):98–104.
108. Kurahashi T, Miyake H, Oka N, et al. Clinical outcome of ureteroscopic lithotripsy for 2,129 patients with ureteral stones. Urol Res. 2007;35(3):149–53.
109. Takazawa R, Kitayama S, Kobayashi S, et al. Transurethral lithotripsy with rigid and flexible ureteroscopy for renal and ureteral stones: results of the first 100 procedures. Hinyokika Kiyo. 2011;57(8):411–6.
110. Tanriverdi O, Silay MS, Kadihasanoglu M, et al. Revisiting the predictive factors for intra-operative complications of rigid ureteroscopy: a 15-year experience. Urol J. 2012;9(2):457–64.
111. Alcaide JRC, Elbers JR, Perez DL, et al. Flexible ureterorenoscopy (URS): technique and results. Arch Esp Urol. 2010;63(10):862–70.
112. Grasso M, Ficazzola M. Retrograde ureteropyeloscopy for lower pole caliceal calculi. J Urol. 1999;162:1904–8.
113. Fuganti PE, Pires S, Branco R, Porto J. Predictive factors for intraoperative complications in semirigid ureteroscopy: analysis of 1235 ballistic ureterolithotripsies. Urology. 2008;72(4):770–4.
114. Baş O, Tuygun C, Dede O, et al. Factors affecting complication rates of retrograde flexible ureterorenoscopy: analysis of 1571 procedures-a single-center experience. World J Urol. 2016;35(5):819–26.
115. El Harrech Y, Abakka N, El Anzaoui J, et al. Ureteral stenting after uncomplicated ureteroscopy for distal ureteral stones: a randomized, controlled trial. Minim Invasive Surg. 2014;2014:892890.
116. Jung GH, Jung JH, Ahn TS, et al. Comparison of retrograde intrarenal surgery versus a single-session percutaneous nephrolithotomy for lower-pole stones with a diameter of 15 to 30 mm: a propensity score-matching study. Korean J Urol. 2015;56(7):525–32.
117. Klingler HC, et al. Stone treatment and coagulopathy. Eur Urol. 2003;43(1):75–9.
118. Al Busaidy SS, Kurukkal SN, Al Hooti QM, et al. Is RIRS emerging as the preferred option for the management of 2 cm-4 cm renal stones: our experience. Can J Urol. 2016;23(4):8364–7.

119. Liu K, Xiao CL, Liu YQ, et al. Management of calyceal diverticular calculi with stenotic infundibulum by flexible ureteroscopic holmium laser infundibulectomy and lithotripsy. Beijing Da Xue Xue Bao. 2015;47(4):618–21.

120. Cohen J, Cohen S, Grasso M. Ureteropyeloscopic treatment of large, complex intrarenal and proximal ureteral calculi. BJU Int. 2013;111(3 Pt B):E127–31.

121. Marguet CG, Springhart WP, Tan YH, et al. Simultaneous combined use of flexible ureteroscopy and percutaneous nephrolithotomy to reduce the number of access tracts in the management of complex renal calculi. BJU Int. 2005;96(7):1097–100.

122. Hamamoto S, Yasui T, Okada A, et al. Developments in the technique of endoscopic combined intrarenal surgery in the prone split-leg position. Urology. 2014;84(3):565–70.

123. Hamamoto S, Yasui T, Okada A, et al. Efficacy of endoscopic combined intrarenal surgery in the prone split-leg position for staghorn calculi. J Endourol. 2015;29(1):19–24.

124. Sternberg KM, Jacobs BL, King BJ, et al. The prone uretero- scopic technique for managing large stone burdens. Can J Urol. 2015;22(2):7758–62.

125. Bernardo N, Lopez-Silva M, Sanguinetti H, et al. Unplanned flexible ureteroscopy during percutaneous nephrolithotomy in the prone position. Actas Urol Esp. 2016;40(2):115–8.

126. Chew BH, Lange D. The future of ureteroscopy. Minerva Urol Nefrol. 2016;68(6):592–7.

127. Fernstrom I, Johansson B. Percutaneous pyelolithotomy, a new extraction technique. Scand J Urol Nephrol. 1976;10:257–9.

128. Alken P, Hutschenreiter G, Gunther R, Marberger M. Percutaneous stone manipulation. J Urol. 1981;125:463–6.

129. Thomas K, Smith NC, Hegarty N, Glass JM. The Guy's stone score—grading the complexity of percutaneous nephrolithot- omy procedures. Urology. 2011;78(2):277–81.

130. Vernez SL, Okhunov Z, Motamedinia P, et al. Nephrolithometric scoring systems to predict outcomes of percutaneous nephroli- thotomy. Rev Urol. 2016;18(1):15–27.

131. Torricelli FC, Padovani GP, Marchini GS, et al. Percutaneous nephrolithotomy in patients with solitary kidney: a critical out- come analysis. Int Braz J Urol. 2015;41(3):496–502.

132. Ishibashi M, Morita S, Rabito CA, et al. Evaluation of the therapeutic effect of percutaneous nephroureterolithot- omy by Tc-99m diethylenetiaminepentaacetic acid (DTPA)

renal scintigraphy--alteration of the renal fraction of blood flow, split-GFR, and renal mean transit time. Kurume Med J. 1990;37(4):285–91.

133. Sharma GR, Maheshwari PN, Sharma AG, et al. Fluoroscopy guided percutaneous renal access in prone position. World J Clin Cases. 2015;3(3):245–64.

134. Valdivia Uria JG, Valle Gerhold J, Lopez Lopez JA, et al. Technique and complications of percutaneous nephroscopy: experience with 557 patients in the supine position. J Urol. 1998;160:1975–8.

135. Ibarluzea G, Scoffone CM, Cracco CM, et al. Supine Valdivia and modified lithotomy position for simultaneous anterograde and retrograde endourological access. BJU Int. 2007;100: 233–6.

136. Serra S, Corona A, De Lisa A. Endoscopic combined intra renal surgery (ECIRS) in prone position. Urologia. 2012;79(Suppl 19): 121–4.

137. Hoznek A, Rode J, Ouzaid I, et al. Modified supine percutaneous nephrolithotomy for large kidney and ureteral stones: technique and results. Eur Urol. 2012;61(1):164–70.

138. Kumar P, Bach C, Kachrilas S, et al. Supine percutaneous nephrolithotomy (PCNL): 'in vogue' but in which position? BJU Int. 2012;110(11 Pt C):E1018–21.

139. Kim SC, Lingeman JE. Percutaneous access to the urinary tract. In: Nakada SY, Pearle MS, editors. Advanced endourology: the complete clinical guide. Totowa, NJ: Humana Press Inc; 2006. p. 43–60.

140. Ko R, Soucy F, Denstedt JD, Razvi H. Percutaneous nephrolithotomy made easier: a practical guide, tips and tricks. BJU Int. 2008;101(5):535–9.

141. Munver R, Delvecchio FC, Newman GE, Preminger GM. Critical analysis of supracostal access for percutaneous renal surgery. J Urol. 2001;166:1242–6.

142. El-Karamany T. A supracostal approach for percutaneous nephrolithotomy of staghorn calculi: a prospective study and review of previous reports. Arab J Urol. 2012;10(4): 358–66.

143. Li J, Xiao B, Hu W, et al. Complication and safety of ultrasound guided percutaneous nephrolithotomy in 8,025 cases in China. Chin Med J (Engl). 2014;127(24):4184–9.

144. Helal M, Black T, Lockhart J, Figueroa TE. The Hickman peel-away sheath: alternative for pediatric percutaneous nephrolithotomy. J Endourol. 1997;11:171–2.

145. Jackman SV, Hedican SP, Peters CA, Docimo SG. Percutaneous nephrolithotomy in infants and preschool age children: experience with a new technique. Urology. 1998;52:697–701.

146. Jackman SV, Docimo SG, Cadeddu JA, Bishoff JT, Kavoussi LR, Jarrett TW. The "mini-perc" technique: a less invasive alternative to percutaneous nephrolithotomy. World J Urol. 1998;16:371–4.

147. Ganpule AP, Desai MR. What's new in percutaneous nephrolithotomy. Arab J Urol. 2012;10(3):317–23.

148. Desai MR, Sharma R, Mishra S, et al. Single-step percutaneous nephrolithotomy (microperc): the initial clinical report. J Urol. 2011;186:140–5.

149. Sabnis RB, Ganesamoni R, Doshi A, et al. Micropercutaneous nephrolithotomy (microperc) vs retrograde intrarenal surgery for the management of small renal calculi: a randomized controlled trial. BJU Int. 2013;112(3):355–61.

150. Kaynar M, Sümer A, Şalvarcı A, et al. Micropercutaneous nephrolithotomy (Microperc®) in a two-year-old with the 'all-seeing needle'. Urol Int. 2013;91(2):239–41.

151. Desai MR, Kukreja RA, Desai MM, et al. A prospective randomized comparison of type of nephrostomy drainage following percutaneous nephrostolithotomy: large bore versus small bore versus tubeless. J Urol. 2004;172(2):565–7.

152. Istanbulluoglu MO, Ozturk B, Gonen M, et al. Effectiveness of totally tubeless percutaneous nephrolithotomy in selected patients: a prospective randomized study. Int Urol Nephrol. 2009;41(3):541–5.

153. Chang CH, Wang CJ, Huang SW. Totally tubeless percutaneous nephrolithotomy: a prospective randomized controlled study. Urol Res. 2011;39(6):459–65.

154. Garofalo M, Pultrone CV, Schiavina R, et al. Tubeless procedure reduces hospitalization and pain after percutaneous nephrolithotomy: results of a multivariable analysis. Urolithiasis. 2013;41(4):347–53.

155. Javali T, Pathade A, Nagaraj HK. A Novel method of ensuring safe and accurate dilatation during percutaneous nephrolithotomy. Int Braz J Urol. 2015;41(5):1014–9.

156. Maheshwari PN, Sharma GR, Wagaskar VG. RE: A Novel method of ensuring safe and accurate dilalation during percutaneous nephrolithotomy. Int Braz J Urol. 2016;42(3):628–9.

157. Kumar S, Singh S, Singh P, Singh SK. Day care PNL using 'Santosh-PGI hemostatic seal' versus standard PNL: a randomized controlled study. Cent European J Urol. 2016;69(2):190–7.

158. Song Y, Ma Y, Song Y, Fei X. Evaluating the learning curve for percutaneous nephrolithotomy under total ultrasound guidance. PLoS One. 2015;10(8):e0132986.

159. Armitage JN, Withington J, van der Meulen J, et al. Percutaneous nephrolithotomy in England: practice and outcomes described in the Hospital Episode Statistics database. BJU Int. 2014;113(5):777–82.

160. Yamaguchi A, Skolarikos A, Buchholz NP, et al. Clinical Research Office Of The Endourological Society Percutaneous Nephrolithotomy Study Group. Operating times and bleeding complications in percutaneous nephrolithotomy: a comparison of tract dilation methods in 5,537 patients in the Clinical Research Office of the Endourological Society Percutaneous Nephrolithotomy Global Study. J Endourol. 2011;25(6):933–9.

161. Meng XJ, Mi QW, Hu T, Zhong WD. Value of CT angiography in reducing the risk of hemorrhage associated with mini-percutaneous nephrolithotomy. Int Braz J Urol. 2015;41(4):690–6.

162. Shokeir AA. Transurethral cystolitholapaxy in children. J Endourol. 1994;8(2):157–9. Discussion 159–60.

163. Comisarow RH, Barkin M. Electrohydraulic cystolitholapaxy. Can J Surg. 1979;22(6):525–6.

164. Teichman JM, Rogenes VJ, McIver BJ, Harris JM. Holmium:yttrium-aluminum-garnet laser cystolithotripsy of large bladder calculi. Urology. 1997;50(1):44–8.

165. Li A, Ji C, Wang H, et al. Transurethral cystolitholapaxy with the AH-1 stone removal system for the treatment of bladder stones of variable size. BMC Urol. 2015;15:9.

166. Gallego Vilar D, Beltran Persiva J, Pérez Mestre M, et al. Giant bladder lithiasis: case report and bibliographic review. Arch Esp Urol. 2011;64(4):383–7.

167. Cohen J, Giuliano K, Sopko N, et al. Cystolitholapaxy in Ileal Conduit. Urol Case Rep. 2015;3(6):185–7.

168. Floyd MS Jr, Stubington SR. Mitrofanoff cystolitholapaxy: an innovative method of stone clearance in a hostile abdomen with an inaccessible urethra. Urol J. 2015;12(2):2115–8.

169. Xiong Y, Yang S, Liao W, et al. Autonomic dysreflexia during cystolitholapaxy in patients with spinal cord injury. Minerva Urol Nefrol. 2015;67(2):85–90.

170. Al-Marhoon MS, Sarhan OM, Awad BA, et al. Comparison of endourological and open cystolithotomy in the management of bladder stones in children. J Urol. 2009;181(6):2684–7. Discussion 2687–8.

171. Gamal W, Eldahshoury M, Hussein M, Hammady A. Cystoscopically guided percutaneous suprapubic cystolitholapaxy in children. Int Urol Nephrol. 2013;45(4):933–7.

172. Metwally AH, Sherief MH, Elkoushy MA. Safety and efficacy of cystoscopically guided percutaneous suprapubic cystolitholapaxy without fluoroscopic guidance. Arab J Urol. 2016;14(3):211–5.

173. Meria P, Milcent S, Desgrandchamps F, et al. Management of pelvic stones larger than 20 mm: laparoscopic transperitoneal pyelolithotomy or percutaneous nephrolithotomy? Urol Int. 2005;75(4):322–6.

174. Basiri A, Tabibi A, Nouralizadeh A, et al. Comparison of safety and efficacy of laparoscopic pyelolithotomy versus percutaneous nephrolithotomy inpatients with renal pelvic stones: a randomized clinical trial. Urol J. 2014;11(6):1932–7.

175. Rui X, Hu H, Yu Y, et al. Comparison of safety and efficacy of laparoscopic pyelolithotomy versus percutaneous nephrolithotomy in patients with large renal pelvic stones: a meta-analysis. J Investig Med. 2016;64(6):1134–42.

176. Sasaki Y, Kohjimoto Y, Nishizawa S, et al. Laparoscopic pyelolithotomy in a horseshoe kidney. Hinyokika Kiyo. 2012;58(2):87–91.

177. Ölçücüoğlu E, Çamtosun A, Biçer S, Bayraktar AM. Laparoscopic pyelolithotomy in a horseshoe kidney. Turk J Urol. 2014;40(4):240–4.

178. Chipde SS, Agrawal S. Retroperitoneoscopic pyelolithotomy: a minimally invasive alternative for the management of large renal pelvic stone. Int Braz J Urol. 2014;40(1):123–4. Discussion 124

179. Agrawal S, Chipde SS, Kalathia J, Agrawal R. Renal stone in crossed fused renal ectopia and its laparoscopic management: case report and review of literature. Urol Ann. 2016;8(2):236–8.

180. Stein RJ, Turna B, Nguyen MM, et al. Laparoscopic pyeloplasty with concomitant pyelolithotomy: technique and outcomes. J Endourol. 2008;22:1251–5.

181. Gandhi HR, Thomas A, Nair B, Pooleri G. Laparoscopic pyelolithotomy: an emerging tool for complex staghorn nephrolithiasis in high-risk patients. Arab J Urol. 2015;13(2):139–45.

182. Agrawal V, Bajaj J, Acharya H, et al. Laparoscopic management of pediatric renal and ureteric stones. J Pediatr Urol. 2013;9(2):230–3.

183. Al-Hunayan A, Abdulhalim H, El-Bakry E, et al. Laparoscopic pyelolithotomy: is the retroperitoneal route a better approach? Int J Urol. 2009;16(2):181–6.
184. Pastore AL, Palleschi G, Silvestri L, et al. Combined laparoscopic pyelolithotomy and endoscopic pyelolithotripsy for staghorn calculi: long-term follow-up results from a case series. Ther Adv Urol. 2016;8(1):3–8.
185. Simforoosh N, Radfar MH, Nouralizadeh A, et al. Laparoscopic anatrophic nephrolithotomy for management of staghorn renal calculi. J Laparoendosc Adv Surg Tech A. 2013;23(4):306–10.
186. Ghani KR, Rogers CG, Sood A, et al. Robot-assisted anatrophic nephrolithotomy with renal hypothermia for managing staghorn calculi. J Endourol. 2013;27(11):1393–8.
187. Ghani KR, Trinh QD, Jeong W, et al. Robotic nephrolithotomy and pyelolithotomy with utilization of the robotic ultrasound probe. Int Braz J Urol. 2014;40(1):125–6. Discussion 126.
188. King SA, Klaassen Z, Madi R. Robot-assisted anatrophic nephrolithotomy: description of technique and early results. J Endourol. 2014;28(3):325–9.
189. Garg M, Singh V, Sinha RJ, et al. Prospective randomized comparison of open versus transperitoneal laparoscopic ureterolithotomy: experience of a single center from Northern India. Curr Urol. 2013;7(2):83–9.
190. Khalil M, Omar R, Abdel-Baky S, et al. Laparoscopic ureterolithotomy; which is better: Transperitoneal or retroperitoneal approach? Turk J Urol. 2015;41(4):185–90.
191. Torricelli FC, Monga M, Marchini GS, et al. Semi-rigid ureteroscopic lithotripsy versus laparoscopic ureterolithotomy for large upper ureteral stones: a meta-analysis of randomized controlled trials. Int Braz J Urol. 2016;42(4):645–54.
192. Şahin S, Aras B, Ekşi M, et al. Laparoscopic ureterolithotomy. JSLS. 2016;20(1):e2016.00004.
193. Ma L, Yu DM, Zhang ZG, et al. Transperitoneal laparoscopic ureterolithotomy for upper ureteral calculi: a report of 1171 cases. Zhonghua Yi Xue Za Zhi. 2013;93(20):1577–9.
194. Verit A, Savas M, Ciftci H, et al. Outcomes of urethral calculi patients in an endemic region and an undiagnosed primary fossa navicularis calculus. Urol Res. 2006;34(1):37–40.
195. Akhtar J, Ahmed S, Zamir N. Management of impacted urethral stones in children. J Coll Physicians Surg Pak. 2012;22(8):510–3.
196. Walker BR, Hamilton BD. Urethral calculi managed with transurethral Holmium laser ablation. J Pediatr Surg. 2001;36(9):E16.

197. Smith MJ, Boyce WH. Anatrophic nephrotomy and plastic calyrhaphy. J Urol. 1968;99(5):521–7.
198. Gil-Vernet JM, Caralps A. Human renal homotransplantation. New surgical technique. Urol Int. 1968;23(3):201–23.
199. Gil-Vernet JM, Carretero P, Caralps A, Ballesteros JJ. New surgical technique for balanitic hypospadias correction. J Urol. 1974;112(5):673.
200. Gil-Vernet JM. A new technique for surgical correction of vesicoureteral reflux. J Urol. 1984;131(3):456–8.
201. Gil-Vernet JM, Gutierrez del Pozo R, Carretero P, et al. Urogenital diaphragm raising maneuver. J Urol. 1988;140(3):555–8.
202. Gil-Vernet JM, Gil-Vernet A, Campos JA. New surgical approach for treatment of complex vesicovaginal fistula. J Urol. 1989;141(3):513–6.
203. Gil-Vernet JM, Gil-Vernet A, Caralps A, et al. Orthotopic renal transplant and results in 139 consecutive cases. J Urol. 1989;142(2 Pt 1):248–52.
204. Gil-Vernet S. Pathologia Urogenital: Biologia y pathologia de la prostata. T.1. Madird: Editorial Paz-Montalvo; 1953.
205. Crosby RW, Cody J. Max Brödel: the man who put art into medicine. New York: Springer; 1991.
206. Brödel M. The intrinsic blood-vessels of the kidney and their significance in nephrotomy. The Johns Hopkins Hospital Bulletin. XII/118; 1901.
207. Latarjet M, Ruiz Liard A. Systema urinario. Riñón. In: Anatomía Humana, vol. 2. 4th ed. Buenos Aires: Editorial Medica Panamericana; 2008. p. 1509–26.
208. Lunardi P, Timsit MO, Roumiguie M, et al. Single procedure treatment of complex nephrolithiasis: about a modern series of anatrophic nephrolithotomy. Prog Urol. 2015;25(2):90–5.
209. Bove AM, Altobelli E, Buscarini M. Indication to open anatrophic nephrolithotomy in the twenty-first century: a case report. Case Rep Urol. 2012;2012:851020.
210. Aminsharifi A, Irani D, Masoumi M, et al. The management of large staghorn renal stones by percutaneous versus laparoscopic versus open nephrolithotomy: a comparative analysis of clinical efficacy and functional outcome. Urolithiasis. 2016;44(6):551–7.
211. Mahran MR, Dawaba MS. Cystolitholapaxy versus cystolithotomy in children. J Endourol. 2000;14(5):423–5.
212. Ma C, Lu B, Sun E. Giant bladder stone in a male patient: a case report. Medicine (Baltimore). 2016;95(30):e4323.
213. Randall A. Giant vesical calculus. J Urol. 1920;5(2):119–25.

214. Moran ME. The largest stone of all! In: Urolithiasis. A comprehensive history. Now York: Springer; 2014. p. 351–63.

215. Pearle MS, Goldfarb DS, Assimos DG, et al. Medical management of kidney stones: AUA guideline. J Urol. 2014;192(2):316–24.

216. Prezioso D, Strazzullo P, Lotti T, et al. Dietary treatment of urinary risk factors for renal stone formation. A review of CLU Working Group. Arch Ital Urol Androl. 2015;87(2):105–20.

217. Bates GP, Miller VS. Sweat rate and sodium loss during work in the heat. J Occup Med Toxicol. 2008;3:4.

218. Godek SF, Peduzzi C, Burkholder R, et al. Sweat rates, sweat sodium concentrations, and sodium losses in 3 groups of professional football players. J Athl Train. 2010;45(4):364–71.

219. Brake DJ, Bates GP. Fluid losses and hydration status of industrial workers under thermal stress working extended shifts. Occup Environ Med. 2003;60(2):90–6.

220. Pak CY, Sakhaee K, Fuller CJ. Physiological and physiochemical correction and prevention of calcium stone formation by potassium citrate therapy. Trans Assoc Am Physicians. 1983;96:294–305.

221. Sakhaee K, Nicar M, Hill K, Pak CY. Contrasting effects of potassium citrate and sodium citrate therapies on urinary chemistries and crystallization of stone-forming salts. Kidney Int. 1983;24(3):348–52.

222. Siener R. Can the manipulation of urinary pH by beverages assist with the prevention of stone recurrence? Urolithiasis. 2016;44(1):51–6.

223. Sorensen MD, Hsi RS, Chi T. Dietary intake of fiber, fruit and vegetables decreases the risk of incident kidney stones in women: a Women's Health Initiative report. J Urol. 2014;192(6):1694–9.

224. Manfredini R, De Giorgi A, Storari A, Fabbian F. Pears and renal stones: possible weapon for prevention? A comprehensive narrative review. Eur Rev Med Pharmacol Sci. 2016;20(3):414–25.

225. Nijenhuis T, Vallon V, van der Kemp AW, et al. Enhanced passive Ca2+ reabsorption and reduced Mg2+ channel abundance explains thiazide-induced hypocalciuria and hypomagnesemia. J Clin Invest. 2005;115:1651–8.

226. Laerum E, Larsen S. Thiazide prophylaxis of urolithiasis. A double-blind study in general practice. Acta Med Scand. 1984;215:383–9. An early RCT to show the effect of HCTZ in the prevention of calcium stone recurrence.

227. Escribano J, Balaguer A, Roqué i Figuls M, et al. Dietary interventions for preventing complications in idiopathic hypercalciuria. Cochrane Database Syst Rev. 2014;(2):CD006022.

228. Escribano J, Balaguer A, Pagone F, et al. Pharmacological interventions for preventing complications in idiopathic hypercalciuria. Cochrane Database Syst Rev. 2009;(1):CD004754.

229. Nicar MJ, Hill K, Pak CY. Inhibition by citrate of spontaneous precipitation of calcium oxalate in vitro. J Bone Miner Res. 1987;2(3):215–20.

230. Barcelo P, Wuhl O, Servitge E, et al. Randomized double-blind study of potassium citrate in idiopathic hypocitraturic calcium nephrolithiasis. J Urol. 1993;150(6):1761–4.

231. Coe FL, Evan A, Worcester E. Pathophysiology-based treatment of idiopathic calcium kidney stones. Clin J Am Soc Nephrol. 2011;6(8):2083–92.

232. Xu H, Zisman AL, Coe FL, Worcester EM. Kidney stones: an update on current pharmacological management and future directions. Expert Opin Pharmacother. 2013;14(4):435–47.

233. Gul Z, Monga M. Medical and dietary therapy for kidney stone prevention. Korean J Urol. 2014;55(12):775–9.

234. Kok DJ. Metaphylaxis, diet and lifestyle in stone disease. Arab J Urol. 2012;10(3):240–9.

235. Carrasco A Jr, Granberg CF, Gettman MT, et al. Surgical management of stone disease in patients with primary hyperoxaluria. Urology. 2015;85(3):522–6.

236. Lorenzo V, Torres A, Salido E. Primary hyperoxaluria. Nefrologia. 2014;34(3):398–412.

237. Holmes RP, Goodman HO, Assimos DG. Contribution of dietary oxalate to urinary oxalate excretion. Kidney Int. 2001;59(1):270–6.

238. Ettinger B, Tang A, Citron JT, et al. Randomized trial of allopurinol in the prevention of calcium oxalate calculi. N Engl J Med. 1986;315:1386–9.

239. Beara-Lasic L, Pillinger MH, Goldfarb DS. Advances in the management of gout: critical appraisal of febuxostat in the control of hyperuricemia. Int J Nephrol Renovasc Dis. 2010;3:1–10.

240. Preminger GM, Sakhaee K, Skurla C, et al. Prevention of recurrent calcium stone formation with potassium citrate therapy in patients with distal renal tubular acidosis. J Urol. 1985;134:20–3.

241. Maalouf NM, Cameron MA, Moe OW, et al. Novel insights into the pathogenesis of uric acid nephrolithiasis. Curr Opin Nephrol Hypertens. 2004;13:181.

242. Biyani CS, Cartledge JJ. Cystinuria: diagnosis and management. EAU-EBU Update Series. 2006;4:175–83.
243. Preminger GM, Assimos DG, Lingeman JE, et al. AUA Nephrolithiasis Guideline Panel. Chapter 1: AUA guideline on management of staghorn calculi: diagnosis and treatment recommendations. J Urol. 2005;173(6):1991–2000.
244. Crawhall JC, Scowen EF, Watts RW. Effect of penicillamine on cystinuria. Br Med J. 1963;1:588–90.
245. Lotz M, Bartter FC. Stone dissolution with D-penicillamine in cystinuria. Br Med J. 1965;2:1408–9.
246. Goldfarb DS, Coe FL, Asplin JR. Urinary cystine excretion and capacity in patients with cystinuria. Kidney Int. 2006;69:1041–7.
247. Fattah H, Hambaroush Y, Goldfarb DS. Cystine nephrolithiasis. Transl Androl Urol. 2014;3(3):228–33.
248. Griffith DP, Gleeson MJ, Lee H, et al. Randomized, double-blind trial of Lithostat (acetohydroxamic acid) in the palliative treatment of infection-induced urinary calculi. Eur Urol. 1991;20:243.
249. Rodman JS, Williams JJ, Jones RL. Hypercoagulability produced by treatment with acetohydroxamic acid. Clin Pharmacol Ther. 1987;42:346.
250. Faridi P, Roozbeh J, Mohagheghzadeh A. Ibn-Sina's life and contributions to medicinal therapies of kidney calculi. Iran J Kidney Dis. 2012;6(5):339–45.
251. Nasim MJ, Bin Asad MH, Durr-e-Sabih, et al. Gist of medicinal plants of Pakistan having ethnobotanical evidences to crush renal calculi (kidney stones). Acta Pol Pharm. 2014;71(1):3–10.
252. Bahmani M, Baharvand-Ahmadi B, Tajeddini P, et al. Identification of medicinal plants for the treatment of kidney and urinary stones. J Renal Inj Prev. 2016;5(3):129–33.
253. Boim MA, Heilberg IP, Schor N. Phyllanthus niruri as a promising alternative treatment for nephrolithiasis. Int Braz J Urol. 2010;36(6):657–64. Discussion 664.
254. Kieley S, Dwivedi R, Monga M. Ayurvedic medicine and renal calculi. J Endourol. 2008;22(8):1613–6.
255. Micali S, Sighinolfi MC, Celia A, et al. Can Phyllanthus niruri affect the efficacy of extracorporeal shock wave lithotripsy for renal stones? A randomized, prospective, long-term study. J Urol. 2006;176(3):1020–2.
256. Erickson SB, Vrtiska TJ, Canzanello VJ, Lieske JC. Cystone® for 1 year did not change urine chemistry or decrease stone burden in cystine stone formers. Urol Res. 2011;39(3):197–203.

257. Erickson SB, Vrtiska TJ, Lieske JC. Effect of Cystone® on urinary composition and stone formation over a one year period. Phytomedicine. 2011;18(10):863–7.

258. Atmani F, Slimani Y, Mimouni M, Hacht B. Prophylaxis of calcium oxalate stones by Herniaria hirsuta on experimentally induced nephrolithiasis in rats. BJU Int. 2003;92(1):137–40.

259. Rodgers AL, Webber D, Ramsout R, Gohel MD. Herbal preparations affect the kinetic factors of calcium oxalate crystallization in synthetic urine: implications for kidney stone therapy. Urolithiasis. 2014;42(3):221–5.

260. Monti E, Trinchieri A, Magri V, et al. Herbal medicines for urinary stone treatment. A systematic review. Arch Ital Urol Androl. 2016;88(1):38–46.

261. Iqbal MW, Shin RH, Youssef RF, et al. Should metabolic evaluation be performed in patients with struvite stones? Urolithiasis. 2017;45(2):185–92.

262. Alamuri P, Eaton KA, Himpsl SD, et al. Vaccination with proteus toxic agglutinin, a hemolysin-independent cytotoxin in vivo, protects against Proteusmirabilis urinary tract infection. Infect Immun. 2009;77(2):632–41.

263. Hoppe B, Groothoff JW, Hulton SA, et al. Efficacy and safety of Oxalobacter formigenes to reduce urinary oxalate in primary hyperoxaluria. Nephrol Dial Transplant. 2011;26(11):3609–15.

264. Jairath A, Parekh N, Otano N, et al. Oxalobacter formigenes: opening the door to probiotic therapy for the treatment of hyperoxaluria. Scand J Urol. 2015;49(4):334–7.

265. Rimer JD, An Z, Zhu Z, et al. Crystal growth inhibitors for the prevention of L-cystine kidney stones through molecular design. Science. 2010;330(6002):337–41.

266. Goldfarb DS. Potential pharmacological treatments for cystinuria and for calcium stones associated with hyperuricosuria. Clin J Am Soc Nephrol. 2011;6(8):2093–7.

267. Sahota A, Parihar JS, Yang M, et al. Novel cystine ester mimics for the treatment of cystinuria-induced urolithiasis in a knock-out mouse model. Urology. 2014;84(5):1249.e9–15.

268. Lee MH, Sahota A, Ward MD, Goldfarb DS. Cystine growth inhibition through molecular mimicry: a new paradigm for the prevention of crystal diseases. Curr Rheumatol Rep. 2015;17(5):33.

269. Wendt-Nordahl G, Sagi S, Bolenz C, et al. Evaluation of cystine transport in cultured human kidney cells and establishment of cystinuria type I phenotype by antisense technology. Urol Res. 2008;36(1):25–9.

Chapter 12
Special Conditions in Urinary Lithiasis

"Effects vary with the conditions which bring them to pass, but laws do not vary. Physiological and pathological states are ruled by the same forces; they differ only because of the special conditions under which the vital laws manifest themselves".

Claude Bernard (1813–1878)

12.1 Management of Urinary Stones in Pregnancy

Urologists are frequently called to assess a pregnant lady presenting with flank pain and found subsequently to have hydronephrosis (HN) after ultrasonography. It should be remembered here that the most common cause of hydronephrosis in pregnancy is physiologic, being mainly due to mechanical causes whereby compression of the ureters by the gravid uterus and the iliac and gonadal vessels has been proposed to be an important contributory factor. The effect of Progesterone in reducing ureteral tone, peristalsis, and contraction pressure appears to be modest [1, 2]. The overall incidence of physiologic hydronephrosis was found to be 90% on the right side and up to 67% on the left side during pregnancy [3]. The predominance of HN on the right side is proposed to be due to the fact that the right ureter crosses the iliac and ovarian vessels at a more acute angle than the left before it enters the pelvis [2]. A further suggested factor is the compressive effect arising from the dextrorotation of the pregnant uterus while the left ureter seems to be protected by

© Springer International Publishing AG 2017   281
S.A. Al-Mamari, *Urolithiasis in Clinical Practice*,
In Clinical Practice, DOI 10.1007/978-3-319-62437-2_12

the gas-filled sigmoid colon [4]. Therefore it has been suggested that the left lateral position may be a therapeutic posture to both relieving pain and allowing a better drainage of the right pelvi-calyceal system, thus preventing pyelonephritis [5].

A ureteric stone should be clinically suspected in presence of moderate to severe ipsilateral colicky pain in association with hydronephrosis, but will hardly be directly visualized by ultrasonography. The presence of macroscopic or microscopic haematuria would be an additional clue to this etiology.

The association of urolithiasis with pregnancy is a controversial topic abundantly discussed in the literature. A large review study of over 21,000 deliveries revealed that 86 women have got symptomatic urolithiasis for an incidence of 1 in 244 pregnancies (0.4%), and the symptoms were most likely to occur in the second or third trimester [6]. However it is generally accepted that this incidence varies widely from 1/200 to 1/2000 women, and is finally not different from the reported incidence in the non-pregnant female population of the child-bearing age (0.03–0.5%) [7–9]. Even when restricting the study to the sole pregnant patients hospitalized for renal colic, it was shown that only 19.4% were ultimately diagnosed to have a renal or ureteric stone, while 28% patients were found to have UTI [10].

If pregnancy does not increase the incidence of urinary stone compared to age-matched non-pregnant women, it has however an influence in the stone composition. As already discussed above (See Chap. 4: Stone composition), calculi in pregnant women are predominantly made of CaP (hydroxyapatite) (74%) while CaOx component is more common in non-pregnant females [11]. More importantly, the combination of urolithiasis with pregnancy represents a challenge to both Gynae-obstetricians and Urologists for their diagnosis and treatment. It has been shown that nephrolithiasis exposes to an increased risk of preterm premature rupture of membranes compared with a control group with values of 7.0% and 2.9% respectively [6]. Flank pain is the most common presentation and the diagnosis is based essentially on Ultrasonography [10]. However when ultrasound study is inconclusive and diagnosis certainty is required before embarking in a high risk surgery, experts panel exceptionally recommend Magnetic Resonance Imaging (MRI) as a second-line imaging modality, while low-dose CT should cautiously be used as a last-line option and care taken not to exceed 0.05 Gy X-ray exposure [12]. Conservative management of renal colic in pregnant patients is effective in 3/4 of cases and should be considered as the first-line management here [4, 9, 13]. It consists of pain control and rehydration. Medical expulsive therapy (MET) with alphablockers or calcium-channel blockers can be safely added in order to increase the rate of stone passage in pregnant women [4, 14].

ESWL is absolutely contra-indicated for urolithiasis in pregnancy and the indications of surgical intervention are restricted to:

• failure of conservative management
• sepsis
• obstruction of a solitary kidney
• bilateral ureteric obstruction.

Surgical intervention consists of a retrograde ureteral DJ stent insertion. This is regarded as a reliable, safe, and stable first-line urological intervention and has been found to be equally effective and safe as percutaneous nephrostomy, with less complications (bleeding and stent dislodgement) and less inconvenience (no external drainage system) [15, 16].

Whether a rigid ureteroscopy should be performed to remove the stone straightaway in pregnant women is a matter of debate. This may be advisable in selected cases under expert hands. Indeed the physiological dilatation of the ureters in pregnancy would plead for this initiative. Definitive treatment of the stone using a Swiss pneumatic lithoclast or Holmium Lasers through a semirigid ureteroscope under general anesthesia was shown to be safe for the foetus [17–19], and the expert panels consider this intervention as a reasonable alternative to avoid long-term stenting or drainage [20, 21]. However a recent study has revived our attention showing that obstetrical risks triggered by ureteroscopy may reach 4% [22], a figure that is higher than in previous studies. Consequently, as a general recommendation before any surgery in pregnant women, the opinion of Gynae-

Obstetricians must always be sought with regard to the probability of complications such as miscarriage and preterm labor [21].

The use of fluoroscopy should also be avoided or reduced to the minimum and restricted to the area of interest while shielding the uterus with a lead apron. Ultrasonography is a safer and effective means to guide ureteroscopy and DJ-stenting in pregnancy to avoid harming the fetus with ionizing radiation exposure [23].

12.2   Management of Urolithiasis in Children

Fifty to eighty-five percent of children with urolithiasis have a family history of stone disease [24–26] and 93.2% of them have metabolic abnormalities detected in a 24-h urine study, hypercalciuria being the most common (75%), followed by hypocitraturia (44%) and hyperuricosuria (30%) (Table 12.1).

TABLE 12.1 Metabolic disorders in the urinary analysis of patients with urolithiasis hospitalized in HUG during the period of 2002–2012 (analysis performed from a 24-h urine or a single urine sample)

Metabolic disorders	N (%)
Hypercalciuria	44 (74.6%)
Hypocitraturia	26 (44.1%)
Hyperuricosuria	18 (30.5%)
Hyperoxaluria	5 (8.5%)
Cystinuria	3 (5.1%)
Hyperphosphaturia	1 (1.7%)
Hypomagnesuria	1 (1.7%)
Hypercalciuria + Hypocitraturia	8 (14.5%)
Hypercalciuria + Hyperuricosuria	7 (12.72%)
Hypercalciuria + Hypocitraturia + Hyperuricosuria	7 (12.72%)

From Amancio et al. [24]. J. Bras. Nefrol. Creative Commons Attribution License.

Metabolic evaluation of urolithiasis in the pediatric population should never be overlooked because the risk of renal stone recurrence in childhood is high, ranging 50–70% within 3 years [25, 27].

Beside metabolic abnormalities, anatomical defects and functional abnormalities are the second most important cause (25%), and include vesico-ureteral reflux, PUJ, neurogenic bladder [25].

A third etiological group is formed by the so-called endemic pediatric bladder stones that are defined as those formed in the absence of obstruction, infection or neurogenic disease. These stones are found in some geographic areas where children are subjected to malnutrition, diarrheal disease, and/or chronic dehydration, such as North and Sub-Saharian African countries, Turkey, Iraq, Iran, India, Pakistan, Afghanistan, Nepal, Thailand, and Indonesia [28]. The pathophysiology proceeds through two major factors: dietary and nutritional deficiencies which promote crystalluria, and chronic dehydratation secondary to diarrhea, hot temperature, and relatively low water intake. These stones are mostly made of ammonium acid urate or mixtures of ammonium acid urate + CaOx and CaP [28, 29]. They are generally found in children younger than 10 year-old with a peak at 2–4 years, and boys are more commonly affected than girls with a male/female ratio of 12–13:1 [30, 31].

The importance of nutritional factors in developing countries has been reemphasized by a recent Indian prospective study conducted in Mumbai which showed only 21% of 24-h urine abnormalities, while there was low calcium intake in 59% resulting in increased intestinal oxalate absorption, and hypocalcemia was seen in 43% of cases. An important associated factor was the low urine volume found in as much as 65% of children [32].

The presenting symptoms of urolithiasis in children vary with their age:

- For infants younger than 60 days, the most common symptom is irritability [26].
- Children of a mean age 10.3 ± 6.1 months present with urinary tract infection and related symptoms in 50%.

Others are admitted after incidentally diagnosed renal stones during imaging for other causes (20%), or after a painful stone passage, hematuria, voiding difficulty, or antenatal detected urinary anomaly [25].

- For older children with a mean age of 8.00 ± 4.25 years, the most common clinical manifestation is diffuse abdominal pain seen in 57%, followed by classic renal colic seen in 44%, then urinary infection, macroscopic haematuria, and vomiting [24] (Table 12.2)

Ultrasonography with a full bladder is the recommended first-line imaging technique to diagnose a urinary stone in children because of his safety: absence of radiation and avoidance of anesthesia [12]. Plain X-ray KUB and NCCT KUB are only indicated when the ultrasound study is inconclusive.

The use of Alpha-1 adrenergic antagonists (either Doxazosin 0.03 mg/kg/day or Tamsulosin >4 years:0.4 mg <4 years:0.1 mg) increase the probability of ureteral calculus

TABLE 12.2 Clinical manifestations of hospitalized patients with urolithiasis between 2002 and 2012	**Clinical manifestations**	**N (%)**
	Abdominal pain	59 (56.7%)
	Classic renal colic	46 (44.2%)
	Urinary infection	39 (37.5%)
	Macroscopic hematuria	33 (31.9%)
	Vomits	29 (27.9%)
	Urinary symptoms	25 (24.0%)
	Stones elimination	25 (24.0%)
	Fever	15 (14.4%)
	Nausea	13 (12.5%)
	Microscopic hematuria	6 (5.8%)
	Other	2 (2.0%)

From Amancio et al. [24]. J. Bras. Nefrol. Creative Commons Attribution License

expulsion in children by 27% and their use is correlated with fewer episodes of pain when compared to ibuprofen alone 10 mg/kg 2–4×/day [33].

When the conservative management of a ureteral stone has failed, a rigid pediatric ureteroscope can safely be introduced and the stone be treated using Holmium Laser. This carries a high stone-free rate (>90%) [34]. However this approach has shown better results with lower and mid-ureteral stones than with upper ureteral calculi [35]. It should also be noticed that cystine stone composition and lower patient's age reduce the one-session stone free achievement, and younger patient's age of less than 5 years expose to an increased complication rate and the need for conversion to open procedure [36].

Old studies have also suggested an affective role of ESWL in the management of pediatric ureteral stones performed under general anesthesia with an overall successful outcome of 87% at 3-month follow-up [37] (Fig. 12.1), however this approach has been supplanted by Ureteroscopy nowadays.

Currently ESWL is reserved for renal stones of small to moderate size. Nonetheless harder stones such as those made of cystine are difficult to clear with this non-invasive technique and generally necessitate the use of a flexible ureteroscope with Holmium Laser, and multiple sessions are expected for larger stones. PCNL is also increasingly used in children for large stones, and the use of smaller nephroscopes (17-Fr) allows reducing bleeding complications [38].

De-novo or post-ESWL/RIRS small residual renal stones can be treated conservatively [39]. However it is notoriously known that spontaneous passage of fragments located in the lower calyces is hindered by the physical law of gravity and these fragments can act as a nidus to promote further stone growth. Herein a recent study evaluated the safety and effectiveness of the so-called "mechanical percussion diuresis and inversion therapy" aiming at clearing such unfavorably located stones in children [40]. This therapy starts by an oral fluid intake to promote diuresis (10 mL/kg of water). Thirty minutes later the child is laid in a prone Trendelenburg posture on a couch angled at 45°, and receives continuous 10-min mechanical percussion applied over the affected flank by a

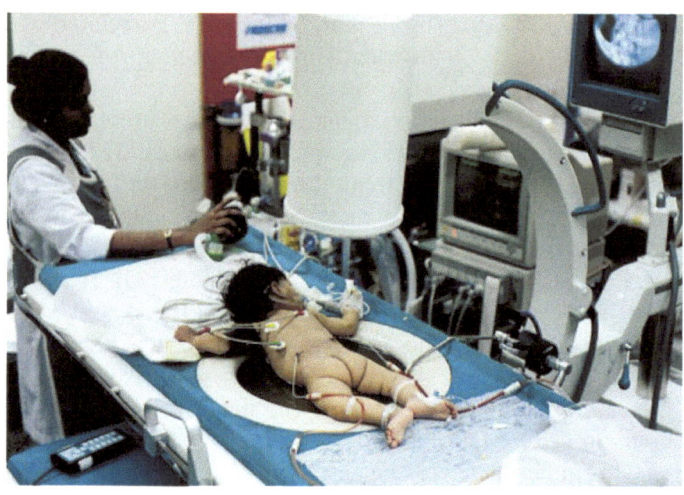

FIGURE 12.1 Positioning of a 6-month-old infant on the Wolf Lithotripter with bilateral nephrostomies due to complete bilateral ureteric calculi. From Al-Busaidy SS et al. [37], with permission from John Wiley and Sons

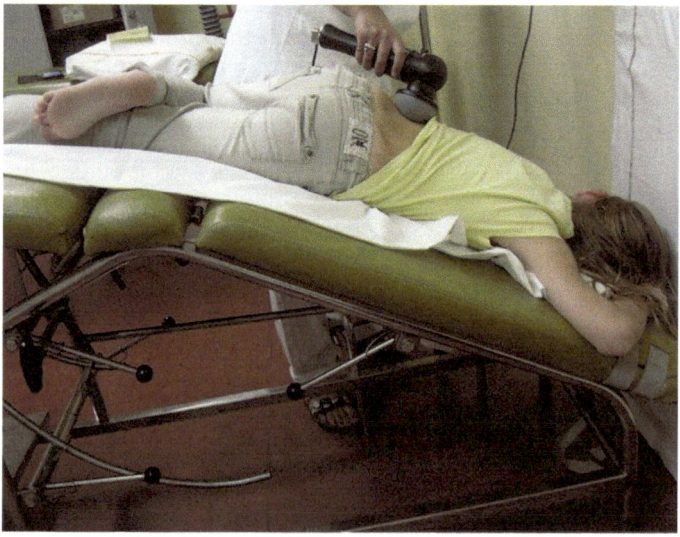

FIGURE 12.2 Application of mechanical percussor on a patient placed in a Trendelenburg position on a 45° couch. From Faure A et al. [40], with permission from Elsevier

physiotherapist (Fig. 12.2). This study showed a good tolerance to the treatment, no adverse effects, an overall stone-free rate of 65%, and a 100% decrease of the stone burden.

Depending on their size, bladder stones are managed either by Cystolitholapaxy preferably using Holmium-Laser [41] (Fig. 12.3a–f) or by cystolithotomy.

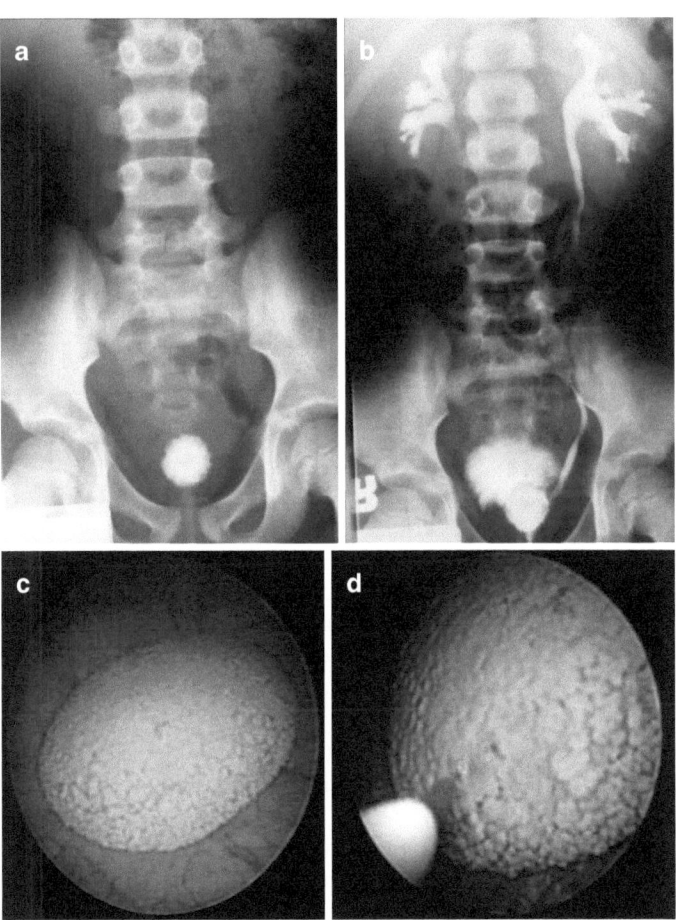

FIGURE 12.3 (**a–f**) Treatment of a large bladder stone with Holmium-Laser resulting in complete clearance. From Ramakrishnan PA et al. [41] with permission from the Canadian Journal of Urology

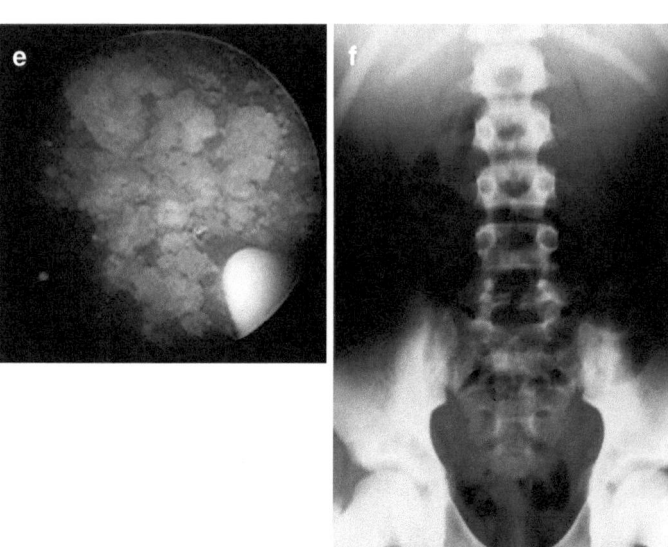

FIGURE 12.3 (continued)

12.3   Stones in Renal Transplant

Stones may be already present in the donated kidney, or form de novo in the graft after transplantation.

Candidates for kidney donation who present with symptomatic renal stones should be turned away while those with incidentally diagnosed small calculi (<1 cm) may be accepted. Several studies have reported successfull ESWL before donor nephrectomy, or removal of small stones from ex-vivo kidneys either through ultrasound-guided nephrotomy, pyelotomy, or ureteroscopies (rigid or flexible) using an iced saline perfusion, just before their successful transplantation [42, 43].

There are multiple potential factors which predispose a transplanted kidney to de-novo formation of a stone. These include secondary hyperparathyroidism with hypercalciuria, hyperuricosuria and hypocitraturia induced by cyclosporine, ureteral complications with possible obstruction, recurrent UTI, post-surgical foreign bodies (sutures, staple, stents, etc.) [44].

However the frequency of urolithiasis in renal transplant recipients in recent publications remains similar to that observed in the general population (1–3%) [45–49], owing to compensatory factors such as the generous fluid intake by transplant patients, the glomerular filtration through only one kidney rather than two, and the mildly impaired urinary concentration ability [44].

The mean interval time to presentation after renal transplantation is 28 ± 22 months [42, 45], but a wide variation from few months to as much as 18 years has been reported in the literature [48]. A very recent meta-analysis showed no gender difference in the frequency of stones in transplant kidney [45].

It should be borne in mind that stones in the denervated renal graft are asymptomatic and the diagnosis is generally incidentally reached during post-transplantation follow-up, while a minority of cases present with oliguria or anuria due to obstructing ureteral stone, or are diagnosed after a failed removal of stone-incrusted DJ stents [46, 47].

The unicity of the functioning kidney and the immune-compromised status of these patients expose them to more serious complications. Therefore a high index of clinical suspicion is required to detect this condition early, and it is strongly recommended to perform U/S or NCCT to rule out calculi in renal transplanted patients presenting with fever of unknown etiology, or in children with unexplained failure to thrive [12].

Metabolic causes of renal stones are probably more frequent in these patients than in the general population (60–80%) with hypocitraturia, hypercalcemia caused by tertiary hyperthyroidism and hyperuricemia being frequently encountered [47–49]. UTI is another important etiological factor seen in 40–50% [47–49]. Associated causal microorganisms are generally E. coli and P. mirabilis. Stone analysis has shown predominance of calcium stones which represent 67% of transplant kidney stones (subdivided as 30% mixed CaOx/CaP, 27%CaOx and 10%CaP), followed by struvite stones and uric acid stones with 20% and 13% respectively [45].

The diagnosis is reached by Ultrasound, X-ray KUB, and/or CT-scan, and the stone size varies considerably as in the general population.

The treatment is multimodal. For obstructed kidney, an urgent percutaneous drainage is required and may be followed by antegrade DJ stent insertion. ESWL treatment in prone position is the first-line treatment for small renal and ureteral stones. PCNL is reserved for multiple pyelocaliceal calculi, and staghorn calculus in the lower calyx [47, 48].

Retrograde URS with laser lithotripsy and/or basket extraction is an effective treatment for small renal transplant stones [50]. Localizing and intubating the transplant ureteric orifice is generally challenging, but may be considerably facilitated by a prior antegrade DJ stent insertion. Open surgery is reserved for cases where the above approaches have failed [45].

When efficiently treated, nephrolithiasis in graft kidneys does not have significant negative impact on the transplant survival [51].

References

1. Au KK, Woo JS, Tang LC, Liang ST. Aetiological factors in the genesis of pregnancy hydronephrosis. Aust N Z J Obstet Gynaecol. 1985;25(4):248–51.
2. Cheung KL, Lafayette RA. Renal physiology of pregnancy. Adv Chronic Kidney Dis. 2013;20(3):209–14.
3. Peake SL, Roxburgh HB, Langlois SL. Ultrasonic assessment of hydronephrosis of pregnancy. Radiology. 1983;146(1):167–70.
4. Celik O, Türk H, Cakmak O, et al. Current approach for urinary system stone disease in pregnant women. Arch Ital Urol Androl. 2016;87(4):280–5.
5. Roberts JA. Hydronephrosis of pregnancy. Urology. 1976;8(1):1–4.

6. Lewis DF, Robichaux AG III, Jaekle RK, et al. Urolithiasis in pregnancy. Diagnosis, management and pregnancy outcome. J Reprod Med. 2003;48(1):28–32.

7. Fligelstone LJ, Datta SN, Evans C, Matthews PN. Problematic renal calculi presenting during pregnancy. Ann R Coll Surg Engl. 1996;78(2):142–5.

8. Gorton E, Whitfeld HN. Renal calculi in pregnancy. Br J Urol. 1997;80(Suppl 1):4–9.

9. Juan YS, Wu WJ, Chuang SM, Wang CJ, et al. Management of symptomatic urolithiasis during pregnancy. Kaohsiung J Med Sci. 2007;23(5):241–6.

10. Fontaine-Poitrineau C, Branchereau J, Rigaud J, et al. Renal colic in pregnancy: series of 103 cases. Prog Urol. 2014;24(5):294–300.

11. Ross AE, Handa S, Lingeman JE, Matlaga BR. Kidney stones during pregnancy: an investigation into stone composition. Urol Res. 2008;36(2):99–102.

12. Türk C, Petřík A, Sarica K, et al. EAU guidelines on diagnosis and conservative management of urolithiasis. Eur Urol. 2016;69(3):468–74.

13. Hendricks SK, Ross SO, Krieger JN. An algorithm for diagnosis and therapy of management and complications of urolithiasis during pregnancy. Surg Gynecol Obstet. 1991;172(1):49–54.

14. Weber-Schoendorfer C, Hannemann D, Meister R, et al. The safety of calcium channel blockers during pregnancy: a prospective, multicenter, observational study. Reprod Toxicol. 2008;26(1):24–30.

15. Evans HJ, Wollin TA. The management of urinary calculi in pregnancy. Curr Opin Urol. 2001;11(4):379–84.

16. Choi CI, Yu YD, Park DS. Ureteral stent insertion in the management of renal colic during pregnancy. Chonnam Med J. 2016;52(2):123–7.

17. Rana AM, Aquil S, Khawaja AM. Semirigid ureteroscopy and pneumatic lithotripsy as definitive management of obstructive ureteral calculi during pregnancy. Urology. 2009;73(5):964–7.

18. Abdel-Kader MS, Tamam AA, Elderwy AA, et al. Management of symptomatic ureteral calculi during pregnancy: experience of 23 cases. Urol Ann. 2013;5(4):241–4.

19. Semins MJ, Trock BJ, Matlaga BR. The safety of ureteroscopy during pregnancy: a systematic review and meta-analysis. J Urol. 2009;181(1):139–43.

20. Türk C, Petřík A, Sarica K, et al. EAU guidelines on interventional treatment for urolithiasis. Eur Urol. 2016;69(3):475–82. doi:10.1016/j.eururo.2015.07.041. Epub 2015 Sep 4.

21. Assimos D, Krambeck A, Miller NL, et al. Surgical management of stones: American Urological Association/Endourological Society Guideline, PART II. J Urol. 2016;196(4):1161–9.

22. Johnson EB, Krambeck AE, White WM. Obstetric complications of ureteroscopy during pregnancy. J Urol. 2012;188(1):151–4.

23. Deters LA, Belanger G, Shah O, Pais VM. Ultrasound guided ureteroscopy in pregnancy. Clin Nephrol. 2013;79(2):118–23.

24. Amancio L, Fedrizzi M, Bresolin NL, Penido MG. Pediatric urolithiasis: experience at a tertiary care pediatric hospital. J Bras Nefrol. 2016;38(1):90–8.

25. Serdaroglu E, Aydogan M, Ozdemir K, Bak M. Incidence and causes of urolithiasis in children between 0-2 years. Minerva Urol Nefrol. 2016.

26. Naseri M. Urolithiasis in the first 2 months of life. Iran J Kidney Dis. 2015;9(5):379–85.

27. Tasian GE, Kabarriti AE, Kalmus A, Furth SL. Kidney stone recurrence among children and adolescents. J Urol. 2016;197(1):246–52.

28. Soliman NA, Rizvi SA. Endemic bladder calculi in children. Pediatr Nephrol. 2016. doi:10.1007/s00467-016-3492-4.

29. Naqvi SAA, Rizvi SAH, Shahjehan S. Analysis of urinary calculi by chemical methods. J Pak Med Assoc. 1984;34:147–53.

30. Thalut K, Rizal A, Brockis JG, et al. The endemic bladder stones of Indonesia—epidemiology and clinical features. Br J Urol. 1976;48(7):617–21.

31. Kamoun A, Daudon M, Abdelmoula J, et al. Urolithiasis in Tunisian children: a study of 120 cases based on stone composition. Pediatr Nephrol. 1999;13(9):920–5. Discussion 926.

32. Gajengi AK, Wagaskar VG, Tanwar HV, et al. Metabolic evaluation in paediatric urolithiasis: a 4-year open prospective study. J Clin Diagn Res. 2016;10(2):PC04–6.

33. Glina FP, Castro PM, Monteiro GG, et al. The use of alpha-1 adrenergic blockers in children with distal ureterolithiasis: a systematic review and meta-analysis. Int Braz J Urol. 2015;41(6):1049–57.

34. Al-Busaidy SS, Prem AR, Medhat M, Al-Bulushi YH. Ureteric calculi in children: preliminary experience with holmium:YAG laser lithotripsy. BJU Int. 2004;93(9):1318–23.

35. Al Busaidy SS, Prem AR, Medhat M. Paediatric ureteroscopy for ureteric calculi: a 4-year experience. Br J Urol. 1997;80(5):797–801.
36. Tiryaki T, Azili MN, Özmert S. Ureteroscopy for treatment of ureteral stones in children: factors influencing the outcome. Urology. 2013;81(5):1047–51.
37. Al Busaidy SS, Prem AR, Medhat M, Giriraj D, Gopakumar P, Bhat HS. Paediatric ureteric calculi: efficacy of primary in situ extracorporeal shock wave lithotripsy. Br J Urol. 1998;82(1):90–6.
38. Celik H, Camtosun A, Altintas R, Tasdemir C. Percutaneous nephrolithotomy in children with pediatric and adult-sized instruments. J Pediatr Urol. 2016;12(6):399.e1–5.
39. Dos Santos J, Lopes RI, Veloso AO. Outcome analysis of asymptomatic lower pole stones in children. J Urol. 2016;195(4 Pt 2):1289–93.
40. Faure A, Dicrocco E, Hery G, et al. Postural therapy for renal stones in children: a Rolling Stones procedure. J Pediatr Urol. 2016;12(4):252.e1–6.
41. Ramakrishnan PA, Medhat M, Al-Bulushi YH, Gopakumar KP, Sampige VP, Al-Busaidy SS. Holmium laser cystolithotripsy in children: initial experience. Can J Urol. 2005;12(6):2880–6. 2015;6(3):114–8.
42. Klingler HC, Kramer G, Lodde M, Marberger M. Urolithiasis in allograft kidneys. Urology. 2002;59(3):344–8.
43. Rashid MG, Konnak JW, Wolf JS Jr, et al. Ex vivo ureteroscopic treatment of calculi in donor kidneys at renal transplantation. J Urol. 2004;171(1):58–60.
44. Gdor Y, Wolf JS Jr. Surgical management of urolithiasis in transplanted kidneys. In: Rao NP, Preminger GM, Kavanagh JP, editors. Urinary tract stone disease. London: Springer; 2011. p. 537–42.
45. Cheungpasitporn W, Thongprayoon C, Mao MA, et al. Incidence of kidney stones in kidney transplant recipients: a systematic review and meta-analysis. World J Transplant. 2016;6(4):790–7.
46. Branchereau J, Thuret R, Kleinclauss F, Timsit MO. Urinary lithiasis in renal transplant recipient. Prog Urol. 2016;26(15):1083–7.
47. Cicerello E, Merlo F, Mangano M, et al. Urolithiasis in renal transplantation: diagnosis and management. Arch Ital Urol Androl. 2014;86(4):257–60.
48. Challacombe B, Dasgupta P, Tiptaft R, et al. Multimodal management of urolithiasis in renal transplantation. BJU Int. 2005;96(3):385–9.

49. Harper JM, Samuell CT, Hallison PC, et al. Risk factors for calculus formation in patients with renal transplants. Br J Urol. 1994;74(2):147–50.
50. Swearingen R, Roberts WW, Wolf JS Jr. Ureteroscopy for nephrolithiasis in transplanted kidneys. Can J Urol. 2015;22(2):7727–31.
51. Rezaee-Zavareh MS, Ajudani R, Ramezani Binabaj M, et al. Kidney allograft stone after kidney transplantation and its association with graft survival. Int J Organ Transplant Med. 2015;6(3):114–8.

Index

© Springer International Publishing AG 2017   297
S.A. Al-Mamari, *Urolithiasis in Clinical Practice*,
In Clinical Practice, DOI 10.1007/978-3-319-62437-2